Prostate Specific Antigen

Prostate Specific Antigen

edited by

Michael K. Brawer

Northwest Prostate Institute
Seattle, Washington

MARCEL DEKKER, INC.   NEW YORK · BASEL

ISBN: 0-8247-0555-6

This book is printed on acid-free paper.

Headquarters
Marcel Dekker, Inc.
270 Madison Avenue, New York, NY 10016
tel: 212-696-9000; fax: 212-685-4540

Eastern Hemisphere Distribution
Marcel Dekker AG
Hutgasse 4, Postfach 812, CH-4001 Basel, Switzerland
tel: 41-61-261-8482; fax: 41-61-261-8896

World Wide Web
http://www.dekker.com

The publisher offers discounts on this book when ordered in bulk quantities. For more information, write to Special Sales/Professional Marketing at the headquarters address above.

Current printing (last digit):
10 9 8 7 6 5 4 3 2 1

PRINTED IN THE UNITED STATES OF AMERICA

This book is lovingly dedicated to the memory of Gerald P. Murphy and to Thomas Alexander Stamey: two men who have contributed volumes to our knowledge of prostate specific antigen and who taught, challenged, and mentored me throughout my career. I am greatly indebted to them for their support over the years.

Preface

It has certainly been established that prostate specific antigen (PSA) has revolutionized the diagnosis, treatment, and monitoring of patients with prostate cancer. Indeed, it is difficult to think of any other diagnostic modality that has so altered our approach to a common condition. PSA has allowed us to identify malignancy at a curable stage in the majority of men, assisted greatly in the selection of therapy, and emerged as the main tool for monitoring established disease.

Over the last several years, I have declined the opportunity to produce a book such as this one. I felt that the PSA story was unfolding too rapidly and any such tome would be outdated before its publication. Now, however, I believe that we are at a place in our understanding of this most important of all tumor markers where a text written by the true experts in the field will be useful to students from a number of disciplines. I was heartened to have agreement from, and am truly indebted to, the contributing authors, most of whom pioneered the area of their chapter.

Many questions remain about PSA. Novel prostate markers are being identified at an increasing rate. PSA will, I believe, remain a major part of our armamentarium and will continue to truly aid in the care of the patients we serve.

Success of a multiauthored text is due in greatest part to the contributions of the individual authors. *Prostate Specific Antigen* will, I believe, represent a great source of information about this most important tumor marker, owing to the expertise of the authors and the excellence of their contributions. I owe them a great deal for their hard work. I also thank Irene Schleicher, who pulled the effort together. She maintained communication between the contributors and kept everyone on time. This text could not have been accomplished without her diligence and skillful organization.

Finally, I wish once again to express my gratitude to my family: Lisa, Alli, Danny, and Patti for their patience and forbearance throughout all my endeavors. You four make it all worthwhile.

Michael K. Brawer

Contents

Contributors

Gerald L. Andriole, M.D.   Division of Urologic Surgery, Washington University, St. Louis, Missouri

Emilia Bagiella, Ph.D.   Department of Biostatistics, Columbia University College of Physicians and Surgeons, New York, New York

Mitchell C. Benson, M.D.   Department of Urology, Columbia University College of Physicians and Surgeons, New York, New York

Ophelia Blake, F.I.B.M.S., M.I.Biol., M.Sc.   Department of Surgery, Mater Misericordiae Hospital, Dublin, Ireland

Michael K. Brawer, M.D.   Northwest Prostate Institute, Seattle, Washington

David Crawford, M.D.   Department of Surgery and Department of Radiation Oncology, Section of Urologic Oncology, University of Colorado Health Sciences Center, Denver, Colorado

Juanita Crook, M.D., F.R.C.P(c)   Radiation Oncology, University of Toronto, Toronto, Ontario, Canada

Gabriela De Angelis, M.D.   Department of Clinical Chemistry and Laboratory Medicine, Westfälische Wilhelms-Universität, Münster, Germany

Bob Djavan, M.D., Ph.D.   Department of Urology, University of Vienna, Vienna, Austria

Jonathan D. Eaton, B.Sc., M.B.B.S., M.R.C.S.   Urology Department, St. George's Hospital, London, United Kingdom

Mark R. Feneley, M.D., F.R.C.S.   Department of Urology, The Johns Hopkins Hospital, Baltimore, Maryland

John M. Fitzpatrick, M.D., M.Ch., F.R.C.S.I., F.R.C.S.   Department of Surgery, Mater Misericordiae Hospital, Dublin, Ireland

Martin E. Gleave, M.D., F.R.C.S.C., F.A.C.S.   The Prostate Centre at Vancouver, General Hospital/University of British Columbia, Vancouver, British Columbia, Canada

S. Larry Goldenberg, M.D., F.R.C.S.C., F.A.C.S.   The Prostate Cancer Centre at Vancouver General Hospital/University of British Columbia, British Columbia, Vancouver, Canada

Celestia Higano, M.D.   Department of Medicine and Urology, University of Washington, Seattle, Washington

Eric H. Holmes, Ph.D.   Northwest Biotherapeutics, Inc. and Northwest Hospital, Seattle, Washington

Faiyaaz M. Jhaveri, M.D.   Department of Urology, Northwest Hospital, Seattle, Washington

Roger S. Kirby, M.D., F.R.C.S.   Urology Department, St. George's Hospital, London, United Kingdom

George G. Klee, M.D., Ph.D.   Department of Laboratory Medicine and Pathology, Mayo Foundation, Rochester, Minnesota

David Knowles, M.D.   Department of Urology, Columbia University College of Physicians and Surgeons, New York, New York

Shane E. LaBianca, M.B., B.S., F.R.A.C.S.   The Prostate Centre at Vancouver General Hospital/University of British Columbia, Vancouver, British Columbia, Canada

Paul H. Lange, M.D.   Department of Urology, University of Washington School of Medicine, Seattle, Washington

Paul E. Li, M.D.   Department of Urology, University of Washington School of Medicine, Seattle, Washington

Kevin McGeeney, M.Sc.   Department of Surgery, Mater Misericordiae Hospital, Dublin, Ireland

Grenville M. Oades, B.Sc., M.B.Ch.B., M.R.C.S.   Urology Department, St. George's Hospital, London, United Kingdom

David K. Ornstein, M.D.   Division of Urologic Surgery, Department of Surgery, University of North Carolina, Chapel Hill, North Carolina

Alan W. Partin, M.D., Ph.D.   Department of Urology, The Johns Hopkins Hospital, Baltimore, Maryland

Hans-Peter Schmid, M.D.   Department of Urology, Westfälische Wilhelms-Universität, Münster, Germany

Axel Semjonow, M.D.   Department of Urology, Westfälische Wilhelms-Universität, Münster, Germany

Ulf-Håkan Stenman, M.D.   Department of Clinical Chemistry, Helsinki University Central Hospital, Helsinki, Finland

Donald Tindall, Ph.D.   Department of Urology Research, Mayo Clinic and Mayo Foundation, Rochester, Minnesota

Andrea Veatch, M.D.   Division of Oncology, Department of Medicine, University of Washington Medical Center; Fred Hutchinson Cancer Research Center, Seattle, Washington

Alfredo Velasco, M.D.   Department of Urology, Catholic University Hospital, Santiago, Chile

Steve Waxman, M.D.   Associated Urologists, Inc., Indianapolis, Indiana

Charles Young, Ph.D.   Department of Urology and Biochemistry/Molecular Biology, Mayo Clinic and Mayo Foundation, Rochester, Minnesota

1
The History of Prostate Specific Antigen

David Crawford
University of Colorado Health Sciences Center, Denver, Colorado

Steve Waxman
Associated Urologists, Inc., Indianapolis, Indiana

As a tumor marker, prostate specific antigen (PSA) has revolutionized the detection and management of adenocarcinoma of the prostate (CAP) like no other marker in the history of oncology. From its discovery in the early 1970s to its application in the 1980s and, finally, its widespread usage in the 1990s, PSA has had a profound impact on the way in which we treat prostate cancer. The contributions to the PSA story are numerous by researchers in basic science and clinical practice. This chapter will review the history of the many people who have brought PSA to the forefront in the diagnosis and treatment of adenocarcinoma of the prostate.

I. THE PRE-PSA ERA

Prior to the 1930s, there were no biochemical markers for adenocarcinoma of the prostate. The diagnosis of adenocarcinoma of the prostate was made by results of clinical history and physical examination. In 1938, Gutman and Gutman discovered that serum acid phosphatase levels were frequently elevated in patients with metastatic adenocarcinoma of the prostate [1]. Huggins and Hodges also showed in 1941 that patients with bony metastases from adenocarcinoma of the prostate had high serum acid phosphatase levels and that these levels decreased significantly with either castration or the administration of estrogen. This decrease

1

in serum acid phosphatase was also accompanied by significant regression of tumor in patients with metastases both clinically and radiologically [2–4]. They also noted that serum alkaline phosphatase activity initially increased following estrogen administration and then declined towards normal levels.

As a tumor marker, serum acid phosphatase was limited in its usefulness due to lack of specificity for prostatic tissue. Acid phosphatase is present in many normal blood components and organs and is elevated in several nonprostatic malignancies including osteosarcoma, carcinoma of the breast, and other disease processes [5,6]. Fishman and Lerner developed an assay for the fraction of acid phosphatase produced by the prostate (prostatic acid phosphate [PAP]) gland, hoping thus to increase the specificity of biochemical detection of prostatic disease [7]. Subsequent research by other investigators, however, showed that early assays for PAP in fact did not completely detect only that acid phosphatase produced by prostatic sources [8].

During the 1960s and 1970s, many researchers worked on improving our knowledge and detection of PAP. Sensitivity and specificity of prostatic acid phosphatase was also limited by the realization that elevations were noted in patients who had undergone digital rectal examination, cystoscopy, transurethral resection of the prostate (TURP), and prostatic infarction. Finally, many series reported elevations of prostatic acid phosphatase occurring in only 20–30% of patients with clinically localized adenocarcinoma of the prostate. This rendered the method very insensitive in the detection of adenocarcinoma of the prostate at a stage when it can be potentially treated in hopes for a cure [5].

Prostatic acid phosphatase was helpful in focusing attention on tumor markers in the detection and treatment of adenocarcinoma of the prostate. However, sensitivity and specificity were still inadequate to detect, stage, and accurately follow treatment of prostate cancer biochemically.

II. EARLY DISCOVERIES

Several groups of investigators claim to have first discovered prostate specific antigen. Working independently, researchers identified prostate antigens in the late 1960s and early 1970s, which upon review were in fact found to be what is now known as prostate specific antigen. Ablin and associates reported on antigens from prostatic tissue in 1970; however this cannot be confirmed as what we now know as PSA [10,11]. Hara and associates in Japan described the protein gamma seminoprotein, which they isolated from seminal plasma and reported these findings in 1971 [12,13].

Li and Beling further isolated and purified this same protein from seminal plasma and reported their findings in 1973 [14]. They reported the molecule to have a weight of 31,000 daltons and called the molecule E1 antigen due to its mobility in conventional electrophoresis. Sensabaugh used immunoelectrophoresis to show that this protein was semen specific and could thus be used as a marker for semen identification. He reported the molecular weight to be 30,000 daltons and thus called the protein P30 based on its molecular weight [15]. Graves et al. proposed that P30 could be used in the identification of semen from rape suspects [16].

Finally, Wang and colleagues reported on the purification of the protein prostate specific antigen from prostate tissue [17]. Papsidero, working with Wang and colleagues, was able to show using rocket immunoelectrophoresis that the protein PSA purified from prostatic tissue was in fact identical to PSA in human serum [18].

Advances in amino acid sequencing have shown that proteins described by all these investigators were in fact probably the same: prostate specific antigen [19–21]. Reigman and associates PSA; described and sequenced the PSA gene in 1989 [22]. The biological function of prostate specific antigen in liquefying the seminal coagulum was discovered by the work of Lilja and associates [23,24]. Lilja and his group were also the first to report how PSA existed in serum mainly bound to alpha-2 macroglobulin (AMG) and alpha-1 antichymotrypsin (ACT) [25].

III. CLINICAL APPLICATIONS OF PSA

The Food and Drug Administration approved the first commercial immunoassay for PSA in 1986. In 1987, Stamey et al. reported the total PSA half-life to be 2.2 ± 0.8 days while Oesterling et al. reported in 1988 the half-life to be 3.2 ± 0.1 days [26,27]. Nadji and colleagues showed PSA to be a useful tumor marker in prostate cancer, which they reported in 1981 [28]. Several PSA assays became commercially available during the 1980s including the Tandem-R PSA, Proscheck PSA, Tandem-E PSA, IRMA-count PSA, and Abbott IMX PSA.

In 1986, Myrtle and associates determined the reference range for the tandem-R PSA assay to be 0.0–4.0 ng./ml [29]. Since their introduction, the commercially available PSA assays have undergone significant scrutiny by investigators to help promote standardization within and between these assays. Graves et al. were the first to call for international standardization of PSA assays [30]. Stamey and associates at Stanford were also one of the first groups to perform a clinical study showing the effectiveness of PSA as a tumor marker in prostate cancer, which they published in 1987 [26].

Several early studies showed the utility of PSA in detecting adenocarcinoma of the prostate when used in conjunction with digital rectal examination and transrectal ultrasound of the prostate. Dr. Cooner was one of the pioneers in the clinical application of transrectal ultrasound of the prostate and was one of the first proponents of the "three-legged stool": digital rectal examination, PSA, and transrectal ultrasound of the prostate [31]. The two early studies that confirm the utility of PSA alone in the detection of prostate cancer were performed by Brawer et al. and Catalona and associates [32,33].

IV. REFINEMENT

Due to the fact that there are many causes for the elevation of serum PSA, investigators have sought to improve PSA's ability to detect, stage, and monitor the progression of prostate cancer. Carter and associates introduced the concept of PSA velocity using sera collected as part of the Baltimore longitudinal aging study. They reported their results in 1992 and 1994 [34,35]. Benson and associates proposed the use of PSA density to increase the sensitivity and specificity of prostate cancer detection by PSA [36,37]. The initial correlation of PSA with increasing prostate gland volume was first shown by Stamey and associates in 1987 and confirmed by Babaian and associates in 1990 [26,38].

Age specific PSA reference ranges were first proposed by Oesterling and associates and by Dalkin and his group [39,40].

The use of either free or bound PSA to improve the sensitivity and specificity of prostate cancer detection was first introduced in the early 1990s by Stenman and his group and by Lilja and his associates [41–44]. Each of these approaches is the subject of a chapter in this book.

Partin and associates showed the clinical usefulness of total PSA in conjunction with the clinical stage and Gleason score to improve the preoperative prediction of the final pathological stage [45].

Prostate specific membrane antigen (PSMA) was first described in 1987 by Horoszewicz and associates [46]. While PSMA is distinct from PSA, it may be helpful in identifying aggressive prostate tumors and is also the antigen detected by the Prostascint imaging scan [47,48]. On the horizon, human kallikrein 2 has approximately 80% sequence homology with PSA and stains positive for virtually all prostatic carcinoma it may be useful in the future for the detection, staging, and monitoring of prostate cancer [49].

V. CONCLUSION

From its discovery in the late 1960s and early 1970s to its widespread usage and application in the 1980s, PSA has radically changed the way we deal with prostate cancer. This marker has profoundly affected our ability to diagnose prostate cancer. It has markedly changed our staging and monitoring of adenocarcinoma of the prostate. Numerous investigators have worked to discover, develop, and advance the prostate specific antigen as a tumor marker for prostate cancer. In no other malignancy has a tumor marker so profoundly affected diagnosis, staging, and management.

VI. MILESTONES IN THE HISTORY OF PSA

1971 Hara et al. describe gamma seminoprotein isolated from seminal plasma [12,13].
1973 Li and Beling purify the protein from seminal plasma [14].
1979 Wang et al. purify the protein from prostate tissue [17].
1981 Nadji et al. report association of PSA and prostate cancer [28].
1985 Lilja and associates describe the function and characteristics of PSA [23,25].
1986 Myrtle determines reference range of PSA [29].
1987 Stamey performs first clinical study showing effectiveness of PSA as tumor marker [26].
1990 Cooner promotes "Three-legged stool" approach to detection of prostate cancer (DRE, PSA, TRUS) [31].
1993 Brawer et al. and Catalona et al. publish studies confirming utility of PSA alone in the detection of CAP [32,33].
1992 Carter introduces concept of PSA velocity [34].
1992 Benson proposes use of PSA density [36].
1993 Oesterling et al. and Dalkin et al. report age specific reference ranges [39,40].
1997 Partin shows clinical application of PSA to final pathologic stage [45].

REFERENCES

1. EB Gutman, AB Gutman. An "acid" phosphatase occurring in the serum of patients with metastasizing carcinoma of the prostate gland. J Clin Invest 17:473, 1938.
2. C Huggins, CV Hodges. Studies on prostatic cancer I. The effect of castration, of estrogen and of androgen injection on serum phosphatases in metastatic carcinoma of the prostate. Cancer Res 1:293, 1941.
3. C Huggins, RE Stevens, CV Hodges. Studies on prostatic cancer III. The effects of fever, desoxycorticosterone and of estrogen on clinical patients with metastatic carcinoma of the prostate. J Urol 46:997, 1941.
4. C Huggins, RE Stevens, CV Hodges. Studies on prostatic cancer II. The effects of castration on advanced carcinoma of the prostate gland. Arch Surg, 43:209, 1941.
5. EL Coodley. Diagnostic Enzymology. Philadelphia: Lea & Febiger, 1970, p 158.
6. GR Prout Jr, EV Macalalag Jr, LJ Denis, LW Preston Jr. Alterations in serum lactic

dehydrogenase and its fourth and fifth isozymes in patients with prostatic carcinoma. J Urol 94:451, 1965.

7. WH Fishman, FA Lerner. A method for estimating serum acid phosphatase of prostatic origin. J Biol Chem 200:89, 1953.

8. TP Maramba Jr. Histochemical differentiation of carcinoma of the prostate gland from other tumors by a modified acid phosphatase reaction. Am J Clin Pathol 43: 319, 1965.

9. WJ Catalona, WW Scott. Carcinoma of the Prostate. In: Campbell's Urology. 4th ed., vol 2. Philadelphia: Williams & Wilkins, 1979, pp: 1085–1124.

10. RJ Ablin, P Bronson, WA Soanes, et al. Tissue- and species-specific antigens of normal human prostatic tissue. J Immunol 104:1329, 1970.

11. RJ Ablin, P Bronson, WA Soanes, et al. Precipitating antigens of the normal prostate. J Reprod Fertil 22:573, 1970.

12. M Hara, Y Koyanagi, T Inogue, et al. Some physicochemical characteristics of "γ-seminoprotein," an antigenic component specific for human seminal plasma. Jpn J Legal Med 25:322, 1971.

13. M Hara, T Innore, T Fukulyama, et al. Some physicochemical characteristics of gamma-seminoprotein, an antigenic component specific for human seminal plasma. Nippon Hoigaku Zasshi 25:322, 1971.

14. TS Li, CG Beling. Isolation and characterization of two specific antigens of human seminal plasma. Fertil Steril 24:134, 1973.

15. GF Sensabaugh: Isolation and characterization of a semen-specific protein from human seminal plasma: A potential new marker for semen identification. J Forensic Sci 23:106, 1978.

16. HCB Graves, GF Sensabaugh, ET Blake. Postcoital detection of a male-specific semen protein: Application to the investigation of rape. N Engl J Med 312:338, 1985.

17. MC Wang, LA Valenzuela, GP Murphy, et al. Purification of a human prostate specific antigen. Invest Urol 17:159, 1979.

18. LD Papsidero, MC Wang, LA Valenzuela, GP Murphy, TM Chu. A prostate antigen in sera of prostatic cancer patients. Cancer Res 40:4828, 1980.

19. A Lundwall, H Lilja. Molecular cloning of human prostate specific antigen cDNA. FEBS Lett 214:317, 1987.

20. J Schaller, K Akiyama, R Tsuda, et al. Isolation, characterization and amino-acid sequence of γ-seminoprotein, a glycoprotein from human seminal plasma. Eur J Biochem 170:111, 1987.

21. KWK Watt, PJ Lee, T M'Timkulu, et al. Human prostate-specific antigen: Structural and functional similarity with serine proteases. Proc Natl Acad Sci USA 83:3166, 1986.

22. PHJ Riegman, RJ Vlietstra, JAGM van der Korpert, et al. Characterization of the prostate-specific antigen gene: A novel human kallikrein-like gene. Biochem Biophys Res Commun 159:95, 1989.

23. H Lilja. A kallikrein-like serine protease in prostatic fluid cleaves the predominant seminal vesicle protein. J Clin Invest 76:1899–1903, 1985.

24. H Lilja, CB Laurell. The predominant protein in human seminal coagulate. Scand J Clin Lab Invest 45:635–641, 1985.

25. A Christensson, C-B Laurell, H Lilja. Enzymatic activity of prostate-specific antigen

and its reactions with extracellular serine proteinase inhibitors. Eur J Biochem 194: 755–763, 1990.

26. TA Stamey, N Yang, AR Hay, et al. Prostate-specific antigen as a serum marker for adenocarcinoma of the prostate. N Engl J Med 317:909, 1987.

27. JE Oesterling, DW Chan, JI Epstein, et al. Prostate specific antigen in the preoperative and postoperative evaluation of localized prostatic cancer treated with radical prostatectomy. J Urol 139:766, 1988.

28. M Nadji, SZ Tabei, A Castro, TM Chu, GP Murphy, MC Wang, et al. Prostatic-specific antigen: An immunohistologic marker for prostatic neoplasms. Cancer 1229–1232, 1981.

29. JF Myrtle, PG Klimley, LP Ivor, JF Brun. Clinical utility of prostate-specific antigen (PSA) in the management of prostate cancer. Adv Cancer Diagn, 1986.

30. HCB Graves, N Wehner, TA Stamey. Comparison of a polyclonal and monoclonal immunoassay for PSA: Need for an international antigen standard. J Urol 144:1516–1522, 1990.

31. WH Cooner, BR Mosley, CL Rutherford Jr, et al. Prostate cancer detection in a clinical urological practice by ultrasonography, digital rectal examination and prostate specific antigen. J Urol 143:1146–1154, 1990.

32. MK Brawer, MP Chetner, J Beatie, DM Buchner, RL Vessella, PH Lange. Screening for prostatic carcinoma with PSA. J Urol 147:841–845, 1992.

33. WJ Catalona, DS Smith, TL Ratliff, et al. Measurement of PSA in serum as a screening test for prostate cancer. NEJM 324:1156–1161, 1991.

34. HB Carter, CH Morrell, JD Pearson, et al. Estimation of prostatic growth using serial prostate-specific antigen measurements in men with and without prostate disease. Cancer Res 52:3323–3328, 1992.

35. JD Pearson, HB Carter. Natural history of changes in prostate specific antigen in early stage prostate cancer. J Urol 152:1743–1748, 1994.

36. MC Benson, IS Whang, CA Olsson, et al. The use of prostate specific antigen density to enhance the predictive value of intermediate levels of serum prostate specific antigen. J Urol 147:817–821, 1992.

37. MC Benson, IS Whang, A Pantuck, et al. Prostate specific antigen density: A means of distinguishing benign prostatic hypertrophy and prostate cancer. J Urol 147:815–816, 1992.

38. RJ Babaian, HA Fritsche, RB Evans. PSA and prostate gland volume: Correlation and clinical application. J Clin Lab 4:135–137, 1990.

39. JE Oesterling, SJ Jacobsen, CG Chute, et al. Serum prostate-specific antigen in a community-based population of healthy men. JAMA 270:860–864, 1993.

40. BL Dalkin, FR Ahmann, JB Kopp. Prostate specific antigen levels in men older than 50 years without clinical evidence of prostatic carcinoma. J Urol 150:1837–1839, 1993.

41. A Christensson, T Bjork, O Nilsson, et al. Serum prostate specific antigen complexed to α1-antichymotrypsin as an indicator of prostate cancer. J Urol 150:100–105, 1993.

42. H Lilja. Significance of different molecular forms of serum PSA: The free, non-complexed form of PSA versus that complexed to α1-antichymotrypsin. Urol Clin N Am 20:681–686, 1993.

43. U Stenman, J Leinonen, H Alfthan, et al. A complex between PSA and α1-antichy-

motrypsin is the major form of prostate-specific antigen in serum of patients with prostatic cancer: Assay of the complex improves clinical sensitivity for cancer. Cancer Res 52:222–226, 1991.

44. H Lilja, A Christensson, U Dahlen, et al. Prostate-specific antigen in serum occurs predominantly in complex with α1-antichymotrypsin. Clin Chem 37:1618–1625, 1991.

45. AW Partin, ENP Subong, PC Walsh, et al. Combination of prostate specific antigen, clinical stage, and Gleason score to predict pathological stage of localized prostate cancer: A multi-institutional update. JAMA 377:1445–1451, 1997.

46. JS Horoszewicz, E Kawinski, GP Murphy. Monoclonal antibodies to a new antigenic marker in epithelial prostatic cells and serum of prostatic cancer patients. Anticancer Res 7:927–935, 1987.

47. RJ Babaian, J Sayer, DA Podoloff, et al. Radioimmunoscintigraphy of pelvic lymph nodes with [111]Indium-labeled monoclonal antibody cyt-356. J Urol 152:1951–1955, 1994.

48. D Kahn, RD Williams, DW Seldin, et al. Radioimmunoscintigraphy with [111]Indium-labeled CYT-356 for the detection of occult prostate cancer recurrence. J Urol 152: 1490–1495, 1994.

49. MF Darson, A Pacelli, P Roche, et al. Human glandular kallikrein 2 (hK2) expression in prostatic intraepithelial neoplasia and adenocarcinoma: A novel prostate cancer marker. Urology 49:857–862, 1997.

2
Biochemistry and Basic Science

Ulf-Håkan Stenman
Helsinki University Central Hospital, Helsinki, Finland

Prostate specific antigen (PSA) was initially isolated from prostate tissue extracts by Chu et al. [1]. The same protein had earlier been purified from seminal fluid and called γ-seminoprotein [2], E1 [3], and P30 [4], but Chu et al. were the first to show that PSA was derived from the prostate and that it could be used as a serum marker for prostate cancer [5,6]. PSA is a serine protease that digests the gel forming after ejaculation [7]. It forms complexes with α_2-macroglobulin (A2M) and α_1-antichymotrypsin (ACT) in vitro [8] and a major part of PSA in serum occurs in complex with ACT. The proportion of complexed PSA is higher and that of free PSA is lower in patients with prostate cancer than in men with benign prostatic hyperplasia (BPH) [9]. PSA is a very useful serum marker for monitoring of prostate cancer [10,11], and it can also be used for screening of this disease [12,13]. The use of PSA determinations for screening is hampered by a high-frequency of false-positive results in men with BPH [12,13]. The frequency of false positive results can be reduced by measurement of the proportion of complexed or free PSA in serum [9,14]. A low percentage of PSA in serum occurs in complex with α_1-trypsin inhibitor (API, also called α_1-antitrypsin) [15] and about 10% consists of PSA-A2M [16]. These forms are also of potential diagnostic utility. The presence of various molecular forms of PSA in serum complicates the determination of PSA [9,17] but it has, on the other hand, facilitated development of assays for the various forms of PSA with improved cancer specificity [18].

I. RELATIONSHIP OF PSA TO OTHER PROTEASES

PSA is a serine protease belonging to the human glandular kallikrein family. Until recently, this family was thought to comprise three members: tissue kallikrein or human kallikrein 1 (hK1), which is mainly expressed in pancreas, kidney, and salivary gland; hK2; and PSA (hK3). The latter two are strongly expressed in the prostate [19]. Low-level expression of PSA and hK2 can be detected in the female breast and in some other organs. Recently, 11 other members of the human kallikrein family have been identified. They are all encoded by genes located on chromosome 19q13.3–13.4 [20]. The kallikreins display considerable homology and that between PSA and hK2 is about 80% both at the protein and mRNA levels [21].

II. STRUCTURE AND ENZYMATIC ACTIVITY OF PSA

A. Chemical Characteristics of PSA in Seminal Fluid

Mature, enzymatically active PSA contains 237 amino acids and the calculated molecular weight of the peptide chain is 26,079 [22,23]. In addition, PSA contains a single biantennary carbohydrate moiety linked to Asn 45. The average molecular weight of the carbohydrate moiety is 2351 and that of the glycosylated protein is 28,430 [23]. The apparent molecular size determined by sodium dodecyl sulfate (SDS) gel electrophoresis is about 33 kDa [24]. Based on the cDNA sequence, PSA is synthesised with a 17 amino acid signal sequence, which is removed during synthesis. PSA is secreted as a 244 amino acid proenzyme (proPSA), which is activated by proteolytic removal of a 7 amino acid propeptide [22].

In seminal fluid PSA mainly occurs in active mature form, but about 30% is inactivated due to cleavage or "nicking" of the peptide bonds after Arg 85, Lys 145, and Lys 182 [8,25]. Due to this and variation in carbohydrate composition, PSA is microheterogeneous, displaying several isoenzymes with isoelectric points (pI) in the range 6.6–7.2. Five isoenzymes named PSA-A to -D can be separated by ion exchange chromatography. PSA-A and B have an intact peptide chain and differ only with respect to sialic acid content, while isoenzymes C, D, and E and are nicked in various ways. The isoelectric point of the major isoenzyme (PSA-B) is 6.9 [26]. About 20% of the apparently intact PSA isolated from seminal (isoenzymes A and B) is enzymatically inactive due to some hitherto unknown modification [27]. The nicked isoenzymes lack enzymatic activity against peptide substrates [8] but they react slowly with A2M, suggesting that they retain some enzyme activity [27].

B. Enzymatic Activity

PSA exerts chymotrypsin-like activity, showing preference for hydrophobic residues such as phenylalanin and leucin. However, the specificity is more restricted than that of chymotrypsin and the specific activity of PSA against synthetic substrates is more than 1000-fold lower than that of chymotrypsin [25]. However, PSA efficiently dissolves the semenogelins, suggesting that its activity against its natural substrates is high [7].

C. Reaction of PSA with Protease Inhibitors

When added to serum, PSA reacts preferentially with A2M and somewhat less with ACT [8,27]. PSA also reacts with protein C inhibitor (PCI), pregnancy zone protein (PZ) [8], and API [28]. About 5% of PSA in seminal plasma consists of PSA-PCI [29], but neither this complex nor PSA-PZ is detected in serum [29,30]. A low percentage of PSA in serum consists of PSA-API [31]. Complex formation between PSA and A2M leads to encapsulation of PSA and loss of immunoreactivity [8,27]. PSA in the PSA-A2M complex can be detected by antibodies after denaturation with SDS [8,32] or by high pH [16].

III. PHYSIOLOGICAL FUNCTION OF PSA

A. Role of PSA in Reproduction

PSA is secreted into seminal fluid at concentrations of 0.5–3 mg/ml (i.e., about 1 million times those in plasma) [33]. In semen, PSA dissolves the gel forming after ejaculation by digesting semenogelin-1 and -2 and fibronectin, causing release of the sperm, which is essential for sperm function [7].

PSA is probably secreted in its zymogen form, proPSA, which can be activated by proteases with trypsin-like activity. Recombinant hK2 activates PSA [34], but seminal plasma contains other enzymes with appropriate activity. Trypsin actually occurs in seminal fluid at concentrations high enough to activate proPSA [35]. Because trypsin also activates prohK2 [36], it may be a key enzyme in a protease cascade comprising several protease acting in concert to activate prohK2 and proPSA.

A minor part of PSA binds to A2M in seminal plasma and the PSA-A2M complex is taken up by the α_2-macroglobulin-receptor/low-density lipoprotein receptor-related protein on sperm [37]. PSA-A2M has been suggested to affect sperm function, and the concentration of A2M in seminal fluid has been found to reflect the motility and quality of sperm [38].

B. Possible Role of PSA in BPH and Prostate Cancer

PSA has been shown to digest partially insulin-like growth factor (IGF)-binding protein-3 (IGFBP-3), which is the major transport protein of IGF-I in plasma. This might stimulate the growth of prostate cancer by inducing local release of IGF-1 [39]. Elevated serum IGF-1 levels have been found in some studies to be associated with later development of prostate cancer [40]. However, other studies have shown an association between serum IGF-1, BPH, and prostate volume [41]. IGF-1 stimulates the growth of prostatic stromal cells in culture [42]. Men with acromegaly and high IGF-1 levels have been found to develop BPH in their fourth decade, whereas successfully treated patients with acromegaly have smaller than average prostate volume [43]. Thus the correlation between IGF-1 and prostate cancer may be related to a higher likelihood that a prostate cancer will be diagnosed clinically in men with an enlarged prostate [41].

Considering the high concentrations of PSA within the prostate and the slow growth of prostate cancer, a tumor-promoting function of PSA seems surprising. Recent findings suggest that PSA exerts antiangiogenic activity that could retard tumor growth. Culture fluid from prostate cancer cells contains protease activity that converts plasminogen to angiostatin, and purified PSA has been shown to be antiangiogenic in cell culture. When infused into mice, PSA has been found to reduce the number of lung colonies formed by melanoma cells [44]. Furthermore, purified PSA has been found to release functional angiostatin from plasminogen. An antiangiogenic function of PSA would be in line with the slow development of prostate cancer [45] and the finding that PSA expression decreases with loss of differentiation and increasing aggressiveness of prostate cancer [46]. The idea that PSA suppresses the growth of malignant prostatic cells is attractive, but the evidence is still circumstantial. The PSA concentrations used have been high and minor contaminants with high specific activity could exert the antiangiogenic activity.

IV. METABOLISM OF PSA

A. Release of PSA from the Prostate into Circulation

The normal prostate excretes the vast majority of the PSA produced into the glandular ducts of the prostate, whereas only a small portion leaks out into circulation [47]. However, prostate cancer tissue releases 30-fold more PSA into circulation than normal prostatic tissue and 10-fold more than BPH tissue [10]. This is probably explained by the loss of tissue architecture in cancer. When the malignant tissue loses connection with the prostatic ducts and the polarization of the cells is deranged, PSA may be actively secreted into the extracellular space and into circulation. From normal prostatic cells PSA has to leak out ''backwards'' into the extracellular space before it can reach circulation (Fig. 1) [47].

Differences in the way PSA reaches circulation could also explain why the proportion of free PSA is lower and that of complexed PSA is higher in serum of patients with prostatic cancer than in normal subjects and patients with BPH [9]. When reaching circulation through the extracellular space from BPH and normal prostatic cells, PSA may be subjected to degradation [18,47]. PSA iso-

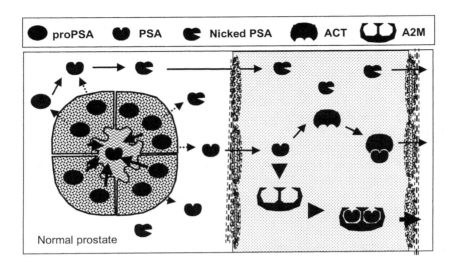

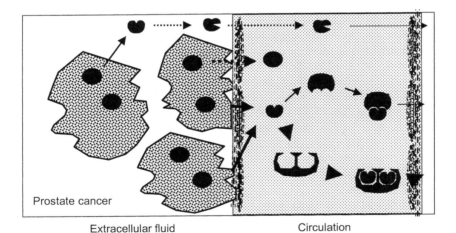

Figure 1 Model for release and secretion of PSA from normal (upper panel) and cancerous (lower panel) prostatic tissue and for the metabolism of the various forms in extracellular fluid and circulation. Within the prostatic cells, PSA exists in its zymogen form, proPSA, which is activated during secretion into seminal fluid, extracellular fluid, and circulation. (Modified with permission from Ref. 47.)

lated from BPH fluid has actually been shown to be extensively nicked (i.e., partially degraded by proteolytic digestion) [48]. Nicked PSA does not react with ACT [27] and free PSA isolated from serum of patients with prostate cancer is less extensively nicked than that isolated from serum of patients with BPH [49]. Thus, PSA secreted from tumor cells probably reaches circulation in an enzymatically more active form than that leaking out from normal and BPH tissue and it may therefore react more extensively with ACT.

The more extensive complexation of serum PSA in prostate cancer than in BPH patients could also be explained by differences in the availability of various inhibitors in the prostate. ACT has been found to be more strongly expressed in cancerous than in hyperplastic prostatic tissue. This could favor formation of PSA-ACT in patients with prostate cancer [50]. However, only free PSA appears to be released into plasma during prostatic surgery [51]. Thus, it is not clear whether prostatic ACT actually contributes to the complexation of PSA in circulation [18].

B.   Clearance of PSA from Circulation

After radical prostatectomy the half-time of PSA is about 3 days [10,11]. With frequent sampling an initial rapid α phase with a half time of 1-2 h has also been observed [52]. The two phases have been interpreted to correspond to the metabolism of free and complexed PSA, respectively. However, recent studies, in which the hemodynamic changes occurring during surgery have been taken into account, suggest that the first rapid phase is mainly caused by changes in plasma volume and redistribution of free PSA released during surgery between the intra- and extravascular spaces [53]. After the initial phase the half-life of free PSA is about 18 hr [51,53], while that of PSA-ACT is about 3 days [53]. PSA released during prostatic surgery may not able to form complexes with ACT and it may thus differ from that released under physiological circumstances [51]. Therefore, studies on the disappearance of PSA after prostatic manipulation may not reflect the physiological metabolism of PSA.

Measurement of the gradient in PSA concentrations over various organs in men indicates that the liver extracts both PSA-ACT and free PSA, while the latter also is extracted by the kidneys [54]. After injection of radiolabeled PSA and PSA complexes into experimental animals, free PSA and PSA-ACT are extracted by the kidneys and the liver while PSA-A2M is taken up by the liver through the α_2-macroglobulin-receptor/low-density lipoprotein receptor-related protein [55]. In rats, the half-life of the human PSA-A2M complex is only 6.7 min. On the basis of the rapid complexation of A2M with enzymatically active PSA [56] and the rapid removal of PSA-A2M, it has been suggested that A2M plays a major role in the metabolism of PSA [18]. This is further supported by the finding that radiolabeled free PSA and PSA-A2M have a similar half-lives in rats [55]. The rate of removal of PSA-A2M is 150-fold that of enzymatically inactive PSA and 600-fold that of PSA-ACT. Thus, the concentrations of PSA-A2M in plasma may be fairly low in vivo even if A2M removes most of the PSA that reaches the circulation [18].

The metabolism of PSA is determined by the rates of complex formation with inhibitors and the half-lives of these and free PSA in circulation. On the basis of presently available data, three major metabolic routes can be envisaged. First, free PSA lacking enzymatic activity due to nicking is removed with a half-life of 18 h. Second, enzymatically active PSA reaching circulation reacts preferentially with A2M and is rapidly removed. Third, part of the enzymatically active PSA reacts with ACT and is slowly removed with a half-time of 3 days.

V. IMMUNOCHEMICAL PROPERTIES AND DETERMINATION OF VARIOUS FORMS OF PSA

A. Factors Affecting Immunoassay of PSA

Immunoassay of PSA is complicated by the heterogeneity of PSA in serum: PSA complexes, various isoenzymes of free PSA, and cross-reaction with hK2. PSA becomes undetectable by conventional immunoassays when bound to A2M [27], while complexation with ACT and API causes loss of some antigenic determinants [9,57]. Although the PSA-A2M complex does not interfere in conventional assays for PSA, complex formation between free PSA and A2M may be responsible for the loss of free PSA during storage of serum [58].

B. Antigenic Regions and Epitopes of PSA

Characterization of the antigenic properties of PSA facilitates development of assays with predefined properties. The binding specificities of 83 widely used monoclonal antibodies to PSA have been characterized in an international collaborative study. Six antigenic regions have been defined, each comprising several overlapping epitopes. Some of the epitopes have been linked to the three-dimensional structure of PSA [59] (Fig. 2). Region 1 is covered by ACT and API in the corresponding complexes. Antibodies reacting with this region are used for specific determination of free PSA and these assays do not recognize hK2. Region 2 surrounds region 1 and antibodies reacting with this region tend to underestimate complexed forms of PSA. Region 2 is surrounded by regions 3, 4, and 5, which further surround region 6. Some epitopes in region 3, 4, and 6 also occur on hk2. Region 6 contains a strong antigenic determinant, which has been mapped to amino acids 3–11 of the N-terminal part of PSA. This epitope appears to be identical on hK2 [57,60]. Most antibodies reacting with regions 4 and 6 enhance the enzymatic activity of PSA, whereas antibodies reacting with the other regions inhibit the activity [61].

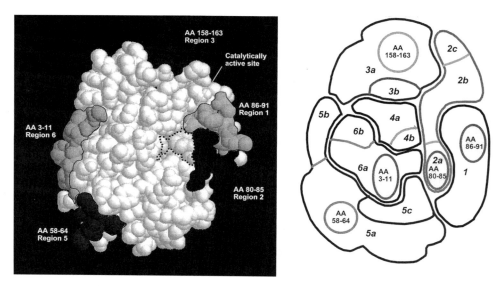

Figure 2 Linkage of the epitope map of PSA to the three-dimensional structure. The right panel shows the epitope map with antigenic regions indicated by numbers. Epitopes that have been linked to defined positions on the peptide chains are indicated by the amino (AA) numbers. The left panel shows a three-dimensional model of PSA, in which the positions of positively identified epitopes and the corresponding antigenic regions are indicated. Region 6 is positioned in the middle of the epitope map but far left on the three-dimensional model. This reflects the limited ability of the two-dimensional map to reflect the three-dimensional structure. Region 5b is probably located on the invisible backside of the model. Region 4 has not been linked to the three-dimensional model. The boundary of the active site is demarcated by a broken line; those of regions 1, 5, and 6 by solid lines. (Modified from Ref. 59 with permission, S. Karger, AG, Basel, Switzerland.)

C. Determination of the Various Forms of PSA in Serum

1. Total PSA

Total PSA comprises free PSA, PSA-ACT, and PSA-API [15]. Many early PSA assays underestimated the complexed forms of PSA, which led to discrepancies between the results from various methods. This was mostly due to the use of polyclonal antibodies, which underestimated complexed PSA [17], but it was also a problem with some assays that used two monoclonal antibodies [62]. This problem can be reduced by using a standard containing free PSA and PSA-ACT in proportions similar to those occurring in serum [63]. However, this is not an ideal solution especially if the assay is used together with an assay for free PSA to estimate the proportion of free PSA. Therefore, most of the assays presently available in United States are based on two monoclonal antibodies, which recognize free and complexed PSA equally. However, very large differences exist between the more than 60 assays available in Europe [64].

2. Free PSA

Monoclonal antibodies have been used to develop very specific assays for free PSA [65]. These antibodies, which recognize epitope region 1, cross-react at a rate of less than 1% with PSA-ACT and PSA-API but they, as well as other monoclonal antibodies, may recognize various nicked PSA isoenzymes quite differently [57]. Several forms of free PSA occur in serum, in addition to the nicked and apparently intact forms, a variant lacking the first N-terminal amino acid [49], and a form resembling proPSA [66]. The isoelectric point of proPSA expressed by LNCaP cells is 8.2–8.4 [67] and a small fraction of free PSA with this pI has been detected in serum [68]. However, proPSA has not been detected in PSA isolated from serum [49,69]. Free PSA in serum from patients with BPH is more extensively nicked than that in prostate cancer serum [49]. It has been suggested that specific determination of certain nicked forms could be utilized to improve the differentiation between prostate cancer and BPH [70]. The heterogeneity of free PSA may explain why assays for this PSA often give different results [71,72].

An assay for γ-seminoprotein has been used as an alternative to free PSA. However, direct comparison between this method and various assays for free PSA has shown that the γ-seminoprotein assay does not specifically measure free PSA [72].

3. PSA-ACT

PSA-ACT can be measured specifically by using a capture antibody recognizing both free and complexed PSA and an antibody specific to ACT as a tracer [9]. This assay is complicated by a variable background caused by nonspecific adsorption of ACT and protease-ACT complexes to the solid phase [56,73]. This causes variation, which may explain why the proportion of PSA-ACT has not been found to be as useful as that of free PSA [73]. The variation can be reduced by measuring PSA-ACT and total PSA simultaneously with a double-label assay. The discrimination between prostate cancer and BPH with such an assay was equal to that obtained with free and total PSA [56]. Being easier to measure accurately than PSA-ACT, free PSA is now routinely used to estimate the proportion of the two major forms of PSA in serum.

4. PSA-API

The PSA-API complex can be determined by a sandwich assay using a catcher antibody to PSA on the solid phase and a detector antibody to API [9]. This assay is also hampered by a nonspecific background caused by adsorption of API to the solid phase [28]. When this background is eliminated, the median serum concentrations of PSA-API are higher in BPH than in prostate cancer (i.e., 1.6% and 0.9%, respectively). Thus, the behavior of PSA-API is opposite to that of PSA-ACT and PSA-API can be used to improve the cancer specificity of free and total PSA [31].

5. PSA-A2M

A2M is the major inhibitor of PSA in plasma [8,16,27] but quantitative assay of this form of PSA has only recently become possible. This method is based on removal of free PSA, PSA-ACT and PSA-API by immunoadsorption and denaturation of PSA-A2M at high pH and measurement of the released PSA immunoreactivity by a conventional PSA assay. Denaturation causes release of some PSA in free, enzymatically active, and fully immunoreactive form, while most of it remains bound but is rendered partially immunoreactive. The median ratio of PSA-A2M to total PSA in sera from patients with prostate cancer and BPH is 8% and 12%, respectively [16] and thus PSA-A2M provides diagnostic information complementary to that of free and total PSA [74]. If one considers the short half-time of PSA-A2M, the serum concentrations are surprisingly high. It is therefore possible that part of the PSA-A2M in serum is formed by reaction with free PSA in vitro after sampling. This could explain why the proportion of PSA-A2M, like that of free PSA, is higher in BPH than in prostate cancer [74].

6. Complexed PSA

The sum of PSA-ACT and PSA-API can be measured together by an assay for ''complexed PSA.'' This assay is based on blocking of the reaction of free PSA with a free-specific PSA antibody [75]. The proportion of complexed PSA (PSA-ACT + PSA-API) is theoretically inferior to the proportion of PSA-ACT because PSA-ACT increases and PSA-API decreases in prostate cancer. However, the first studies have provided promising results [76]. Complexed PSA is extensively described in Chapter 8.

D. Distribution of the Various Forms of PSA in Serum in Prostatic Disease

About 60–95% of the immunoreactive PSA in serum consists of PSA-ACT, free PSA represents 5–40%, and PSA-API about 0.5–5%. Together these forms of PSA make up the so-called total PSA [15]. However, what is generally called ''total PSA'' does not include PSA-A2M, because this form is not measured by conventional PSA assays. PSA may actually constitute more than 20% of PSA in serum [16]. The proportion of PSA-ACT is higher whereas that of free PSA,

PSA-API, and PSA-A2M are lower in men with than without prostate cancer. The proportion of PSA-ACT tends to increase and that of free PSA decrease with increasing PSA concentrations because of the increasing contribution of prostate cancer tissue to the serum concentration of PSA [9].

Figure 3 shows how the proportions of free PSA, PSA-ACT, and PSA-API are affected by the contribution of various tissues to serum PSA in different patients with total PSA concentrations of 4 ng/ml. The concentration can be raised to this level by a relatively small tumor (1 g) in a normal gland. The tumor contributes most of the PSA and the proportion of free PSA is low. This situation

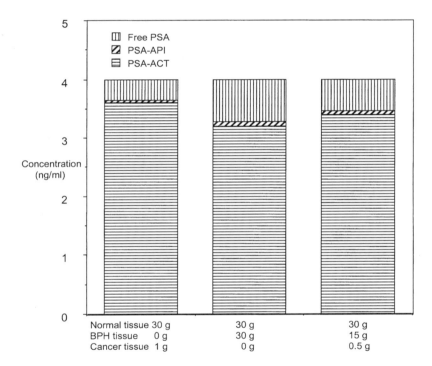

Figure 3 Distribution of PSA-ACT, PSA-API, and free PSA in patients with a border-line PSA value of 4 ng/ml caused by a 1 g tumor in a normal gland (left column), a gland enlarged due to BPH (middle), and a small tumor (0.5 g) in a gland containing BPH tissue. The proportion of free PSA provides the best discrimination when most of the PSA is derived from cancer tissue. If a substantial part of PSA is derived from BPH tissue, a smaller tumor will increase serum PSA to 4 ng/ml, but the effect of the cancer on the proportion of free PSA will be intermediate between that of pure BPH and a cancer in a small gland.

is typical of early prostate cancer in relatively young men. Longitudinal studies of men who later develop prostate cancer have shown that a decrease in the proportion of free PSA often is observed more than a decade before clinical presentation [77]. When the PSA level is increased by a large BPH gland, which contributes most of the PSA, the proportion of free PSA will be low. When a small prostate cancer together with an enlarged BPH gland cause the PSA elevation, free PSA levels will be intermediate. Therefore, free PSA is less useful in men with a large prostate and a higher cutoff for the proportion is indicated for them [78,79]. However, a more rational approach is to use logistic regression or neural networks to estimate the probability of prostate cancer on the basis of the combined impact of free and total PSA, digital rectal examination, and prostate volume [80,81] (see Sec. VII).

VI. ASSAY STANDARDIZATION

Appropriate standardization of immunoassays requires the use of standards and reference methods [62]. A preparation containing 90% PSA-ACT and 10% free PSA has recently been accepted by the World Health Organization (WHO) as an international standard [63]. The standard has already been used by kit manufacturers, and this appears to have contributed to improved comparability of the most commonly used assays [82], but results for free PSA still show large variation [72]. Although the general agreement between some assays is excellent, considerable difference may be observed in some patients. Therefore, use of the same assay during monitoring of individual patients is strongly recommended.

VII. INTERPRETATION OF RESULTS FOR PSA

A cut-off level of 4 ng/ml has become widely used as a decision limit although it does not correspond to any reference value. The PSA concentrations in serum increase with age [83] and, therefore, the reference values are age-dependent. The upper reference limits determined on the basis of the 95th percentile are 2.5 ng/ml in the age group 40–49 years, 3.5 ng/ml at age 50–59 years, 4.5 ng/ml at age 60–69 years, and 6.5 ng/ml at age 70–79 years [84]. The value of using age-specific reference ranges is debated, and this aspect is reviewed in Chapter 20. The probability of finding a prostate cancer in a man with a serum PSA of 4 ng/L is about 20% and it is similar when PSA is in the range 2.6–4 ng/ml [85]. In a screening setting the use of lower decision limits may nearly double the number of biopsies, which, however, can be reduced by determining the proportion of free PSA [85,86]. So far there is no consensus on which cutoff to use for free PSA and it is furthermore dependent on the assay method.

An alternative method of deciding the need to confirm or exclude prostate cancer by biopsy is to estimate of the combined impact of total and free PSA by logistic regression or neural networks [80,81,87]. The relative impact of various input variables on prostate cancer risk can be estimated by logistic regression, and this shows that free PSA actually affects the risk much more strongly than total PSA in the concentration range 3–20 ng/ml [80,81]. When total PSA is 4 ng/ml the average prostate cancer risk is 15–20%, but the risk varies considerably depending on the proportion of free PSA. The commonly used cutoff of 4 ng/ml for total PSA is a very crude estimate of the need to perform a biopsy (Table 1). When free PSA is 40% the risk is only 3%, whereas it is 50% when the proportion is 5%. Even when total PSA is 20 ng/ml, the risk is below 10% when

Table 1 Probability of Finding Prostate Cancer with Various Combinations of Free and Total PSA in Men with Normal (A) or Abnormal Findings on Digital Rectal Examination (B)

Proportion of free PSA	Probability of prostate cancer in biopsy			
A. Normal DRE				
0.40	0.02	0.03	0.05	0.12
0.35	0.03	0.04	0.09	0.19
0.30	0.04	0.07	0.15	0.29
0.25	0.07	0.12	0.24	0.42
0.20	0.12	0.19	0.35	0.56
0.15	0.19	0.28	0.49	0.69
0.10	0.30	0.42	0.63	0.79
0.05	0.52	0.64	0.81	0.90
Total PSA (ng/ml)	4	10	20	30
B. Abnormal DRE				
0.40	0.08	0.12	0.25	0.43
0.35	0.13	0.20	0.37	0.57
0.30	0.21	0.30	0.51	0.70
0.25	0.32	0.43	0.65	0.80
0.20	0.45	0.57	0.76	0.88
0.15	0.59	0.70	0.84	0.92
0.10	0.72	0.80	0.90	0.95
0.05	0.86	0.91	0.96	0.98
Total PSA (ng/ml)	4	10	20	30

The calculations are based on data from the Dutch prostate cancer screening trial [80]. Free and total PSA were determined by the Delfia Prostatus PSA assay (Wallac, Turku, Finland). The probabilities may be different in other populations (cf. 81) and are also affected by differences between the assay methods used. The cancer probability is affected by prevalence and tends to be higher in referred patients.

free PSA is 35% [80] (Table 1). This shows that much more emphasis should be placed on the proportion of PSA, but the probability estimate is preferable because it takes into account the impact of all significant input variables.

An abnormal finding on digital rectal examination is associated with a substantial increase in prostate cancer probability (Table 1, part B) and the impact of this result can be taken into account in the probability calculation. A further refinement in the probability estimate can be obtained by including prostate volume and an optimized neural network rather than logistic regression [81]. So far there is no consensus on which cutoff for prostate cancer probability should be used and the acceptable probability may vary from one case to another depending on age, life expectancy, and personal preferences. Nevertheless, the estimated probability is a more valid basis for making the decision to perform biopsy than the presently used decision limits. Furthermore, the meaning of cancer probability is easy to understand for the patient.

VIII. PREANALYTICAL FACTORS AFFECTING THE PSA CONCENTRATIONS IN SERUM

A. Biological Variation

There is considerable intraindividual variation in the serum concentrations of PSA, with a coefficient of variation for total PSA over time of 10–20% [88] and a larger variation for free PSA [89]. Little is known about the cause of this variation. Ejaculation has been shown to cause a slight but significant increase in the concentrations of free PSA for some hours and a smaller increase of total PSA peaking around 1 day later. However, ejaculation explains only a minor part of the physiological variation; the major causes are not yet known [90]. Various types of prostatic manipulation cause smaller or larger increases in serum PSA levels. The effect of digital rectal examination is mostly negligible [91,92], but because it occasionally has a notable effect, samples for PSA determinations should be drawn before or at least one day after clinical examinations of the prostate [18]. Prostate biopsy and surgery cause a strong increase in serum PSA and the effect may last for weeks [10].

B. Stability of PSA in Serum During Storage

The concentrations of PSA in serum tend to decrease during storage of serum [56]. During short-term storage the main effect is loss of free PSA. This is probably due to complex formation between free PSA and A2M and possibly to proteolytic degradation [58,93]. Nearly 10% of both free and total PSA is lost when serum is stored for 2 years at $-20°C$ [94] and 30–40% is lost after 20 years [95]. Total PSA is unaffected and less than 5% of free PSA is lost when serum is stored at $-70°C$ for 2 years [94]. Therefore, blood samples used for assay of PSA should be separated within 2 h, serum should be kept for no more than 1 day at 4°C and for less than a month at $-20°C$. Long-term storage should be at $-70°C$.

IX. CONCLUSIONS

Through the use of PSA and its derivatives, better markers are available for prostate cancer than for any other common malignant tumor. Total and free PSA are now widely used and further improvement appears possible through the use of new markers. Of these, hK2, PSA-API, and PSA-A2M appear to be the most promising.

REFERENCES

1. MC Wang, LA Valenzuela, GP Murphy, TM Chu. Purification of a human prostate specific antigen. Invest Urol 17:159–163, 1979.
2. M Hara, Y Koyanagi, T Inoue, T Fukuyama. [Some physico-chemical characteristics of ''γ-seminoprotein,'' an antigenic component specific for human seminal plasma. Forensic immunological study of body fluids and secretion. VII]. Nippon Hoigaku Zasshi 25:322–324, 1971.
3. TS Li, CG Beling. Isolation and characterization of two specific antigens of human seminal plasma. Fertil Steril 24:134–144, 1973.
4. GF Sensabaugh. Isolation and characterization of a semen-specific protein from human seminal plasma: A potential new marker for semen identification. J Forensic Sci 23:106–115, 1978.
5. M Kuriyama, MC Wang, LD Papsidero, CS Killian, T Shimano, L Valenzuela, T Nishiura, GP Murphy, TM Chu. Quantitation of prostate-specific antigen in serum by a sensitive enzyme immunoassay. Cancer Res 40:4658–4662, 1980.
6. MC Wang, LD Papsidero, M Kuriyama, LA Valenzuela, GP Murphy, TM Chu. Prostate antigen: A new potential marker for prostatic cancer. Prostate 2:89–96, 1981.
7. H Lilja: A kallikrein-like serine protease in prostatic fluid cleaves the predominant seminal vesicle protein. J Clin Invest. 76:1899–1903, 1985.
8. A Christensson, CB Laurell, H Lilja. Enzymatic activity of prostate-specific antigen and its reactions with extracellular serine proteinase inhibitors. Eur J Biochem 194: 755–763, 1990.
9. UH Stenman, J Leinonen, H Alfthan, S Rannikko, K Tuhkanen, O Alfthan. A complex between prostate-specific antigen and alpha 1-antichymotrypsin is the major form of prostate-specific antigen in serum of patients with prostatic cancer: assay of the complex improves clinical sensitivity for cancer. Cancer Res 51:222–226, 1991.
10. TA Stamey, N Yang, AR Hay, JE McNeal, FS Freiha, E Redwine. Prostate-specific

antigen as a serum marker for adenocarcinoma of the prostate. N Engl J Med 317: 909–916, 1987.

11.   JE Oesterling, DW Chan, JI Epstein, AW Kimball, Jr., DJ Bruzek, RC Rock, CB Brendler, PC Walsh. Prostate specific antigen in the preoperative and postoperative evaluation of localized prostatic cancer treated with radical prostatectomy. J Urol 139:766–772, 1988.

12.   WJ Catalona, DS Smith, TL Ratliff, KM Dodds, DE Coplen, JJ Yuan, JA Petros, GL Andriole. Measurement of prostate-specific antigen in serum as a screening test for prostate cancer [published erratum appears in N Engl J Med 325:1324, 1991]. N Engl J Med 324:1156–1161, 1991.

13.   MK Brawer, MP Chetner, J Beatie, DM Buchner, RL Vessella, PH Lange. Screening for prostatic carcinoma with prostate specific antigen. J Urol 147:841–845, 1992.

14.   A Christensson, T Bjork, O Nilsson, U Dahlen, MT Matikainen, AT Cockett, PA Abrahamsson, H Lilja. Serum prostate specific antigen complexed to alpha 1-antichymotrypsin as an indicator of prostate cancer. J Urol 150:100–105, 1993.

15.   W-M Zhang, P Finne, J Leinonen, S Vesalainen, S Nordling, U-H Stenman. Measurement of the complex between prostate-specific antigen and alpha 1-protease inhibitor in serum. Clin Chem 45:814–821, 1999.

16.   WM Zhang, P Finne, J Leinonen, S Vesalainen, S Nordling, S Rannikko, UH Stenman. Characterization and immunological determination of the complex between prostate-specific antigen and alpha2-macroglobulin. Clin Chem 44:2471–2479, 1998.

17.   HC Graves. Standardization of immunoassays for prostate-specific antigen. A problem of prostate-specific antigen complexation or a problem of assay design? Cancer 72:3141–3144, 1993.

18.   UH Stenman, J Leinonen, WM Zhang, P Finne. Prostate-specific antigen. Semin Cancer Biol 9:83–93, 1999.

19.   PH Riegman, RJ Vlietstra, L Suurmeijer, CB Cleutjens, J Trapman. Characterization of the human kallikrein locus. Genomics 14:6–11, 1992.

20.   EP Diamandis, GM Yousef, I Luo, I Magklara, CV Obiezu. The new human kallikrein gene family: implications in carcinogenesis. Trends Endocrinol Metab 11:54–60, 2000.

21.   LJ Schedlich, BH Bennetts, BJ Morris. Primary structure of a human glandular kallikrein gene. DNA 6:429–437, 1987.

22.   A Lundwall, H Lilja. Molecular cloning of human prostate specific antigen cDNA. FEBS Lett 214:317–322, 1987.

23.   A Belanger, H van Halbeek, HC Graves, K Grandbois, TA Stamey, L Huang, I Poppe, F Labrie. Molecular mass and carbohydrate structure of prostate specific antigen: studies for establishment of an international PSA standard. Prostate 27:187–197, 1995.

24.   M Wang, L RM., S-L Li, T Chu. Physico-chemical characterization of prostate antigen purified from human prostate gland and seminal plasma. IRCS J Med Sci 11: 327–328, 1983.

25.   KW Watt, PJM Lee, T Timkulu, WP Chan, R Loor. Human prostate-specific antigen: structural and functional similarity with serine proteases. Proc Natl Acad Sci USA. 83:3166–3170, 1986.

26.   WM Zhang, J Leinonen, N Kalkkinen, B Dowell, UH Stenman. Purification and

characterization of different molecular forms of prostate-specific antigen in human seminal fluid. Clin Chem 41:1567–1573, 1995.

27. J Leinonen, WM Zhang, UH Stenman. Complex formation between PSA isoenzymes and protease inhibitors. J Urol 155:1099–1103, 1996.

28. WM Zhang, J Leinonen, N Kalkkinen, UH Stenman. Prostate-specific antigen forms a complex with and cleaves alpha 1-protease inhibitor in vitro. Prostate 33:87–96, 1997.

29. A Christensson, H Lilja. Complex formation between protein C inhibitor and prostate-specific antigen in vitro and in human semen. Eur J Biochem 220:45–53, 1994.

30. F Espana, J Sanchez-Cuenca, CD Vera, A Estelles, J Gilabert. A quantitative ELISA for the measurement of complexes of prostate-specific antigen with protein C inhibitor when using a purified standard. J Lab Clin Med 122:711–719, 1993.

31. P Finne, W-M Zhang, A Auvinen, J Leinonen, L Määttänen, S Rannikko, T Tammela, U-H Stenman. Use of the complex between prostate-specific antigen and α_1-protease inhibitor in screening for prostate cancer. J Urol 164:1956–1960, 2000.

32. AM Zhou, PC Tewari, BI Bluestein, GW Caldwell, FL Larsen. Multiple forms of prostate-specific antigen in serum: differences in immunorecognition by monoclonal and polyclonal assays. Clin Chem 39:2483–2491, 1993.

33. TJ Wang, HG Rittenhouse, RL Wolfert, CM Lynne, NL Brackett. PSA concentrations in seminal plasma. Clin Chem 44:895–896, 1998.

34. J Lovgren, K Rajakoski, M Karp, a Lundwall, H Lilja. Activation of the zymogen form of prostate-specific antigen by human glandular kallikrein 2. Biochem Biophys Res Commun 238:549–555, 1997.

35. A Lukkonen, Z-W Ming, S Nordling, A Bjartell, U-H Stenman. Purification and characterisation of trypsiongen from human seminal fluid and prostate. Eur Urol 37 (S2) Abstr. 309, 2000.

36. SD Mikolajczyk, LS Millar, KM Marker, LS Grauer, A Goel, MM Cass, A Kumar, MS Saedi. Ala217 is important for the catalytic function and autoactivation of prostate-specific human kallikrein 2. Eur J Biochem 246:440–446, 1997.

37. G Birkenmeier, E Usbeck, A Schafer, A Otto, HJ Glander. Prostate-specific antigen triggers transformation of seminal alpha2-macroglobulin (alpha2-M) and its binding to alpha2-macroglobulin receptor/low-density lipoprotein receptor-related protein (alpha2-M-R/LRP) on human spermatozoa. Prostate 36:219–225, 1998.

38. HJ Glander, J Kratzsch, C Weisbrich, G Birkenmeier. Insulin-like growth factor-I and alpha 2-macroglobulin in seminal plasma correlate with semen quality. Hum Reprod 11:2454–2460, 1996.

39. P Cohen, HC Graves, DM Peehl, M Kamarei, LC Giudice, RG Rosenfeld. Prostate-specific antigen (PSA) is an insulin-like growth factor binding protein-3 protease found in seminal plasma. J Clin Endocrinol Metab 75:1046–1053, 1992.

40. JM Chan, MJ Stampfer, E Giovannucci, PH Gann, J Ma, P Wilkinson, CH Hennekens, M Pollak. Plasma insulin-like growth factor-I and prostate cancer risk: a prospective study. Science 279:563–566, 1998.

41. P Finne, A Auvinen, H Koistinen, W-M Zhang, L Määttänen, S Rannikko, T Tammela, M Seppälä, M Hakama, U-H Stenman. Insulin-like growth factor-i is not a useful marker of prostate cancer in men with elevated levels of prostate-specific antigen. J Clin Endocrinol Metab, 85:2744–2747, 2000.

42. DM Sutkowski, RL Goode, J Baniel, C Teater, P Cohen, AM McNulty, HM Hsiung, GW Becker, BL Neubauer. Growth regulation of prostatic stromal cells by prostate-specific antigen. J Natl Cancer Inst 91:1663–1669, 1999.
43. A Colao, P Marzullo, S Spiezia, D Ferone, A Giaccio, G Cerbone, R Pivonello, SC Di, G Lombardi. Effect of growth hormone (GH) and insulin-like growth factor I on prostate diseases: An ultrasonographic and endocrine study in acromegaly, GH deficiency, and healthy subjects. J Clin Endocrinol Metab 84:1986–1991, 1999.
44. AH Fortier, BJ Nelson, DK Grella, JW Holaday. Antiangiogenic activity of prostate-specific antigen. J Natl Cancer Inst 91:1635–1640, 1999.
45. HH Heidtmann, DM Nettelbeck, A Mingels, R Jager, HG Welker, RE Kontermann. Generation of angiostatin-like fragments from plasminogen by prostate-specific antigen. Br J Cancer 81:1269–1273, 1999.
46. PA Abrahamsson, H Lilja, S Falkmer, LB Wadstrom. Immunohistochemical distribution of the three predominant secretory proteins in the parenchyma of hyperplastic and neoplastic prostate glands. Prostate 12:39–46, 1988.
47. UH Stenman. Prostate-specific antigen, clinical use and staging: An overview. Br J Urol 79:53–60, 1997.
48. Z Chen, H Chen, TA Stamey. Prostate specific antigen in benign prostatic hyperplasia: purification and characterization. J Urol 157:2166–2170, 1997.
49. H Hilz, J Noldus, P Hammerer, F Buck, M Luck, H Huland. Molecular heterogeneity of free PSA in sera of patients with benign and malignant prostate tumors. Eur Urol 36:286–292, 1999.
50. A Bjartell, T Bjork, MT Matikainen, PA Abrahamsson, A di Sant'Agnese, H Lilja. Production of alpha-1-antichymotrypsin by PSA-containing cells of human prostate epithelium. Urology 42:502–510, 1993.
51. H Lilja, A Haese, T Bjork, MG Friedrich, T Piironen, K Pettersson, E Huland, H Huland. Significance and metabolism of complexed and noncomplexed prostate specific antigen forms, and human glandular kallikrein 2 in clinically localized prostate cancer before and after radical prostatectomy. J Urol 162:2029–2034, 1999.
52. J van Straalen, M Bossens, T de Rejke, G Sanders. Biological half-life of prostate specific antigen after radical prostatectomy. Eur J Clin Chem Biochem 32:53–55, 1994.
53. E Brandle, O Hautmann, M Bachem, K Kleinschmidt, HW Gottfried, A Grunert, RE Hautmann. Serum half-life time determination of free and total prostate-specific antigen following radical prostatectomy—a critical assessment. Urology 53:722–730, 1999.
54. AH Agha, E Schechter, JB Roy, DJ Culkin. Prostate specific antigen is metabolized in the liver. J Urol 155:1332–1335, 1996.
55. G Birkenmeier, F Struck, R Gebhardt. Clearance mechanism of prostate specific antigen and its complexes with alpha2-macroglobulin and alpha1-antichymotrypsin. J Urol 162:897–901, 1999.
56. J Leinonen, T Lovgren, T Vornanen, UH Stenman. Double-label time-resolved immunofluorometric assay of prostate-specific antigen and of its complex with alpha 1-antichymotrypsin. Clin Chem 39:2098–2103, 1993.
57. J Leinonen, WM Zhang, E Paus, UH Stenman. Reactivity of 77 antibodies to prostate

specific antibody with isoenzymes and complexes of PSA. Tumor Biol 20:S1:28–34, 1999.

58. J Leinonen, UH Stenman. Reduced stability of prostate-specific antigen after long-term storage of serum at −20 degrees C. Tumour Biol 21:46–53, 2000.

59. U-H Stenman, E Paus, WJ Allard, I Andersson, C Andrés, TR Barnett, C Becker, A Belenky, L Bellanger, CM Pellegrino, OP Börmer, G Davis, B Dowell, LS Grauer, DC Jette, B Karlsson, FT Kreutz, TM van Der Kwast, L Lauren, M Leinimaa, J Leinonen, H Lilja, HJ Linton, M Nap, O Nilsson, PC Ng, K Nustad, A Peter, K Pettersson, T Piironen, J Rapp, HG Rittenhouse, PD Rye, P Seguin, J Slota, RL Sokoloff, MR Suresh, DL Very, TJ Wang, I Wigheden, RL Wolfert, KK Yeung, W Zhang, Z Zhou, J Hilgers. Summary Report of the TD-3 Workshop: Characterization of 83 antibodies against prostate-specific antigen. Tumour Biol 20:S1:1–12, 1999.

60. T Piironen, BO Villoutreix, C Becker, K Hollingsworth, M Vihinen, D Bridon, X Qiu, J Rapp, B Dowell, T Lovgren, K Pettersson, H Lilja. Determination and analysis of antigenic epitopes of prostate specific antigen (PSA) and human glandular kallikrein 2 (hK2) using synthetic peptides and computer modeling. Protein Sci 7:259–269, 1998.

61. O Nilsson, I Andersson, A Peter, B Karlsson. Characterization of antibodies to prostate-specific antigen. Tumour Biol 20 (SI):43–51, 1999.

62. UH Stenman, J Leinonen, WM Zhang. Standardization of PSA determinations. Scand J Clin Lab Invest Suppl 221:45–51, 1995.

63. TA Stamey, Z Chen, AF Prestigiacomo. Reference material for PSA: The IFCC standardization study. International Federation of Clinical Chemistry. Clin Biochem 31:475–481, 1998.

64. A Semjonow, B Brandt, F Oberpenning, S Roth, L Hertle. Discordance of assay methods creates pitfalls for the interpretation of prostate-specific antigen values. Prostate Suppl 7:3–16, 1996.

65. H Lilja, A Christensson, U Dahlen, MT Matikainen, O Nilsson, K Pettersson, T Lovgren. Prostate-specific antigen in serum occurs predominantly in complex with alpha 1-antichymotrypsin. Clin Chem 37:1618–1625, 1991.

66. SD Mikolajczyk, LS Grauer, LS Millar, TM Hill, A Kumar, HG Rittenhouse, RL Wolfert, MS Saedi. A precursor form of PSA (pPSA) is a component of the free PSA in prostate cancer serum. Urology 50:710–714, 1997.

67. V Väisänen, J Lövgren, J Hellman, T Piironen, H Lilja, K Pettersson. Characterization and processing of prostate specific antigen (hK3) and human glandular kallikrein 2 (hK2) secreted by LNCaP cells. Prostate Cancer Prostat Dis 7:1–7, 1999.

68. PR Huber, HP Schmid, G Mattarelli, B Strittmatter, GJ van Steenbrugge, A Maurer. Serum free prostate specific antigen: Isoenzymes in benign hyperplasia and cancer of the prostate. Prostate 27:212–219, 1995.

69. J Noldus, Z Chen, TA Stamey. Isolation and characterization of free form prostate specific antigen (f-PSA) in sera of men with prostate cancer. J Urol 158:1606–1609, 1997.

70. SD Mikolajczyk, LS Millar, TJ Wang, HG Rittenhouse, RL Wolfert, LS Marks, W Song, TM Wheeler, KM Slawin. ''BPSA,'' a specific molecular form of free prostate-specific antigen, is found predominantly in the transition zone of patients with nodular benign prostatic hyperplasia. Urology 55:41–45, 2000.

71. A de la Taille, A Houlgatte, P Houdelette, ET Goluboff, P Berlizot, I Ricordel. Influence of free-to-total prostate specific antigen variability on the early diagnosis of prostate cancer: a comparative study of three immunoassays. Br J Urol 82:389–392, 1998.

72. M Kuriyama, H Uno, K Ueno, Y Hamamoto, PQ Vihn, Y Ban. Comparative study of assays for prostate-specific antigen molecular forms. Jpn J Clin Oncol 29:303–307, 1999.

73. K Pettersson, T Piironen, M Seppala, L Liukkonen, A Christensson, MT Matikainen, M Suonpaa, T Lovgren, H Lilja. Free and complexed prostate-specific antigen (PSA): in vitro stability, epitope map, and development of immunofluorometric assays for specific and sensitive detection of free PSA and PSA-alpha 1-antichymotrypsin complex. Clin Chem 41:1480–1488, 1995.

74. W-M Zhang, P Finne, J Leinonen, S Nordling, U-H Stenman. Determination of prostate specific antigen complexed to α_2-macroglobulin in serum increases the specificity of free to total PSA for prostate cancer. Urology 56:267–272, 2000.

75. WJ Allard, Z Zhou, KK Yeung. Novel immunoassay for the measurement of complexed prostate-specific antigen in serum. Clin Chem 44:1216–1223, 1998.

76. MK Brawer, GE Meyer, JL Letran, DD Bankson, DL Morris, KK Yeung, WJ Allard. Measurement of complexed PSA improves specificity for early detection of prostate cancer. Urology 52:372–378, 1998.

77. HB Carter, AW Partin, AA Luderer, EJ Metter, P Landis, DW Chan, JL Fozard, JD Pearson. Percentage of free prostate-specific antigen in sera predicts aggressiveness of prostate cancer a decade before diagnosis. Urology 49:379–384, 1997.

78. WJ Catalona, DS Smith, RL Wolfert, TJ Wang, HG Rittenhouse, TL Ratliff, RB Nadler. Evaluation of percentage of free serum prostate-specific antigen to improve specificity of prostate cancer screening. JAMA 274:1214–1220, 1995.

79. U-H Stenman, J Leinonen, W-M Zhang. Problems of PSA determinations. Eur J Clin Chem Clin Biochem 34:735–740, 1996.

80. A Virtanen, M Gomari, R Kranse, UH Stenman. Estimation of prostate cancer probability by logistic regression: free and total prostate-specific antigen, digital rectal examination, and heredity are significant variables. Clin Chem 45:987–994, 1999.

81. P Finne, R Finne, A Auvinen, H Juusela, J Aro, L Määttänen, M Hakama, S Rannikko, T Tammela, U-H Stenman. Predicting the outcome of prostate biopsy in screen-positive men by a multilayer perceptron network. Urology, in press.

82. CH Bangma, R Kranse, BG Blijenberg, FH Schroder. Free and total prostate-specific antigen in a screened population. Br J Urol 79:756–762, 1997.

83. RJ Babaian, H Miyashita, RB Evans, EI Ramirez. The distribution of prostate specific antigen in men without clinical or pathological evidence of prostate cancer: Relationship to gland volume and age. J Urol 147:837–840, 1992.

84. JE Oesterling, SJ Jacobsen, GG Klee, K Pettersson, T Piironen, PA Abrahamsson, UH Stenman, B Dowell, T Lovgren, H Lilja. Free, complexed and total serum prostate specific antigen: The establishment of appropriate reference ranges for their concentrations and ratios. J Urol 154:1090–1095, 1995.

85. WJ Catalona, DS Smith, DK Ornstein. Prostate cancer detection in men with serum PSA concentrations of 2.6 to 4.0 ng/mL and benign prostate examination. Enhancement of specificity with free PSA measurements. JAMA 277:1452–1455, 1997.

86. CH Bangma, R Kranse, BG Blijenberg, FH Schroder. The value of screening tests in the detection of prostate cancer. Part II: Retrospective analysis of free/total prostate-specific analysis ratio, age-specific reference ranges, and PSA density. Urology 46: 779–784, 1995.

87. GD Carlson, CB Calvanese, AW Partin. An algorithm combining age, total prostate-specific antigen (PSA), and percent free PSA to predict prostate cancer: Results on 4298 cases. Urology 52:455–461, 1998.

88. K Komatsu, N Wehner, AF Prestigiacomo, Z Chen, TA Stamey. Physiologic (intra-individual) variation of serum prostate-specific antigen in 814 men from a screening population. Urology 47:343–346, 1996.

89. RG Nixon, JD Lilly, RJ Liedtke, JD Batjer. Variation of free and total prostate-specific antigen levels: the effect on the percent free/total prostate-specific antigen. Arch Pathol Lab Med 121:385–391, 1997.

90. DK Ornstein, DS Smith, GS Rao, JW Basler, TL Ratliff, WJ Catalona. Biological variation of total, free and percent free serum prostate specific antigen levels in screening volunteers. J Urol 157:2179–2182, 1997.

91. GN Collins, PJ Martin, DA Wynn, PJ Brooman, PH O'Reilly. The effect of digital rectal examination, flexible cystoscopy and prostatic biopsy on free and total prostate specific antigen, and the free-to-total prostate specific antigen ratio in clinical practice. J Urol 157:1744–1747, 1997.

92. DK Ornstein, GS Rao, DS Smith, TL Ratliff, JW Basler, WJ Catalona. Effect of digital rectal examination and needle biopsy on serum total and percentage of free prostate specific antigen levels. J Urol 157:195–198, 1997.

93. T Piironen, K Pettersson, M Suonpaa, UH Stenman, JE Oesterling, T Lovgren, H Lilja. In vitro stability of free prostate-specific antigen (PSA) and prostate-specific antigen (PSA) complexed to alpha 1-antichymotrypsin in blood samples. Urology 48:81–87, 1996.

94. D Woodrum, L York. Two-year stability of free and total PSA in frozen serum samples. Urology 52:247–251, 1998.

95. UH Stenman, M Hakama, P Knekt, A Aromaa, L Teppo, J Leinonen. Serum concentrations of prostate specific antigen and its complex with alpha 1-antichymotrypsin before diagnosis of prostate cancer. Lancet 344:1594–1598, 1994.

3

Variability of Immunoassays for PSA

Axel Semjonow, Gabriela De Angelis, and Hans-Peter Schmid
Westfälische Wilhelms-Universität, Münster, Germany

Prostate specific antigen (PSA) initially served only for monitoring patients in whom prostate cancer (PCa) had already been diagnosed. In recent years, however, it has been increasingly used for the diagnosis of PCa (see Chap. 9) [1–5] and is currently the most widely used parameter in uro-oncologic laboratory diagnostics [6]. The availability of numerous different assays for the determination of various forms of PSA has created substantial problems in the interpretation of PSA concentrations. Well over 80 assays for the detection of PSA are currently available commercially worldwide. The majority of the assays for total PSA (T-PSA) are based on the commonly used reference range (<4 ng/ml), although this has rarely been verified. Some manufactures avoid specifying the reference range altogether, while others derive the data from very small populations. Some reference ranges have been established with sera of young males, or even with an unspecified proportion of female sera. Since T-PSA concentrations may vary in identical samples by a factor of two depending on the assay used [7], the clinician in charge of interpreting the results needs to be aware of the method used, and must have detailed information on the assay-specific reference range. Usually the physician remains unaware of the name of the assay used. Apart from unnecessarily causing anxiety to the subject investigated, the results may be overlooked PCa or biopsies unnecessarily performed [8].

To increase the predictive value of T-PSA in the detection of clinically relevant PCa confined to the organ, detailed studies have been carried out to establish reference ranges, but only very few of the available assays have been thoroughly investigated [7,9,17].

I. ATTEMPTS TO INCREASE THE SPECIFICITY OF T-PSA FOR THE DIAGNOSIS OF PCa

A number of possibilities have been explored for increasing the specificity of T-PSA for the detection of PCa. Besides combining T-PSA with rectal palpation and transrectal sonography [1,12], these include determination of the T-PSA/prostate volume ratio (see Chap. 4) [18–22], age-dependent T-PSA decision points (see Chap. 6) [14,23–25], the change in T-PSA concentration over time (see Chap. 5) [26], and the selective determination of free (F-PSA), complexed or T-PSA in the same sample (see Chap. 7) [25,27–44].

Utilizing the change of T-PSA over time for diagnosis [26] or therapy control [45] requires long-term follow-up to reduce the influence of intraindividual fluctuations [46–48]. The time course of T-PSA levels must be determined without any change in the assay method used [7,8,13,49]. Otherwise a putative T-PSA rise could merely be the result of discordance between the assays [7,50]. Given the current availability of numerous T-PSA assays and related frequent changes of methods in laboratories, recognizing this in daily practice is usually problematic [7,51] (Fig. 1).

II. VARIOUS PSA ASSAY METHODS

PSA concentrations should be interpreted in combination with the related clinical findings and an understanding of the limitations of the assay [34,52]. The cut-

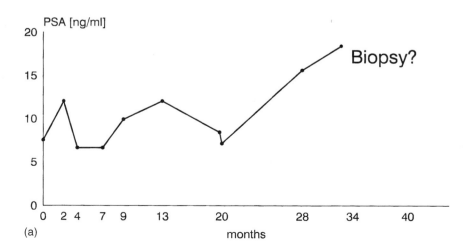

(a)

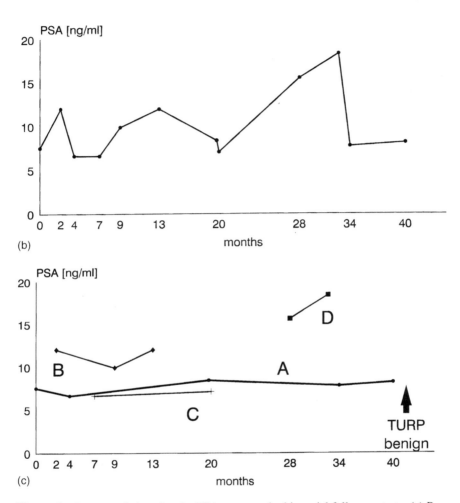

Figure 1 Dangers of changing the PSA assay method in serial follow-up tests. (a) Presentation of a 63-year-old patient with the depicted PSA values for prostate biopsy on the basis of a ''rapid PSA rise'' with normal digital rectal examination. (b) Serial PSA values, including two PSA determinations prior to the suggested prostate biopsy. (c) Serial PSA values differentiated according to the four PSA assay methods involved (A–D). Prostate biopsy was not performed. Transurethral resection of the prostate, performed to relieve obstructive micturition symptoms (month 41), revealed BPH without appreciable inflammatory changes. (From Ref. 7. Reprinted by permission of Wiley-Liss, Inc., a subsidiary of John Wiley and Sons, Inc.)

off quoted for one PSA assay cannot necessarily be transferred to another assay [13,34,53–57]. All the methods for increasing the specificity of PSA for the detection of PCa mentioned in the previous section and in several chapters of this book are of little or no use if the assay method applied and the specific reference range for the assay in use are not known to the clinician in charge of interpreting the PSA values. Because interassay variability may account for a factor of two [7,13,58–62], the existence of various assays for PSA poses substantial problems for the interpretation of individual PSA values [7,8,58,59,63–72]. This problem is especially likely when using PSA to diagnose PCa, since the reference range of <4 ng/ml for detecting PCa is not valid for many of the commercially available assay methods. Without knowledge of the assay-specific reference range, misinterpretations of PSA values will occur [73].

Less problematic are differences between assays used for monitoring patients with PCa, since in this case each individual represents his own reference. Again, a prerequisite is that the method is not changed in the course of the determinations (Fig. 1).

III. REASONS FOR THE MEASUREMENT OF DISCORDANT CONCENTRATIONS IN IDENTICAL SAMPLES

Apart from gross errors, such as the confounding of samples or mistakes in pipetting, two basic situations arise in which immunoassays yield discordant results. First, in well-correlated assays that yield nearly identical values, large deviations are found for the same sample from one assay to another. Usually these deviant findings cannot be satisfactorily explained or eliminated [74–78]. A possible underlying reason may be cross-reactivity of the employed antibodies with substances that yield a high amino acid sequence homology with PSA such as human kallikrein 2 (hK2) (see Chap. 16) [79,80]. Second, two assays may measure differently over the entire measurement range and generally produce higher or lower values. Variation may result from differential calibration of the assays or length of incubation time in nonequilibrium assays.

The choice of test principle also has a decisive influence on the accuracy of the method. In the presence of very high analyte concentrations, the "high-dose hook effect" of so-called sandwich assays may lead to incorrectly low results [50,58,81–85].

IV. A SPECIAL PROBLEM IN T-PSA ASSAYS: THE MOLAR RESPONSE RATIO

In T-PSA assays there is an additional possible source of discordancy: equimolar or nonequimolar detection of various PSA forms (Fig. 2). Assays that preferen-

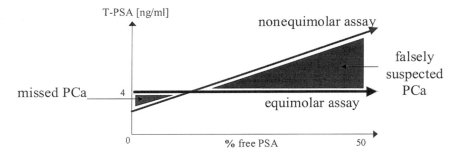

Figure 2   Clinical impact of nonequimolar measurement and calibration of T-PSA assays. Assays that preferentially detect F-PSA may overreport the actual T-PSA in patients with BPH, since BPH leads to a higher average proportion of F-PSA in serum, than PCa. Depending on the calibration of a nonequimolar assay, the result may be falsely suspected or missed PCa. (From Ref. 102.)

tially detect F-PSA may overreport the actual T-PSA in benign prostatic hyperplasia (BPH) [8,53,70,86,87], since BPH leads to a higher average proportion of F-PSA in serum than PCa [29]. Evidence is mounting that the calculation of the ratio of F/T PSA permits an improvement in the specificity for the detection of PCa (see Chap. 7) [42]. According to preliminary studies, this ratio appears to be of significant clinical value in men in whom the T-PSA level is in an intermediate range (e.g., 4–10 ng/ml) [25,41,88] or even between 2.51 and 4 ng/ml [89]. This is of considerable interest since the incidence of BPH clearly exceeds the incidence of PCa and often leads to T-PSA values in these ranges.

PSA circulates in a free form and also in complexes with protease inhibitors. First, PSA is produced as an inactive protease, which is converted to the active enzyme by release of a small propeptide [90]. This activation is apparently dependent on the action of hK2 [79]. The enzymatic action may be inactivated by the reaction of PSA with several abundant extracellular protease inhibitors, such as $\alpha 2$-macroglobulin, $\alpha 1$-antichymotrypsin (ACT), $\alpha 1$-antitrypsin, or protein C inhibitor. The site of complexation of PSA to protease inhibitors is uncertain. To date also the molecular characterization of F-PSA in the serum remains unknown. However, it is assumed that F-PSA in serum is enzymatically inactive, whereas active serum PSA is predominantly bound to protease inhibitors (see Chap. 2) [27,36,37]. Most assays contain antibodies against active F-PSA derived from seminal plasma. Antibodies against F-PSA usually have a lower affinity for complexed PSA. The affinity of antibodies against various PSA forms varies from one assay to the other [50,57]. The polyclonal antibody conjugates used in some commercial assays typically include a subpopulation of antibodies that bind to the region of the PSA molecule to which ACT binds. As a result, ACT will block the epitopes and preclude binding of this antibody subpopulation to the

Table 1 Methodological Reasons for Discordance of PSA Measurements between Assays in the Same Serum Sample

---

Antibodies: affinity and specificity for various epitopes of PSA forms [50,56,57] or crossreactivity to PSA homologous antigens [79]

Calibration of the assay method

Procedure of the assay: incubation time, equilibrium or kinetics, adjuvants, "high-dose hook" effect [50,81–85,91]

Lot-to-lot variations in assays [103]

Interferences: autoanti-PSA-antibodies [56]

---

complex. The result of this epitope shielding is that fewer polyclonal antibodies will bind to each molecule of ACT-PSA than to F-PSA, thus attenuating the response to ACT-PSA [37]. Identical measurements have been achieved only with assays in which equimolar reactions occur with F-PSA as well as with PSA complexes, whereas nonequimolar responding assays overreport the F-PSA.

Another factor contributing to a nonequimolar response in T-PSA assays may be the length of incubation time. In nonequilibrium assays, quantification of T-PSA is influenced by the rate of reaction, which can be different for each PSA form. For each form to be measured equally, the assay should be allowed to approach equilibrium. The shorter the incubation time, the more likely the assay will not reach equilibrium and thus exhibit a nonequimolar response [91].

Another reason underlying the measurement of different PSA levels may lie in the calibration of the assays. Assays that do not detect all aforementioned PSA forms on an essentially equimolar basis are most accurate with the PSA composition that corresponds to that of the calibration standards.

Table 1 lists possible causes underlying discordant results of PSA measurements obtained with different assays. Figure 2 shows the influence of nonequimolar PSA measurement on the reported T-PSA concentration.

V. PSA ASSAY STANDARDIZATION

Standardization of T-PSA assay methods is especially desirable in the concentration range of the greatest overlap between BPH and PCa, since the greatest difficulties in differentiating between the two conditions are encountered in this range. Suggestions for standardization presuppose a method of purifying PSA and characterizing the molecule, whereby agreement must be reached on the form of PSA on which the standardization is to be based. With the help of such a PSA standard substance it would be possible to standardize the calibration of the individual assay methods [54]. However, the problem posed by the existence of different complexed or uncomplexed forms of PSA remains unsolved, since various assays are capable to different degrees of detecting the individual forms (e.g., owing to differences in the antibodies used) [92]. At the 2nd Standardization Conference in Stanford in 1994 [93], a standard substance was therefore presented for discussion. This substance contains a mixture of 90% complexed PSA (bound to ACT) and 10% F-PSA and thus corresponds to the distribution typically found in PCa. This mixture ratio is supposed to be advantageous in that, due to the smaller proportion of F-PSA, assays that overreport F-PSA become more similar to assays that measure on an equimolar basis. In contrast to results published by Brawer and co-workers [94], recent studies by Blijenberg et al. [95,96] investigating three equimolar assays before and after recalibration with two standard substances ("Stanford 90 : 10"; "Certified Reference Material 613 Prostate-Specific Antigen") conclude that after recalibration even equimolar assays for T-PSA are still not completely interchangeable. These results are in concordance with the results of the Assay Comparison Study for PSA, demonstrating that assay modifications using recalibration alone do not lead to a "standardization" of T-PSA assays [73].

However, since the serum of patients with BPH contains markedly higher proportions of F-PSA, it is to be expected, despite recalibration, that assays preferentially measuring F-PSA overreport T-PSA values in benign prostatic disease and underreport T-PSA values in PCa [8]. This causes only an ostensible standardization of the assays, since they would produce comparable values only in an arbitrarily selected subpopulation, namely in samples having an F/T PSA ratio of 10%. However, the assays continue to differ with regard to the population of men with BPH owing to the high proportion of F-PSA, and it is precisely this population that presents problems in terms of differential diagnosis. So far it remains questionable whether complexed PSA is superior to F-PSA as an assay calibrator [50]. As a consequence, recent recommendations of the Committee on PSA Standardization and Quality Assessment at the World Health Organization First International Consultation on Prostate Cancer stated that F-PSA, isolated from seminal fluid, should be used as primary standard for F- and T-PSA immunoassays [54]. The use of recombinant PSA was not recommended since such preparations do not include the various isoforms of PSA [54].

VI. CONVERSION OF T-PSA CONCENTRATIONS IN VARIOUS ASSAYS

A comparison of the assays may reveal considerable discordance in the T-PSA concentrations measured in the same sample [7,8,13,58,86]. T-PSA concentrations measured with different assays cannot simply be converted by applying a factor. A whole series of different factors along a concentration-dependent scale must be applied. Yet, such an approach still does not consider shifts due to differences in the ability of various assays to detect F- and T-PSA since the deviations inherent in the methods depend on the proportion of F-PSA and therefore on the nature of the underlying prostatic disease. This means that the conversion factors between different assay methods differ according to the proportion of patients with PCa in the population examined, because the various PSA forms are present in different proportions. Converting a diagnostic parameter that is supposed to aid in finding the correct diagnosis obviously is not practical if the conversion of the parameter presupposes knowledge of the diagnosis that is supposed to be found with the help of this parameter [55]. Assays that preferentially detect F-PSA (nonequimolar assays) will reveal relatively higher T-PSA concentrations in patients with BPH than in patients with PCa [8].

VII. IMPORTANCE OF THE REFERENCE RANGE

The problems associated with the reference range lie primarily in the definition of a normal or reference population. A correctly determined reference range for T-PSA and the F/T PSA ratio is of crucial importance for the primary diagnosis of PCa. There are few other situations in which invasive diagnostic measures are initiated solely on the basis of measured elevation of a serum marker. Irrespective of the outcome of the prostate biopsy, the suspected diagnosis of PCa alone is enough to invoke a mental and social crisis in the patient. Moreover, the biopsy and follow-up tests are associated with considerable costs.

VIII. REFERENCE RANGES OF THE FIRST COMMERCIAL ASSAYS

The first two commercially available assays were the polyclonal Pros-Check PSA (Yang Laboratories) [97] and the monoclonal Tandem-R PSA (Hybritech Inc.) [98]. Since the two assays differ considerably, the evaluating clinician was usually informed of the assay method and the related reference range (Pros-Check <2.5; Tandem-R <4.0 ng/ml). In 1991 there were still only two commercially available PSA assays in the United States [99]. More than 80 assays for PSA forms are currently available worldwide. Since not all assay methods measure the same T-PSA concentration, yet are interpreted on the basis of the clinically established reference range of the first widely used assay (Hybritech, Tandem-R), the result may be superfluous biopsies and follow-up tests with unnecessary distress caused to the patient due to the unfounded suspicion of carcinoma.

The reference range originally determined for the Hybritech assay on a moderately large population of men [9] has become generally established. Its upper limit was defined as the concentration that included 97% of 207 allegedly healthy men over 40 years of age. Large-scale series have meanwhile confirmed the validity of this reference range [12,14].

IX. REFERENCE RANGES OF MORE RECENT ASSAYS

For the more recent assays, the reference ranges are often determined on the basis of very small populations. Even if sufficiently large populations were studied, there is still the danger that an assay has a cut-off value similar to the Hybritech reference range in healthy men but deviates markedly in its discrimination between BPH and PCa. Whereas, for example, the reference range of the T-PSA assay ACS (Chiron/Ciba Corning) did not differ greatly from that of the Hybritech assay, the upper limit of the ACS assay with respect to BPH needed to be nearly doubled in comparison to the Hybritech assay in order to achieve the same specificity for the detection of PCa [8,13]. This recently led to a modification of the respective assay by the manufacturer. The modified assay ACS2 now in general reports lower T-PSA concentrations than the old assay ACS. However, in contrast to Brawer et al. [94], who found a "substantial equivalence of the restandardized ACS assay" and the Tandem-R assay (Hybritech), our results still demonstrate a significant nonequimolar response of the new ACS2 assay despite its modification (Fig. 3); PCa patients with a low proportion of F-PSA will show relatively low T-PSA concentrations when determined with this assay. It can be expected that a shift from fewer unnecessary biopsies in patients with BPH to more missed PCa may be the result of the assay modification [100]. Recognizing this problem, other manufacturers of nonequimolar assays modified their assays so that the new assays now produce an equimolar response to complexed and F-PSA. Whereas the polyclonal T-PSA assay produced by Abbott gives a nonequimolar response [71,73], the monoclonal modification of this assay does not underestimate the T-PSA in sera with a low proportion of F-PSA [73,100]. Within the time frame of the Assay Comparison Study, another manufacturer succeeded in eliminating nonequimolar response characteristics of their T-PSA assay in the clinically relevant concentration range. The new Vidas PSA (bioMérieux), in contrast to the older version, now detects complexed and F-PSA in the range of 2–20 ng/ml on an equimolar basis [73].

X. F/T PSA RATIO IN VARIOUS ASSAY COMBINATIONS

Assays that preferentially detect F-PSA tend to overestimate the T-PSA in patients with BPH, since BPH is associated with a higher average proportion of F-PSA in serum than PCa. Conversely, this may yield relatively low T-PSA values

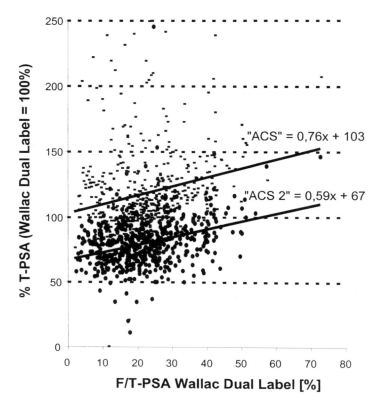

Figure 3 T-PSA concentrations measured in identical samples by the Chiron/Ciba Corning T-PSA assay before (brand name ''ACS'') and after modification (brand name: ''ACS 2''). All samples derived from the PSA Assay Comparison Study [73]. Sample characteristics: n = 529 (cancer n = 91; noncancer n = 438), T-PSA range 0.1–101 ng/ml (Wallac Dual Label), linear regression. The modified assay reports, on average, lower T-PSA concentrations than the unmodified assay but still displays a nonequimolar response to complexed and F-PSA (i.e., PCa patients with a relatively low proportion of F-PSA do reveal lower T-PSA concentrations when determined with this assay compared to equimolar assays; see also Fig. 2). (From Ref. 102.)

in PCa, since less F-PSA is expressed. If the F/T PSA ratio is used to enhance the specificity for PCa detection it is of utmost importance to ensure that the molecular response of the T-PSA assay employed is studied. Within the Assay Comparison Study for PSA, 10 assays for F-PSA were evaluated [73]. Dependent on the assay characteristics of the T-PSA assays as well as the T-PSA range in which the ratio was applied, a large variance in the performance of the possible

Table 2 Possible Results of Combining F- and T-PSA Assays
from Different Manufacturers

T-PSA range (ng/ml)	Assay with which T-PSA range determined	F-PSA/T-PSA- assay combination	Specificity at sensitivity >85% (%)
2–10	A	A/A	50
0–10	A	A/A	37
2–10	B	A/A	20
2–10	B	C/D	0

Influence of the T-PSA range and various combinations of F- and T-PSA assays on the diagnostic performance: specificity for the detection of PCa at a fixed sensitivity of >85% investigated using receiver operating characteristic curves [104]. Assays are anonymized, since even well-performing assays may lose their discriminative power when combined with an assay of a different manufacturer or used in an inappropriate T-PSA range.
Source: Adapted from Ref. 102.

assay combinations used to calculate the F/T PSA ratio was observed. It is not so much the assays itself but the mode of combination that diminishes the performance of the F/T PSA ratio. Assays are therefore anonymized in Table 2. A necessary conclusion to be drawn in this situation is that the T-PSA range in which the F/T PSA ratio should be calculated needs to be determined for each assay combination individually. Also, each assay combination needs to be evaluated by itself; it is not feasible to conclude that two well-correlated T-PSA assays will show equally good performance when exchanged in the denominator of the F/T PSA ratio. Decision points for the F/T PSA ratio need to be generated for each assay combination individually.

XI. MANUFACTURER'S INFORMATION ON THE ASSAY METHOD

The informational content of the package inserts accompanying PSA test kits varies to a great extent. This is especially apparent with regard to the information on the valid reference range. For more than half of the assays marketed, no information on the age distribution of the individuals studied is given or the subjects were all younger than 45 years of age. In about a quarter of the assays no information whatsoever is given on the reference range, or the proportion of women in the population is apparently unknown. Only one-third of the assays provide a reference range that was determined on the basis of more than 100 men over 40 years of age [7].

Usually the manufacturer points out that the respective laboratory should establish its own reference ranges for the method used. However, this is hardly possible, since the laboratories do not have access to serum samples from healthy subjects and therefore continue to use the reference range of <4 ng/ml.

Some manufacturers recommend in their package leaflets that PSA should be used only for monitoring PCa that has already been diagnosed. In practice, however, the physician is rarely aware of this advice [51,101]. Separate determination of PSA using two different assays, one for the diagnosis of PCa and the other for follow-up, is hardly feasible. About half of the manufacturers emphasize in their inserts that the PSA concentrations determined by their method is not always comparable to that obtained by other techniques and request laboratories to state the name of the method in the laboratory report. In our experience, however, laboratories rarely quote the assay method used in the laboratory report, and when they do they limit the information to the format of the assay (e.g., enzyme immunoassay [EIA], immunoradiometric assay [IRMA]), without actually identifying the assay method for the physician.

XII. WHAT ARE THE CONSEQUENCES OF DISCREPANCIES IN THE ASSAY METHODS FOR THE PHYSICIAN?

First, different assays report different PSA concentrations in a given serum sample. These differences are of a magnitude that is clinically significant. Second, the PSA forms that occur in serum are detected to different degrees by the various assay methods. As a consequence, deviations between assays depend on the nature of the underlying prostatic disease.

Because sufficiently validated reference ranges are not known for most of the T-PSA assays on the market, physicians are advised to obtain the information listed in Table 3 from their laboratory in order to avoid causing harm to patients

Table 3 Information to Request from Your Laboratory on the PSA Assay Method

Assay method used: The brand name of the assay used must be given in every laboratory report to alert you to any change in the assay method (see Fig. 1)

Validity of reference range: The reference range determined by the laboratory or the manufacturer for this method, including the number, gender, and age of the subjects examined, and the percentage of men with BPH or untreated PCa

Molar response ratio: The ratio by which complexed and F-PSA is detected by the method

Analytical sensitivity

and increasing the resulting costs. This is also a prerequisite for correct interpretation of the F/T PSA ratio but, unfortunately, a correctly determined reference range for this ratio is the exception since large numbers of well-defined samples are needed in a restricted T-PSA range.

XIII. SUMMARY

PSA cannot replace rectal palpation or prostate biopsy as a diagnostic method. However, it does enhance diagnostic sensitivity. PSA can improve the efficiency of interventions that are both expensive and distressing for the patient. However, this presupposes an interpretation of the PSA levels based on knowledge of the assay method used and the assay-specific reference range. The problem is not readily obvious to the physician, since there is evidently no obligation for laboratories to specify the assay method in the laboratory report. Taking into account up to twofold assay-dependent differences in PSA concentrations in a given sample, the need for a reliably determined reference range for each method is obvious. The responsibility of the laboratory practitioner is to clarify the assay method used and provide precise information on the reference collective used by the manufacturer.

The uncritical transfer of the established decision points of "<4.0 ng/ml" (for T-PSA) or ">15%" (for the F/T PSA ratio) to other assays or assay combinations can lead not only to superfluous, cost-intensive and distressing tests but also to overlooked PCa, thus unnecessarily diminishing the value of PSA.

The introduction of new assays for the selective determination of F-PSA further increases the variety of assay methods available. Most suppliers who wish to produce an assay for F-PSA but whose T-PSA assay does not detect the PSA forms on an equimolar basis will try to modify the T-PSA assay. In the absence of a well-working standardization procedure, it can only be hoped that the modified assays will be sufficiently validated by the manufacturers in cooperation with clinicians recognizing that PSA is one of the very few tumor markers that prompts invasive consequences if a concentration above the decision point is found.

REFERENCES

1. WH Cooner, BR Mosley, CL Rutherford Jr, JH Beard, HS Pond, WJ Terry, TC Igel, DD Kidd. Prostate cancer detection in a clinical urological practice by ultrasonography, digital rectal examination and prostate specific antigen. J Urol 143:1146–1152, 1990.
2. WJ Catalona, DS Smith, TL Ratliff, JW Basler. Detection of organ-confined prostate cancer is increased through prostate-specific antigen-based screening. JAMA 270:948–954, 1993.

3. P Lodding, G Aus, S Bergdahl, R Frosing, H Lilja, CG Pihl, J Hugosson. Characteristics of screening detected prostate cancer in men 50 to 66 years old with 3 to 4
    ng./ml. prostate specific antigen. J Urol 159:899–903, 1998.
4. FH Schröder, CH Bangma. The European Randomized Study of Screening for Prostate Cancer (ERSPC). Br J Urol 79:68–71, 1997.
5. A Reissigl, W Horninger, K Fink, H Klocker, G Bartsch. Prostate carcinoma screening in the country of Tyrol, Austria: Experience and results. Cancer 80:1818–1829,
    1997.
6. G De Angelis, B Brandt, HP Schmid, A Semjonow. Vom Antigen zum Tumormarker, Forschungsergebnisse zu PSA und ihre klinische Umsetzung. [From
    antigen to tumor marker. Clinical application of PSA research results.]. Urologe
    A 39:309–312, 2000.
7. A Semjonow, B Brandt, F Oberpenning, S Roth, L Hertle. Discordance of assay
    methods creates pitfalls for the interpretation of prostate-specific antigen values.
    Prostate 7:3–16, 1996.
8. A Semjonow, F Oberpenning, B Brandt, C Zechel, W Brandau, L Hertle. Impact
    of free prostate-specific antigen on discordant measurement results of assays for
    total prostate-specific antigen. Urology 48:10–15, 1996.
9. JF Myrtle, PG Klimley, IP Ivor, JF Bruni. Clinical utility of prostate specific antigen
    (PSA) in the management of prostate cancer. Adv Cancer Diagn 1, 1986.
10. BG Blijenberg, CH Bangma, R Kranse, I Eman, FH Schröder. Analytical evaluation
    of the new Prostatus PSA Free/Total assay for prostate-specific antigen as part of
    a screening study for prostate cancer. Eur J Clin Chem Clin Biochem 35:111–114,
    1997.
11. WJ Catalona, DS Smith, TL Ratliff, KM Dodds, DE Coplen, JJJ Yuan, JA Petros,
    GL Andriole. Measurement of prostate-specific antigen in serum as a screening test
    for prostate cancer. N Engl J Med 324:1156–1161, 1991.
12. WJ Catalona, JP Richie, FR Ahmann, MA Hudson, PT Scardino, RC Flanigan, JB
    deKernion, TL Ratliff, LR Kavoussi, BL Dalkin, WB Waters, MT MacFarlane, PC
    Southwick. Comparison of digital rectal examination and serum prostate specific
    antigen in the early detection of prostate cancer: Results of a multicenter clinical
    trial of 6,630 men. J Urol 151:1283–1290, 1994.
13. CM Schambeck, N Schmeller, P Stieber, HM Jansen, H Pahl, W Schneider,
    A Fateh-Moghadam. Methodological and clinical comparison of the ACS prostate-
    specific antigen assay and the Tandem-E prostate-specific antigen assay in prostate
    cancer. Urology 46:195–199, 1995.
14. BL Dalkin, FR Ahmann, JB Kopp, WJ Catalona, TL Ratliff, MA Hudson, JP Richie, PT Scardino, RC Flanigan, JB Dekernion, WB Waters, LR Kavoussi, MT
    MacFarlane. Derivation and application of upper limits for prostate specific antigen
    in men aged 50–74 years with no clinical evidence of prostatic carcinoma. Br
    J Urol 76:346–350, 1995.
15. AP Wilson, A Van Dalen, PE Sibley, LA Kasper, AP Durham, AS el Shami. Multi-
    centre tumour marker reference range study. Anticancer Res 19:2749–2752, 1999.
16. W Horninger, A Reissigl, H Rogatsch, H Volgger, M Studen, H Klocker, G Bartsch.
    Prostate cancer screening in Tyrol, Austria: Experience and results. Eur Urol 35:
    523–538, 1999.

17. C Becker, T Piironen, K Pettersson, T Björk, KJ Wojno, JE Oesterling, H Lilja. Discrimination of men with prostate cancer from those with benign disease by measurements of human glandular kallikrein 2 (HK2) in serum. J Urol 163:311–316, 2000.
18. RJ Babaian, HA Fritsche, RB Evans. Prostate-specific antigen and prostate gland volume: correlation and clinical application. J Clin Lab Anal 4:135–137, 1990.
19. S Veneziano, P Pavlica, R Querzé, G Nanni, MG Lalanne, F Vecchi. Correlation between prostate-specific antigen and prostate volume, evaluated by transrectal ultrasonography: Usefulness in diagnosis of prostate cancer. Eur Urol 18:112–116, 1990.
20. M Benson, IS Whang, CA Olsson, DJ McMahon, WH Cooner. The use of prostate specific antigen density to enhance the predictive value of intermediate levels of serum prostate specific antigen. J Urol 147:817–821, 1992.
21. A Semjonow, M Hamm, P Rathert, L Hertle. Prostate-specific antigen corrected for prostate volume improves differentiation of benign prostatic hyperplasia and organ-confined prostatic cancer. Br J Urol 73:538–543, 1994.
22. CH Bangma, DE Grobbee, FH Schröder. Volume adjustment for intermediate prostate-specific antigen values in a screening population. Eur J Cancer 31A:12–14, 1995.
23. JE Oesterling, WH Cooner, SJ Jacobsen, HA Guess, MM Lieber. Influence of patient age on the serum PSA concentration. An important clinical observation. Urol Clin North Am 20:671–680, 1993.
24. C Mettlin, PJ Littrup, RA Kane, GP Murphy, F Lee, A Chesley, R Badalament, FK Mostofi. Relative sensitivity and specificity of serum prostate specific antigen (PSA) level compared with age-referenced PSA, PSA density, and PSA change. Data from the American Cancer Society National Prostate Cancer Detection Project. Cancer 74:1615–1620, 1994.
25. CH Bangma, R Kranse, BG Blijenberg, FH Schröder. The value of screening tests in the detection of prostate cancer. Part II: Retrospective analysis of free/total prostate-specific analysis ratio, age-specific reference ranges, and PSA density. Urology 46:779–784, 1995.
26. HB Carter, JD Pearson, EJ Metter, LJ Brant, DW Chan, R Andres, JL Fozard, PC Walsh. Longitudinal evaluation of prostate-specific antigen levels in men with and without prostate disease. JAMA 267:2215–2220, 1992.
27. H Lilja, A Christensson, U Dahlen, MT Matikainen, O Nilsson, K Pettersson, T Lövgren. Prostate-specific antigen in serum occurs predominantly in complex with alpha-1-antichymotrypsin. Clin Chem 37:1618–1625, 1991.
28. T Björk, A Bjartell, PA Abrahamson, S Hulkko, A Santagnese, H Lilja. Alpha 1-antichymotrypsin production in PSA-producing cells is common in prostate cancer but rare in benign prostatic hyperplasia. Urology 43:427–434, 1994.
29. UH Stenman, M Hakama, P Knekt, A Aromaa, L Teppo, J Leinonen. Serum concentrations of prostate specific antigen and its complex with alpha 1-antichymotrypsin before diagnosis of prostate cancer. Lancet 344:1594–1598, 1994.
30. PR Huber, HP Schmid, G Mattarelli, B Strittmatter, GJ van Steenbrugge, A Maurer. Serum free prostate specific antigen: Isoenzymes in benign hyperplasia and cancer of the prostate. Prostate 27:212–219, 1995.

31. W Reiter, P Stieber, N Schmeller, D Nagel, A Fateh-Moghadam. Alpha 1-antichy-motrypsin-PSA (ACT-PSA): A useful marker in the differential diagnosis of benign hyperplasia and cancer of the prostate? Anticancer Res 17:4767–4770, 1997.

32. WJ Allard, Z Zhou, KK Yeung. Novel immunoassay for the measurement of com-plexed prostate-specific antigen in serum. Clin Chem 44:1216–1223, 1998.

33. MK Brawer, GE Meyer, JL Letran, DD Bankson, DL Morris, KK Yeung, WJ Al-lard. Measurement of complexed PSA improves specificity for early detection of prostate cancer. Urology 52:372–378, 1998.

34. MK Brawer, MC Benson, DG Bostwick, B Djavan, H Lilja, A Semjonow, S Su, Z Zhou. Prostate-specific antigen and other serum markers: Current concepts from the World Health Organization Second International Consultation on Prostate Can-cer. Semin Urol Oncol 17:206–221, 1999.

35. K Jung, B Brux, M Lein, A Knabich, P Sinha, B Rudolph, D Schnorr, SA Loening. Determination of alpha1-antichymotrypsin–PSA complex in serum does not im-prove the differentiation between benign prostatic hyperplasia and prostate cancer compared with total PSA and percent free PSA. Urology 53:1160–1167, 1999.

36. A Christensson, CB Laurell, H Lilja. Enzymatic activity of prostate-specific antigen and its reactions with extracellular serine proteinase inhibitors. Eur J Biochem 194: 755–763, 1990.

37. UH Stenman, J Leinonen, H Alfthan, S Rannikko, K Tuhkanen, O Alfthan. A com-plex between prostate-specific antigen and alpha 1-antichymotrypsin is the major form of prostate-specific antigen in serum of patients with prostatic cancer: Assay of the complex improves clinical sensitivity for cancer. Cancer Res 51:222–226, 1991.

38. WG Wood, E van der Sloot, A Böhle. The establishment and evaluation of lumines-cent-labelled immunometric assays for prostate-specific antigen-alpha 1-antichy-motrypsin complexes in serum. Eur J Clin Chem Clin Biochem 29:787–794, 1991.

39. J Leinonen, T Lövgren, T Vornanen, UH Stenman. Double-label time-resolved im-munofluorometric assay of prostate-specific antigen and of its complex with alpha-1-antichymotrypsin. Clin Chem 39:2098–2103, 1993.

40. C King, J Friese, L Lauren, B Dowell, N Shaw, H Lilja, UH Stenman, T Piironen, K Pettersson. Measurement on the IMx immunoassay system of free and total forms of prostate specific antigen for differentiation of patients with benign prostatic hy-perplasia and prostate cancer. Clin Chem 40:1006 (Abstract 0096), 1994.

41. WJ Catalona, DS Smith, RL Wolfert, TJ Wang, HG Rittenhouse, TL Ratliff, RB Nadler. Evaluation of percentage of free serum prostate-specific antigen to improve specificity of prostate cancer screening. JAMA 274:1214–1220, 1995.

42. WJ Catalona, AW Partin, KM Slawin, MK Brawer, RC Flanigan, A Patel, JP Ri-chie, JB deKernion, PC Walsh, PT Scardino, PH Lange, EN Subong, RE Parson, GH Gasior, KG Loveland, PC Southwick. Use of the percentage of free prostate-specific antigen to enhance differentiation of prostate cancer from benign prostatic disease: A prospective multicenter clinical trial. JAMA 279:1542–1547, 1998.

43. DL Woodrum, MK Brawer, AW Partin, WJ Catalona, PC Southwick. Interpretation of free prostate specific antigen clinical research studies for the detection of prostate cancer. J Urol 159:5–12, 1998.

44. M Lein, F Koenig, K Jung, FJ McGovern, SJ Skates, D Schnorr, SA Loening. The

percentage of free prostate specific antigen is an age-independent tumour marker for prostate cancer: Establishment of reference ranges in a large population of healthy men. Br J Urol 82:231–236, 1998.

45. HP Schmid, A Semjonow, R Maibach. Prostate-specific antigen doubling time: A potential surrogate end point in hormone-refractory prostate cancer. J Clin Oncol 17:1645–1646, 1999.

46. M Riehmann, PR Rhodes, TD Cook, GS Grose, RC Bruskewitz. Analysis of variation in prostate-specific antigen values. Urology 42:390–397, 1993.

47. CG Roehrborn, GJ Pickens, T Carmody 3rd. Variability of repeated serum prostate-specific antigen (PSA) measurements within less than 90 days in a well-defined patient population. Urology 47:59–66, 1996.

48. HB Carter, JD Pearson, Z Waclawiw, EJ Metter, DW Chan, HA Guess, PC Walsh. Prostate-specific antigen variability in men without prostate cancer: Effect of sampling interval on prostate-specific antigen velocity. Urology 45:591–596, 1995.

49. HLP van Duijnhoven, NCV Pequeriaux, JPHM van Zon, MA Blankenstein. Large discrepancy between prostate-specific antigen results from different assays during longitudinal follow-up of a prostate cancer patient. Clin Chem 42:637–641, 1996.

50. HC Graves. Standardization of immunoassays for prostate-specific antigen. A problem of prostate-specific antigen complexation or a problem of assay design? Cancer 72:3141–3144, 1993.

51. MW Plawker, JM Fleisher, VW Nitti, RJ Macchia. Primary care practitioners: An analysis of their perceptions of voiding dysfunction and prostate cancer. J Urol 155:601–604, 1996.

52. A Semjonow, W Albrecht, P Bialk, A Gerl, R Lamerz, HP Schmid, H van Poppel. Tumour markers in prostate cancer: EGTM recommendations. European Group on Tumour Markers. Anticancer Res 19:2799–2801, 1999.

53. HC Graves. Issues on standardization of immunoassays for prostate-specific antigen: A review. Clin Invest Med 16:415–424, 1993.

54. RM Nakamura, S Akimoto, HCB Graves, K Griffiths, A Semjonow, H Lilja, H Neels, UH Stenman, JT Wu. PSA standardization and quality assessment. Consensus Committee #4. In: G Murphy, K Griffiths, L Denis, S Khoury, C Chatelain, AT Cockett, eds. Proceedings of the 1st International Consultation on Prostate Cancer. Paris: Scientific Communication International, 1997, pp 141–143.

55. A Semjonow. Importance of standardization of prostate-specific antigen immunoassays in the clinical environment. Consensus Committee #4. In: G Murphy, K Griffiths, L Denis, S Khoury, C Chatelain, AT Cockett, eds. Proceedings of the 1st International Consultation on Prostate Cancer. Paris: Scientific Communication International, 1997, pp 153–156.

56. RL Vessella, PH Lange. Issues in the assessment of PSA immunoassays. Urol Clin North Am 20:607–619, 1993.

57. AM Zhou, PC Tewari, BI Bluestein, GW Caldwell, FL Larsen. Multiple forms of prostate-specific antigen in serum: Differences in immunorecognition by monoclonal and polyclonal assays. Clin Chem 39:2483–2491, 1993.

58. HC Graves, N Wehner, TA Stamey. Comparison of a polyclonal and monoclonal immunoassay for PSA: Need for an international antigen standard. J Urol 144:1516–1522, 1990.

59. MK Brawer, P Daum, JC Petteway, MH Wener. Assay variability in serum prostate-specific antigen determination. Prostate 27:1–6, 1995.

60. TA Stamey, N Yang, AR Hay, JE McNeal, FS Freiha, E Redwine. Prostate-specific antigen as a serum marker for adenocarcinoma of the prostate. N Engl J Med 317: 909–916, 1987.

61. HB Carter, JD Pearson, Z Waclawiw, EJ Metter, DW Chan, HA Guess, PC Walsh. Prostate-specific antigen variability in men without prostate cancer: Effect of sampling interval on prostate-specific antigen velocity. Urology 45:591–596, 1995.

62. K Komatsu, N Wehner, AF Prestigiacomo, Z Chen, TA Stamey. Physiologic (intra-individual) variation of serum prostate-specific antigen in 814 men from a screening population. Urology 47:343–346, 1996.

63. DW Chan, DJ Bruzek, JE Oesterling, RC Rock, PC Walsh. Prostate specific antigen as a marker for prostatic cancer: A monoconal and a polyclonal immunoassay compared. Clin Chem 33:1916–1920, 1987.

64. GL Hortin, RR Bahnson, M Daft, KM Chan, WJ Catalona, JH Ladenson. Differences in values obtained with 2 assays of prostate specific antigen. J Urol 139: 762–765, 1988.

65. UH Stenman, H Alfthan, U Turpeinen. Method dependence of interpretation of immunoassay results. Scand J Clin Lab Invest 51 (Suppl 205):86–94, 1991.

66. R Cattini, D Robinson, O Gill, N Jolley, T Bacarese Hamilton. Measurement of prostate-specific antigen in serum using four different immunoassays. Eur J Clin Chem Clin Biochem 32:181–185, 1994.

67. CH Bangma, BG Blijenberg, FH Schröder. Variabiliteit van uitslagen van prostaatspecifiek antigeen met 6 bepalingsmethoden. [Variability of values of prostate-specific antigen determined with 6 methods.]. Ned Tijdschr Geneeskd 138:813–817, 1994.

68. R Junker, B Brandt, A Semjonow, C Zechel, G Assmann. 12 different assays for the measurement of PSA and free PSA (f-PSA)—a clinical comparison study. Anticancer Res 15:2401, 1995.

69. JE Oesterling, MA Moyad, GLJ Wright, GR Beck. An analytical comparison of the three most commonly used prostate-specific antigen assays: Tandem-R, Tandem-E, and IMx. Urology 46:524–532, 1995.

70. SA Strobel, RL Sokoloff, RL Wolfert, HG Rittenhouse. Multiple forms of prostate-specific antigen in serum measured differently in equimolar- and skewed-response assays. Clin Chem 41:125–127, 1995.

71. MK Brawer, MH Wener, HG Rittenhouse, RL Wolfert. Proportion of free form of PSA explains the majority of bias between the IMx (Abbott) and Tandem (Hybritech) PSA assays. Eur Urol 30 (Suppl 2):20, Abstract #15, 1996.

72. S Strobel, K Smith, R Wolfert, H Rittenhouse. Role of free PSA in discordance across commercial PSA assays. Clin Chem 42:645–647, 1996.

73. A Semjonow, C Weining, F Oberpenning, A Heinecke, B Brandt, HJ Terpe, L Hertle, M Hamm, P Stieber. Application of assay-specific cut-off values can improve performance of PSA tests: Results of the assay comparison study. Tumor Biol 19 (Suppl 2):22, O–20, 1998.

74. G Aumüller, J Seitz, H Lilja, PA Abrahamsson, H von der Kammer, KH Scheit.

Species- and organ-specificity of secretory proteins derived from human prostate and seminal vesicles. Prostate 17:31–40, 1990.

75. X Bosch, O Bernadich. Increased serum prostate-specific antigen in a man and a woman with hepatitis A. N Engl J Med 337:1849–1850, 1997.

76. E Geisler, S Andaz, D Nirmul, P Gheewala, A Sehonanda, PH Gerst. False-positive prostatic-specific antigen in the serum of a man with renal cell carcinoma. Br J Urol 79:299–300, 1997.

77. WJ Glenski, RS Malek, JF Myrtle, JE Oesterling. Sustained, substantially increased concentration of prostate-specific antigen in the absence of prostatic malignant disease: An unusual clinical scenario. Mayo Clin Proc 67:249–252, 1992.

78. K Pummer, G Wirnsberger, P Pürstner, H Stettner, G Wandschneider. False positive prostate specific antigen values in the sera of women with renal cell carcinoma. J Urol 148:21–23, 1992.

79. HG Rittenhouse, JA Finlay, SD Mikolajczyk, AW Partin. Human Kallikrein 2 (hK2) and prostate-specific antigen (PSA): Two closely related, but distinct, kallikreins in the prostate. Crit Rev Clin Lab Sci 35:275–368, 1998.

80. E Corey, KR Buhler, RL Vessella. Cross-reactivity of ten anti-prostate-specific antigen monoclonal antibodies with human glandular kallikrein. Urology 50:567–571, 1997.

81. JF Myrtle. More on "hook effects" in immunometric assays for prostate-specific antigen. Clin Chem 35:2154–2155, 1989.

82. G Bodor, BA Wolf, B Hinds, MH Nahm, MG Scott. More on "hook effects" in immunometric assays for prostate-specific antigen. Clin Chem 35:1262–1263, 1989.

83. A Charrie, G Charriere, A Guerrier. Hook effect in immunometric assays for prostate-specific antigen. Clin Chem 41:480–481, 1995.

84. HC Vaidya, BA Wolf, N Garrett, WJ Catalona, RV Clayman, MH Nahm. Extremely high values of prostate-specific antigen in patients with adenocarcinoma of the prostate; demonstration of the "hook effect." Clin Chem 34:2175–2177, 1988.

85. BA Wolf, NC Garrett, MH Nahm. The "hook effect": High concentrations of prostate-specific antigen giving artifactually low values on one-step immunoassay. N Engl J Med 320:1755–1756, 1989.

86. DD Bankson, ME Lyon, LV Costales, VM Haver. The response of assays for total prostate specific antigen to changing proportions of "free" and alpha1-antichymotrypsin bound PSA. Clin Chem 40:1009, 1994.

87. K Jung, M Lein, D Schnorr, B Brux, W Henke, S Loening. Comparison between equimolar- and skewed-response assays of prostate specific antigen: Is there an influence on the clinical significance when measuring total serum prostate specific antigen? Ann Clin Biochem 33:209–214, 1996.

88. H Lilja. Significance of different molecular forms of serum PSA. The free, noncomplexed form of PSA versus that complexed to alpha 1-antichymotrypsin. Urol Clin North Am 20:681–686, 1993.

89. WJ Catalona, AW Partin, JA Finlay, DW Chan, HG Rittenhouse, RL Wolfert, DL Woodrum. Use of percentage of free prostate-specific antigen to identify men at

high risk of prostate cancer when PSA levels are 2.51 to 4 ng/mL and digital rectal examination is not suspicious for prostate cancer: An alternative model. Urology 54:220–224, 1999.

90. A Lundwall, H Lilja. Molecular cloning of human prostate specific antigen with cDNA. FEBS Lett 214:317–322, 1987.

91. RT McCormack, HG Rittenhouse, JA Finlay, RL Sokoloff, TJ Wang, RL Wolfert, H Lilja, JE Oesterling. Molecular forms of prostate-specific antigen and the human kallikrein gene family: A new era. Urology 45:729–744, 1995.

92. HG Rittenhouse, RL Wolfert, TJ Wang. Editorial Comment on: Corey E, Buhler KR, Vessella RL: Cross-reactivity of ten anti-prostate-specific antigen monoclonal antibodies with human glandular kallikrein. Urology 50:567–571, 1997.

93. TA Stamey. Second Stanford Conference on International Standardization of Prostate-Specific Antigen Immunoassays: September 1 and 2, 1994. Urology 45:173–184, 1995.

94. MK Brawer, DD Bankson, VM Haver, JC Petteway. Comparison of three commercial PSA assays: Results of restandardization of the Ciba Corning method. Prostate 30:269–273, 1997.

95. BG Blijenberg, BN Storm, AE Kruger, FH Schröder. On the standardization of total prostate-specific antigen: An exercise with two reference preparations. Clin Chem Lab Med 37:545–552, 1999.

96. BG Blijenberg, BN Storm, BD Van Zelst, AE Kruger, FH Schröder. New developments in the standardization of total prostate-specific antigen. Clin Biochem 32: 627–634, 1999.

97. N Yang. Diagnostic and prognostic application of prostate-specific tissue markers: Prostate antigen (PA) and prostatic acid phosphatase (PAP). Clin Chem 30:1057, 1984.

98. JF Myrtle, W Shackelford, R Bartholomew, J Wampler. Prostate-specific antigen: Quantitation in serum by immunoradiometric assay. Clin Chem 29:1216, 1983.

99. JE Oesterling. Prostate specific antigen: A critical assessment of the most useful tumor marker for adenocarcinoma of the prostate. J Urol 145:907–923, 1991.

100. A Semjonow, C Weining, F Oberpenning, A Heinecke, A Terpe, HP Schmid, L Hertle, B Brandt, M Hamm, P Stieber. Application of assay-specific cut-off values: Results of the assay comparison study for PSA. Europ Urol 35 (suppl 2):18, 1999.

101. DB Burlington. FDA advises labs regarding off-label use of PSA assays. Clin Lab News 21:5, 1995.

102. A Semjonow, G De Angelis, F Oberpenning, HP Schmid, B Brandt, L Hertle. Clinical impact of different assays for prostate specific antigen. Br J Urol Int 86:590–597, 2000.

103. MH Wener, P Daun, B Close, M Brawer. Method-to-method and lot-to-lot variation in assays for prostate-specific antigen. Am J Clin Pathol 101:387–388, 1994.

104. JA Hanley, BJ McNeil. A method of comparing the areas under receiver operating characteristic curves derived from the same cases. Radiology 148:839–843, 1983.

4

PSA Density: Does It Still Have Utility?

David Knowles, Emilia Bagiella, and Mitchell C. Benson
Columbia University College of Physicians and Surgeons, New York, New York

Serum prostate specific antigen (PSA) has had a dramatic and profound impact on the diagnosis and management of prostate cancer. There is no question that the frequency of organ-confined prostate cancer is increasing and the identification of newly diagnosed, untreated metastatic cancer is plummeting [1,2]. Survival is being increased and we are probably decreasing the death rate from prostate cancer, although the last remains to be definitively proven. If a decrease in the death rate is documented by results of continuing trials, PSA will have satisfied the tenets of a screening tool and will be widely and universally acknowledged as a significant step forward in the diagnosis of prostate cancer. Unfortunately, despite all the advances in the diagnosis of prostate cancer that have emanated from the widespread use of serum PSA as a screening and/or diagnostic tool, the specificity of isolated PSA determinations remains low. Accordingly, it is our practice to perform a prostate biopsy on any and all otherwise healthy patients with an "abnormal" level of serum PSA. Prostate biopsy is expensive in patient anxiety and medical cost. As a result, laboratory research has focused on the discovery of new markers and clinical research has focused on refining serum PSA determinations through the use of PSA derivatives.

The PSA derivatives that are permutations of total serum PSA that have been tested in clinical practice include PSA density (PSAD) [2], the focus of this chapter; PSA velocity (PSAV) [4] (Chap. 5); and age specific PSA (AS-PSA) [5] (Chap. 6). The ratio of free to total PSA (F:T PSA) is not a PSA derivative: it is the first of the "new" markers [6,7]. F:T PSA has been widely tested and is now approved by the Food and Drug Administration (FDA) for use to refine further the risk of prostate cancer in men with total serum PSA levels between 4.1 and 10.0 ng/ml. F:T PSA is discussed in Chapter 7. This chapter will focus on PSA density and what we believe to be its utility.

It is our current opinion that neither PSAD nor any other PSA derivative or new serum marker is capable of eliminating the need for biopsy in a patient who would be considered a candidate for therapy if prostate cancer was diagnosed. It has been suggested that F:T PSA be used to avoid biopsy for those with PSA levels between 4.1 and 10, but the safety of this approach remains to be documented [8–10]. Utilizing an F:T PSA strategy, 5–10% of patients with elevated PSA levels and prostate cancer will not undergo an initial biopsy. In our opinion, before these patients can be safely spared a biopsy it must be proven that the delay in diagnosis has no adverse effect on our ability to intervene with curative intent and, as a result, no adverse effect on prognosis.

Given what we believe to be the current limitations of PSA and the PSA derivatives, the issue is not the sensitivity, specificity, and accuracy of PSA. The issue is: When is a negative biopsy a true negative biopsy? Which patient with a negative biopsy can be assured that all is well and which patient will require either an early or delayed repeat biopsy? Can any parameter assessed either prior to or at the time of biopsy be informative regarding the accuracy of a negative (no malignancy present) result?

This chapter will not review all of the PSAD studies performed. This task has been performed in other chapters [11]. PSAD continues to perform well in our hands and we believe that PSAD adds unique and informative information on the risk of prostate cancer in patients with a normal digital rectal exam and a PSA level between 4.1 and 10 ng/ml. Despite PSAD's performance in our hands and those of some others, these results have not been consistently reproduced and, as a result, PSAD has not attained universal acceptance.

I. PSA DENSITY

PSA density was conceived of in 1990 and first described by the author in 1991 [3]. The concept of PSAD was based on the observation that there was a relationship between serum PSA levels and prostatic hyperplasia and hypertrophy. PSAD was conceived to normalize serum PSA for prostate volume, assuming that a given volume of prostate cancer would cause a greater elevation of serum PSA than a given volume of benign prostatic hyperplasia (BPH). This occurs because cancer cells secrete PSA directly into the stroma and not into the excretory ducts of the prostate. This results in more systemic absorption of PSA per cell and because, cancer in general will have a greater epithelial concentration per unit volume of prostate tissue. Prostate cancer cells do not produce more PSA per cell than benign prostate cells, rather the opposite is true: on average, a cancer cell produces less PSA because of a lack of differentiation. Others have tried to refine PSAD by creating transition-zone PSA density (PSAD-TZ) [12,13]. PSAD-TZ was an attempt to normalize serum PSA directly to the hyperplastic portion of the prostate gland: the transition zone. Like PSAD, some have found PSAD-TZ to be superior to PSA and PSAD, while others have found that it has not added to PSA determinations.

It is our belief that either unintentional selection biases in the patient populations under study or a failure to determine prostate or TZ volume diligently can explain many of the inconsistent results with PSAD and PSAD-TZ. We do not believe that the inconsistent results occur secondary to failure of principle. In this chapter, we will describe where we believe that PSAD is headed, describe our study population, and comment on the results of others with respect to new applications of PSAD.

II. PSAD AND PROSTATE BIOPSY

If one accepts the stipulation that all patients with ''elevated'' serum PSA levels require a prostate biopsy, the postbiopsy dilemma is: How do you evaluate and what do you do with a patient with an ''abnormal'' PSA (increased statistical risk of prostate cancer) and negative results of an initial biopsy? The finding of high-grade prostatic intraepithelial neoplasia (PIN) at the time of biopsy necessitates a repeat prostate biopsy. However, PIN should not be considered a normal biopsy result. For those with negative biopsies, some investigators have suggested a repeat biopsy in all patients. Others repeat the biopsy if a follow-up PSA determination remains ''abnormal.'' Still others place the patient on surveillance and follow PSA velocity. Can any PSA derivative or new PSA marker predict who will be found to have prostate cancer at the time of later biopsy, or even predict which patients will require repeat prostate biopsy by virtue of a rising level of serum PSA?

Since 1991, we have prospectively followed all patients presenting for evaluation of an intermediate PSA elevation (4.1–10.0 ng/ml). Prebiopsy PSA levels were measured and PSAD prospectively calculated at time of prostate ultrasound examination and biopsy. In 1995, with the advent of F:T PSA as a potentially discriminating new marker, we incorporated these values into our routine evaluation. For the purpose of this study, we selected from our database all patients with a PSA level between 4.1 and 10 ng/ml who underwent an initial biopsy between March 1991 and March 1995 that proved negative for prostate cancer. We identified 148 men who presented with a negative initial biopsy who were then followed until the present. All patients had complete information including all laboratory values, biopsy results, and ultrasound results. These patients have been evaluated with measurement of total serum PSA, digital rectal examination, and F:T PSA at least every 6 months. All initial PSA determinations (Hybritech) were performed in our hospital laboratory. F:T PSA determinations were performed by Dianon Laboratories. All ultrasound determinations of prostate volume, prostate biopsies, and digital rectal examinations (DRE) were performed by one author (MCB). A repeat biopsy was performed in those patients who exhibited one of the following: a PSA level rise greater than 1.0 ng/ml/per year, a PSA level rise to greater than 10 ng/ml, and/or abnormal results of DRE during follow-up.

Patients were stratified according to those who required a repeat biopsy and those who did not progress to a second biopsy. We further stratified the group who required a repeat biopsy based on the results of the second biopsy. Thus, we had three groups: those not requiring a repeat biopsy, those whose repeat biopsy showed prostate cancer, and those whose repeat biopsy showed benign disease. These groups were analyzed for their PSA, PSAD, and F:T PSA at initial presentation and at the time of their repeat biopsy (groups 2 and 3). We performed Bonferroni t tests for all variables, and all groups. The Medical Statistics Department of Columbia–Presbyterian Medical Center performed the statistical analysis.

III. PERSONAL RESULTS

Among the 148 patients with an initial negative biopsy, 97 (65.6%) have not progressed to require a second biopsy (Table 1). The average age for this group was 61.5 years, with a minimum of 49 and a maximum of 79. The mean PSA

Table 1 Parameters at Presentation

	Age (years)	PSA (ng/ml)	Prostate volume (cc)	PSAD (cc)	F:T PSA (%)
Group 1 (n = 97)	61.5 ± 16	6.9 ± 4.2	65.1 ± 42.2	0.119 ± 0.06	18.5 ± 8.5
Group 2 (n = 43)	60.0 ± 6.7	7.5 ± 3.7	59.1 ± 21.7	0.128 ± 0.07	16 ± 6.9
Group 3 (n = 8)	65.7 ± 7.1	7.0 ± 4.3	50.7 ± 21.0	0.173 ± 0.08	12 ± 17.1

Distribution of the age, prostate volume, PSA, PSAD, F:T PSA in means given as ± standard deviation at the time of the patient's initial transrectal ultrasound. There is no significant difference between the groups. PSAD trended higher in the group requiring a repeat biopsy, but did not reach statistical significance.
PSA, prostate specific antigen; PSAD, prostate specific antigen density; F:T PSA, free:total prostate specific antigen. Group 1, no repeat biopsy; group 2, repeat biopsy BPH; group 3, repeat biopsy prostate cancer.

within this group was 6.9 ng/ml, the mean PSAD was 0.119, the mean F:T PSA was 18.5%, and the mean prostatic volume 65.1 cc. Fifty-one of the 148 patients (34%) have required a repeat biopsy based upon the above criteria. In 43 of the 148 patients (29%), the repeat biopsy was benign. The average age for this group was 60 years with a minimum of 42 and a maximum of 73. At initial presentation, the mean PSA for this group of 43 patients was 7.5 ng/ml, the mean PSAD was 0.128, the mean F:T PSA was 16%, and the mean prostate volume 59.1 cc. Eight of the 148 patients (5.4%) underwent a second biopsy that revealed prostate cancer. The average age for this group was 65.7 years, with a minimum of 60 and a maximum of 73. At initial presentation, their mean PSA level was 7.0 ng/ml, the mean PSAD was 0.173, the mean F:T PSA was 12%, and the mean prostate volume 50.7 cc (Table 1).

The patients requiring a repeat biopsy underwent transrectal ultrasound re-evaluation. The PSA and PSAD parameters at the time of re-evaluation are shown in Table 2. As expected, the mean PSA at second biopsy was higher for all groups, since a rise in PSA was an indication for biopsy. The 43 patients whose repeat biopsy was benign had a mean PSA level at rebiopsy of 10.9 ng/ml, the mean PSAD was 0.151, the mean F:T PSA was 19%, and the mean prostate volume 64.1 cc. The average age for this group at the time of repeat biopsy was 62 years with a minimum of 43 and a maximum of 73. The 8 patients (5.4%) within the original 148 found to have cancer at repeat biopsy had an average age at rebiopsy of 66.5 years, with a minimum of 61 and a maximum of 74. Within this group the mean PSA at rebiopsy was 8.60 ng/ml, the mean PSAD was 0.180, the mean F:T PSA was 24%, and the mean prostate volume 52.7 cc (Table 2).

In comparing the three different groups for age, prostate volume, PSA, PSAD, and F:T PSA levels, there were no statistically significant differences noted between the various groups for any of the variables analyzed either at the time of initial presentation or rebiopsy. In comparing the group of prostate cancer patients with those with BPH found in the repeat biopsy, there was still no sig-

Table 2 Parameters at the Time of Rebiopsy

	Age (years)	PSA (ng/ml)	Prostate volume (cc)	PSAD (cc)	F:T PSA (%)
Group 1 (n = 97)	61.5 ± 16	6.9 ± 4.2	65.1 ± 42.2	0.119 ± 0.06	18.5 ± 8.5
Group 2 (n = 43)	60.0 ± 6.7	10.9 ± 3.9	64.1 ± 21.7	0.151 ± 0.07	19 ± 6.9
Group 3 (n = 8)	65.7 ± 7.1	8.6 ± 4.3	52.7 ± 21.0	0.180 ± 0.08	24 ± 17.1

Distribution of the age, prostate volume, PSA, PSAD, F:T PSA in means ± standard deviation. We can verify that there is no significant difference between the groups. Although the F:T PSA on the prostate cancer group was clearly higher, the standard deviation was significant.
Abbreviations as in Table 1.

nificant difference between the values obtained and probability levels of 95% (p > 0.05) were not reached. Only PSAD trended towards significance: p = 0.09. However, the study is limited by its relatively small sample size and it is impossible to know if, given a larger sample, any parameter would have proven significant.

These results indicate that none of the currently available PSA derivatives or new markers (F:T PSA) can identify which patients with a first biopsy that is negative for malignancy will require a second biopsy based upon a rise in their serum PSA level or change in findings on a digital rectal examination. PSA density performed best but, given the small sample size, did not reach statistical significance. F:T PSA was found to be of no value. In fact, utilizing the Dianon PSA, the highest F:T ratios were found in those patients with a second biopsy that proved to be malignant (24%). Furthermore, none of the derivatives will identify which patients requiring a second biopsy will be found to have cancer on their second biopsy. As a result, all patients with an elevated serum PSA level and results that are negative for malignancy require careful follow-up. Based on this evaluation scheme, approximately one-third will require a repeat biopsy during an average follow-up of 7 years.

IV. OVERVIEW

The continuing debate about which PSA derivative or new marker will prove to be most useful is ample evidence that there is currently no consensus on how to best utilize the most accurate tumor marker for prostate cancer. Although serum PSA may be the best tumor marker yet employed in any tumor system, it is clear that the discovery or development of a marker that will be more specific than PSA in screening for prostate cancer in the general population would be welcome. Such a marker might also help predict the risk of prostate cancer in men who had a prior negative biopsy. The most confounding to us today is the population of men with an elevated serum PSA who have undergone a prior biopsy that proved negative. This is discussed in detail in Chapter 10. The patient diagnosed with prostate cancer is in many ways much less ambiguous. Those with negative biopsies continue to be labeled as having "abnormal" findings, but without a definitive diagnosis. A marker that would assist in the correct classification of such individuals would vastly decrease the anxiety among patients currently being evaluated based on abnormal results of a digital rectal examination or PSA level. Furthermore, a more accurate marker would decrease the numerous transrectal ultrasound examinations, often with one or more transrectal ultrasound guided biopsies on each occasion, which cause in these patients significant anxiety and discomfort. While this is our goal, we are left with the imperfect markers currently available in our practice.

The dilemma of how to manage the patient with a negative initial prostate biopsy is not new. Ohori et al. [14] analyzed a comparison of total serum PSA and PSAD in a group of 244 patients who were undergoing an initial prostate biopsy prompted by elevated serum PSA levels. The population was diverse (PSA 0.2–1320 ng/ml), and cancer was detected in 110 of the 244 patients (45%). A subset of 82 patients had a PSA level >10 ng/ml and in this group, 50 of the 82 patients (61%) were found to have cancer. Among these 82 patients, cancer was detected in 49 of the 70 patients (70%) with a PSAD >0.150 but in only 1 of the 12 (8%) with a PSAD <0.150. The authors concluded that when serum PSA was high (>10 ng/ml) but the PSAD was low (<0.150), cancer was rarely detected. They suggested that this subset of patients with a PSAD <0.150 (not definitively defined owing to the relatively small number of patients) might be suitable candidates for surveillance rather than an early repeat biopsy.

The value of PSAD and PSA slope or velocity in predicting the detection of prostate cancer on subsequent biopsies in men with an initially negative biopsy was reported by Keetch et al. in 1996 [15]. Using the Washington University PSA-1 database, they identified 327 men over the age of 50 who had a persistently elevated serum PSA level after an initial negative biopsy. Of the 327 men, 81 (25%) were found to have cancer on a subsequent biopsy. The authors found that both PSAD (p < 0.0001) and PSA slope (p = 0.03) were statistically significant in predicting the risk of cancer on a subsequent biopsy. Unfortunately, the authors did not provide information on the serum PSA distribution of the population, and the number of patients with PSA levels above 10 is not known. Since patients with significant PSA elevations undergo repeat biopsy in almost all instances, their inclusion in this study may bias the analysis. However, a combination of PSAD < 0.150 and a PSA slope <0.75 ng/ml per year missed only 11 of the 81 cancers detected. The authors concluded that a significant number of cancers would be missed (9%) if PSAD and PSA slope were used as the only determinants for repeat biopsy. The combination of PSAD and PSA slope as a determinant for avoiding a second biopsy was considered to be reasonable if the patient was not a candidate for aggressive therapy.

With the advent of serum free PSA, Catalona et al. reanalyzed in 1997 the value of PSAD and compared it to F:T PSA in predicting the presence of prostate cancer in men with prior negative biopsies [16]. In this study, they analyzed 163 men with a serum PSA levels between 4.1 and 10 ng/ml who were advised to undergo a repeat prostate biopsy. Ninety-nine of the 163 men consented to a repeat biopsy and 20 were found to have prostate cancer. As expected, the detection of prostate cancer was associated with a lower free PSA and a higher PSAD. PSA slope was not useful in this subset of patients in determining the presence of cancer on a subsequent biopsy. The PSAD cut-offs found to be useful were lower than those previously reported. This study demonstrated that PSAD cut-offs of 0.100 and 0.080 would have detected 90 and 95% of the diagnosed cancers while avoiding 31 and 12% of the repeat biopsies, respectively. In contrast, F:T PSA cut-offs of 28 and 30% would have similarly detected 90 and 95% of the diagnosed cancers but would have spared only 13 and 12% of the repeat biopsies. The authors concluded that both parameters may be used to avoid unnecessary second biopsies. They suggested that F:T PSA has the advantage of not requiring a repeat transrectal ultrasound. It has been our experience that the initial PSAD is equally efficacious so a repeat ultrasound may not necessary.

Djavan et al. introduced a permutation of PSAD, which they called the PSA density of the transition zone [12] (PSA-TZ). The rationale for this approach comes from the fact that it is the transition zone that is enlarging and not the total prostate. Therefore, they believe that PSA-TZ would be a better "normalization" for total PSA than PSAD. They also find TZ volume easier to calculate since, in their hands, TZ length is easier to measure. We have found the exact opposite to be true but this may be due to one being better at what one performs more often. Their initial studies focused on the value of PSA-TZ, which they find to be a powerful parameter for differentiating benign from malignant elevations of serum PSA [13]. Subsequently, in a multi-institutional study, Djavan et al. examined the ability of PSA-TZ, PSAD, and F:T PSA to predict prostate cancer on a repeat biopsy [17]. They analyzed a population of 1051 men prospectively accrued as part of a prostate cancer screening study. Prostate cancer was detected in 231 at the time of their initial biopsy, leaving 820 patients subject to further analysis. All patients had a serum PSA level between 4.1 and 10 ng/ml. Prostate cancer was detected in 83 of the 820 patients (10%) at the time of their repeat biopsy. The authors found that F:T PSA and PSA-TZ were the most accurate predictors of prostate cancer on repeat biopsy. A cut-off of 30% free PSA would have detected 90% of the cancers and eliminated 50% of the repeat biopsies. PSA-TZ with a cut-off of 0.26 detected 78% of the cancers and spared 52% of the biopsies. However, in this multi-institutional study, none of the PSA derivatives fared well; F:T PSA was statistically superior to total PSA, PSAD, and PSA-TZ.

Bangma et al. examining the relative performance of F:T PSA ratio, age specific PSA, and PSA density in a large screening population, found that F:T PSA performed favorably with respect to maintaining cancer detection while decreasing the number of unnecessary biopsies [18]. However, these authors could not determine in their study how many of the prostate cancers missed at the initial screening would be diagnosed subsequently, and if this delay would affect the outcome in the population followed.

In 1999, Noguchi et al., examined a series of 218 consecutive men undergoing prostate biopsy for suspected cancer [19]. They found 114 cases of prostate cancer, 99 (87%) diagnosed on the initial biopsy and 15 (13%) on the repeat biopsy. In this somewhat small study, a comparison of the 15 men in whom cancer was found in the repeat biopsy with those 89 men with a negative repeat biopsy, DRE, PSA, prostate volume, PSA density, and PSA slope were considered to be of no utility. These authors failed to find any significant differences that would stratify those patients in whom a cancer was detected on the second biopsy.

Fowler et al. recently examined the utility of the PSA derivatives in a consecutive series of 298 men with suspected stage T1c–T2 prostate cancer undergoing a repeat biopsy who had an initial biopsy that was benign at a single institution from 1992 to 1999 [20]. This population was derived from a series of 1740 men seen at the Veterans Affairs Medical Center in Jackson (MI). The authors analyzed the relative value of total PSA, PSA density, annualized interbiopsy PSA change in all patients, and percentage free PSA (201 patients) and PSA velocity (171 patients) in the noted subsets. The initial cancer detection rate was 34% (587/1740). Patients with an initially negative biopsy (1153; 66%) underwent a repeat biopsy if their initial serum PSA level was greater than the age-adjusted reference range established by Oesterling et al. [21], if their PSA level rose to above the age-adjusted reference range, or if they had a palpable abnormality to their prostate regardless of PSA level. For the 298 men undergoing a repeat biopsy, the indications for repeat biopsy were initial PSA greater than the age-specific range (199/298; 67%), PSA that rose above the reference range (30/298; 10%), and a prostate that was highly suspicious for carcinoma (69/298; 23%). A repeat biopsy was not performed in another 358 similar patients for unknown reasons and was refused by 23 patients. The results demonstrated that, after univariate analysis, patient age, PSA density, percentage free PSA, and PSA velocity were significant predictors of cancer on repeat biopsy. For the entire group, only patient age (p = 0.002) and PSA density (p = 0.0002) remained significant, with PSA density being the single most important parameter. However, multivariate logistic regression analysis of the 201 patients for whom F:T PSA was available revealed that PSA density was no longer a significant predictor and only patient age (p = 0.002) and percentage free PSA (p = 0.0001) were significant. For the subset in whom PSA velocity was available, age (p = 0.02) and percentage free PSA (p = 0.0003) remained significant but PSA density and PSA velocity were not significant predictors of second biopsy outcome. Interesting, in this study, was that high-grade PIN was not a predictor of for detecting cancer on a repeat biopsy and there appeared to be no difference in PSA fluctuations among men with PIN who did and did not have cancer.

Since the advent of PSAD, there has been waxing and waning enthusiasm for the concept within the literature. The use of PSA density as part of the cancer detection algorithm has been criticized by several authors for not improving sensitivity or specificity, even though some others have found that it does increase sensitivity and specificity compared with PSA alone [3,20–23]. When using PSA density for detection of prostate cancer among patients with intermediate PSA serum levels (4.1–10.0 ng/ml), the goal of PSAD had been to detect significant cancer by immediate biopsy (PSAD of 0.15 or greater). Those patients with a low PSAD (<0.150) not undergoing an initial biopsy have in general been found to harbor low-volume cancer. As a result, it was postulated that a delayed biopsy would not expose them to a significant risk. This strategy had the advantage of diagnosing significant cancers while not exposing the entire population to unnecessary biopsies. Although subject to some criticism, our results published in previous series and those of others suggest that PSAD reasonably fulfills the goal of improving specificity while maintaining sensitivity and allowing for the classification of some patients as having low risk for development of prostate cancer [21–25]. Catalona et al., analyzing 99 volunteer patients who had a previous negative biopsy and a serum PSA level of 4.1–10.0 ng/ml, found 20 (20%) patients with prostate cancer in their second biopsy. This group had significantly lower free PSA levels and higher PSA density values, with 83% overlap in the cases. In their analysis, they concluded that for a detection rate of 90 and 95% of the prostate cancers, they should use 28 and 30% as the percentage free PSA cut-off and a PSA density cut-off of 0.10 and 0.08, avoiding 31 and 12% of the unnecessary biopsies [15,16].

Our attempt to use age, prostate volume, PSA density, and F:T PSA ratio to stratify the large group of patients with an initial negative biopsy into those whose initial biopsy was a false-negative result and those for whom there truly is no cancer has not succeeded. There have been attempts to refine further the application of PSAD by applying age specific reference ranges and correcting for transition zone volume, but these studies tend not to be individually predictive. The ability to salvage patients not undergoing an initial biopsy remains unknown [26,27]. For all the above-mentioned reasons, more and more authors have questioned the utility of PSAD and F:T PSA as improved markers [18,28,29]. We agree with these individuals and have found that the improved specificity resulting from PSAD or F:T PSA does not allow us to avoid an initial biopsy in an individual patient. It remains our opinion that if a patient is candidate for therapy, he must be considered a candidate for diagnosis, and a biopsy should be performed.

V. CONCLUSION

Although the PSA derivative (PSAD) and the marker F:T PSA have proven to have greater specificity than serum PSA levels alone, they do so at the expense of sensitivity. Neither derivative has been *proven* to limit safely the number of biopsies performed due to an abnormal PSA level. The results of this and other studies demonstrate that, to date, PSA and the PSA derivatives cannot be utilized to determine which patients had a true negative initial biopsy and which patients will be at high risk for requiring repeat prostate biopsy. All patients must be closely monitored for evidence of a change in status and new markers for this purpose are urgently needed. At the current time, it remains our opinion and practice to perform a biopsy in any patient who would be deemed a candidate for therapy if prostate cancer were discovered.

REFERENCES

1. SL Parker, T Tong, S Bolden, PA Wingo. Cancer statistics 1997. CA 47:53, 1997.
2. WJ Catalona, DS Smith, TL Ratliff, JW Basler. Detection of organ confined prostate cancer is increased through prostate specific antigen-based screening. JAMA 271: 192–197, 1993.
3. MC Benson, IS Whang, CA Olsson, DJ McMahon, WH Cooner. The use of prostate specific antigen density to enhance the predictive value of intermediate levels of serum prostate specific antigen. J Urol 147:817, 1992.
4. HB Carter, CH Morrel, JD Pearson, JL Brant, CC Plato, EJ Matter, DW Chan, JL Fozard, PL Walsh. Estimation of prostatic growth using serial prostate-specific antigen measurements in men with and without prostate disease. Cancer Res 52:3323, 1992.
5. JE Oesterling, SJ Jacobsen, CG Chute, HH Guess, CJ Girman, LA Panzer, MM Lieber. Serum prostate-specific antigen in a community-based population of healthy men. Establishment of age-specific reference ranges. JAMA 270:860–865, 1993.
6. H Lilja, T Bjork, D Abrahamsson, UH Stenman, N Shaw, B Dowell, J Oesterling, K Petterson, T Tuhkanen, O Alfthan. Improved separation between normals, benign prostatic hyperplasia (BPH) and carcinoma of the prostate (CAP) by measuring free (F), complexed (C) and total concentrations (T) of prostate specific antigen (PSA). J Urol 151 (abstract):400A, 1994.
7. UH Stenman, J Leinonen, J Alfthan, S Rannikkos, K Tuhkanen, O Alfthan. A complex between prostate-specific antigen and alpha 1-antichymotripsin is the major form of prostate-specific antigen in serum of patients with prostate cancer: Assay of the complex improves clinical sensitivity for cancer. Cancer Res 51:222–226, 1991.
8. WJ Catalona, DS Smith, RL Wolfert, TJ Wang, HG Rittenhouse, TL Ratliff, RB Nader. Evaluation of percentage of free serum prostate-specific antigen to improve specificity of prostate cancer screening. JAMA 274:1214–1220, 1995.
9. AA Luderer, YT Chen, TF Soriano, WK Kramp, G Carlson, C Cuny, T Sharp, W Smith, J Petkeway, MK Brawer. Measurement of the proportion of free to total prostate specific antigen improves diagnostic performance of prostate-specific antigen in the diagnostic gray zone of total prostate-specific antigen. Urology 46:187–194, 1995.
10. G Alivizatos, C Deliveliotis, D Mitropoulos, G Raptides. Does free to total ratio of prostate-specific antigen alter decision-making on prostatic biopsy? Urology 48(suppl):71–75, 1996.
11. E Seaman, M Whang, CA Olsson, A Katz, WH Crooner, MC Benson. PSA Density: Role in patient evaluation and management. Urol Clin North Am 20:653–664, 1993.
12. B Djavan, AR Zlotta, G Byttebier, et al. Prostate specific antigen density of the transition zone for early detection of prostate cancer. J Urol 160:411–419, 1998.

13. B Djavan, AR Zlotta, M Remzi, K Ghawidel. Total and transition zone prostate volume and age: How they affect the utility of PSA-based diagnostic parameters for early prostate cancer detection? Urology 54:846–852, 1999.
14. M Ohori, JK Dunn, PT Scardino. Is prostate specific antigen density more useful than prostate specific antigen levels in the diagnosis of prostate cancer? Urology 45:666–671, 1995.
15. DW Keetch, JM McMurtry, DS Smith, GL Andriole, WJ Catalona. Prostate specific antigen density versus prostate specific antigen slope as predictors of prostate cancer in men with initially negative prostate biopsies. J Urol 156:428–431, 1996.
16. WJ Catalona, JA Beiser, DS Smith. Serum free prostate specific antigen and prostate specific antigen density measurements for predicting cancer in men with prior negative prostate biopsies. J Urol 158:2162–2167, 1997.
17. B Djavan, AR Zlotta, M Remzi, G Kramer. Optimal predictors of prostate cancer on repeat prostate biopsy: A prospective study of 1051 men. J Urol 163:1144–1149, 2000.
18. CH Bangma, R Kranse, BG Blijenberg, FH Schroder. The free to total serum prostate specific antigen ratio for staging prostate carcinoma. J Urol 157:544–547, 1997.
19. M Noguchi, J Yahara, H Koga, O Nakashima, S Noda. Necessity of repeat biopsies in men for suspected prostate cancer. Int J Urol 6:7–12, 1999.
20. JE Fowler, Jr., SA Bigler, D Miles, DA Yalkut. Predictors of first repeat biopsy cancer detection with suspected local stage prostate cancer. J Urol 163:813–818, 2000.
21. MC Benson, IS Whang, A Pantuck, K Ring, SA Kaplan, CA Olsson, WH Cooner. Prostate specific antigen density: A means of distinguishing benign prostatic hypertrophy and prostate cancer. J Urol 147(Pt. 2):815–816, 1992.
22. J Ramon, L Boccon-Gibod, T Billebaud, et al. Prostate-specific antigen density: A means to enhance detection of prostate cancer. Eur Urol 25:288–294, 1994.
23. A Semjonow, M Hamm, P Rathert. The quotient of prostate-specific antigen and prostate volume. Improved differentiation between benign prostatic hyperplasia and locally circumscribed prostate cancer. Urologie A 32:250–253, 1993.
24. MC Benson, CA Olsson. Prostate specific antigen and prostate specific antigen density. Roles in patient evaluation and management. Cancer 15:1667–1673, 1994.
25. MC Benson, DJ McMahon, WH Cooner, CA Olsson. An algorithm for prostate cancer detection in a patient population using prostate-specific antigen and prostate-specific antigen density. World J Urol 11:206–213, 1993.
26. AW Eshref, M Bazinet, C Trudel, et al. Role of prostate-specific antigen density after applying age-specific prostate-specific antigen reference ranges. Urology 45:972–979, 1995.
27. JB Rietbergen, R Kranse, RF Hoedmaeker, et al. Comparison of prostate-specific antigen corrected for total prostate volume and transition zone volume in a population based screening study. Urology 52:237–246, 1998.
28. TH Douglas, TO Morgan, DG McLeod, et al. Comparison of serum prostate specific membrane antigen, prostate specific antigen, and free prostate specific antigen levels in radical prostatectomy patients. Cancer 80:107–114, 1997.
29. E Shin, S Kazuho, S Shigehiro. Inadequacy of free prostate-specific antigen parameters in the prediction of pathologic extent of prostate cancer in Japanese men. Urology 52:230–236, 1998.

5
PSA Velocity

Faiyaaz M. Jhaveri
Northwest Hospital, Seattle, Washington

Prostate specific antigen (PSA) velocity, which is the serial elevation of serum PSA over time, is among the earliest approaches used to help enhance the specificity of PSA to detect prostate cancer. Given the elevation of serum PSA in most men with carcinoma, it seems reasonable that the rate of increase of PSA over time would be greater in men who have carcinoma than in those who do not.

I. DETERMINING THE OPTIMAL PSA VELOCITY CUT-OFF

The concept of PSA velocity was first demonstrated by Carter et al. in their Baltimore Longitudinal Aging Study [1,2]. Their study indicated that men with a PSA velocity of 0.75 mg/ml per year have a greater chance of carcinoma than those with a slower rise in PSA over time. In their archival serum study, using the PSA velocity cutoff of 0.75 ng/ml per year gave a sensitivity of 75% and specificity of greater than 90%. However, this longitudinal study was limited by its retrospective nature, the small number of cancer patients [18], the very long interval of testing (7–25 years), and the fact that the men were younger than 70 years with normal PSA levels at the time of entry into the study. Studies have shown an approximate 10% variation in PSA levels when measured a few weeks apart and suggest that short-term estimates of PSA velocity can be misleading [3,4].

Other investigators in Seattle [5,6] were unable to reproduce the results of Carter et al. with relatively short-term PSA intervals of 1 and 2 years. PSA velocity did not help to stratify men with and without cancer in their studies. In their study, men were biopsied based on change in PSA regardless of PSA level. Interesting was that 19% of men with PSA levels of 4.0 ng/ml or less who had a greater than 20% increase in PSA level during the previous year (and an abnormal digital rectal examination if the PSA was less than 1.5 ng/ml) had cancer. The majority of men with cancer detected through the PSA change-driven protocol had normal PSA levels at biopsy.

II. TIMING OF PSA DETERMINATIONS

Smith and Catalona [7] examined prospectively the usefulness of shorter-term measurements (5 years or less) of the serum PSA rate of change in detecting prostate cancer in a serial PSA-based screening study. Similar to Brawer et al.'s findings, they did not show significant enhancement in test accuracy using the PSA velocity cut-off of 0.75 ng/ml/year. They measured PSA every 6 months for 982 cases without prostate cancer at the first visit for screening. Using PSA velocity cut-offs of 0.75 ng/ml per year and 0.4 ng/ml per year, the diagnostic accuracy was good in the cases with PSA levels of 4.0 ng/ml or lower and 4.1 ng/ml or higher, respectively. There study did show two new findings. First, the PSA velocity cut-off point is different in men whose initial values are normal compared with those whose initial levels are elevated. Second, in those whose initial PSA levels are normal the PSA velocity is more predictive of cancer in younger men than in older men.

In a previous study by Keetch et al. [8], approximately 75% of the men with detectable prostate cancer are removed from the study population during the initial screening. In the remaining men with initially normal PSA values, the PSA velocity cutoff of 0.75 ng/ml per year resulted in a sensitivity of 79% and specificity of 66% in predicting cancer. These values are much less than that reported initially by Carter et al. [1].

Carter et al. [9] subsequently, showed that PSA velocity is useful if a minimum of three consecutive measurements are taken over a 2 year period. They also concluded that this was most significant in men who had a PSA level greater than 4.0 ng/ml. The optimal cutoff recommended was 0.75 ng/ml with excellent sensitivity and specificity levels of 72% and 95%, respectively. They classified the cases without prostate cancer with PSA levels lower than 10 ng/ml into three groups: a clinical benign prostatic hypertrophy (BPH) group whose PSA measurement interval was 3 months, and a histological BPH group and a noncancer group whose PSA measurement interval was 2 years. The proportion of cases that exceeded PSA velocity levels of 0.75 ng/ml per year or higher was only 1% in the histological BPH group and noncancer group. However, in the clinical BPH group it was higher at 28% and 17% with the PSA measurement interval of 3 and 6 months, respectively. Therefore, they concluded that PSA should be measured more than three times during a 2 year period with an optimal PSA velocity cut-off of 0.75 ng/ml.

The sensitivity of PSA velocity unfortunately remains too low to avoid prostate biopsy in a patient with elevated PSA levels who is otherwise healthy and could be considered a candidate for therapy if prostate cancer were diagnosed. Mettlin et al. [10] reported that the sensitivity was 55% and the specificity was 96% when the cut-off value of prostate specific antigen velocity was set at 0.75 ng/ml for 84 cases of prostate cancer and 1473 cases of nonprostate cancer. They concluded that the sensitivity of PSA velocity was too low and the specificity was high when compared with PSA, PSA density, and age-referenced PSA.

III. REPEAT BIOPSIES OR LOW INITIAL PSA LEVELS AND PSA VELOCITY

There may be two cohorts of patients for whom PSA velocity may be more clinically applicable. It may be useful in the 20–30% of men who may harbor prostate cancer despite an initially negative prostate biopsy, or the approximately 25% of men found to have cancer with initial PSA levels less than 4.1 ng/ml. Smith and Catalona suggested that using their lower PSA velocity cut-off of 0.4 ng/ml per year in men with elevated PSA levels of 4.0 ng/ml or greater may be viewed as an optimal cut-off point for men with an initially negative biopsy.

For the cohort of men with initial PSA levels less than 4.0 ng/ml, the limitation of using PSA velocity is the physiological (intraindividual) variation of serum PSA. This intraindividual variation of the screening samples has been found to be several times larger than the interassay variation [11]. This may especially be true for very low initial PSA levels. However, if the cut-off of PSA velocity was sufficiently high, the PSA velocity may be clinically applicable, especially in PSA levels of 2.0–4.0 ng/ml. Studies looking at this cohort are forthcoming.

IV. LIMITATIONS OF PSA VELOCITY

The limitations of PSA velocity are the day-to-day variation in serum PSA recently demonstrated [12,13]. This would explain, in part, the relative inability to of PSA velocity to be clinically useful with short intervals between PSA testing, since the biological variation could mask any significant change in PSA that actually may reflect prostate cancer. In addition to the long-term follow-up needed to reduce the influence of intraindividual fluctuations, it is important not to change the assay method used to test PSA [14]. Otherwise the rise in PSA observed would be merely the result of discordance between different assays.

Due to the current availability of numerous PSA assays and the related frequent changes of laboratory methods, recognizing this in daily practice is becoming more difficult.

V. CONCLUSION

PSA velocity, when used during longer intervals, and depending on the initial PSA level measured, may be a useful parameter in determining prostate cancer. However, the sensitivity appears to be too low to avoid consideration of initial prostate biopsy in men with elevated PSA levels. Its usefulness may be greatest in men who initially may have a negative biopsy or in those with PSA levels less than 4.0 ng/ml.

REFERENCES

1. H Carter, CH Morrell, JD Pearson, LJ Brant, CL Plato, EJ Metter, DW Chan, JL Fozard, PC Walsh. Estimation of prostatic growth using serial PSA measurements in men with and without prostatic disease. Cancer Res 52:3323–3328, 1992.
2. H Carter, JD Pearson, J Metter, LJ Brant, DW Chan, R Andres, JL Fozard, PC Walsh. Longitudinal evaluation of prostate specific antigen levels in men with and without prostate disease. JAMA 267:2215, 1992.
3. J Yuan, D Coplen, J Petros, RS Figenshau, TL Ratliff, DS Smith, WJ Catalona. Effects of rectal examination, prostate massage, ultrasonography, and needle biopsy on serum prostate specific antigen levels. J Urol 147:810, 1992.
4. J Oesterling, D Rice, W Glenski, EJ Bergstralh. Effect of cystoscopy, prostate biospy, and transurethral resection of the prostate on serum prostate specific antigen levels. Urology 42:276, 1993.
5. M Brawer, J Beatie, M Wener, RL Vessella, SD Pearson, PH Lange. Screening for prostatic carcinoma with PSA: Results of the second year. J Urol 150(1):106–109, 1993.
6. JR Porter, R Hayward, M Brawer. The significance of short-term PSA change in men undergoing ultrasound guided prostate biopsy. J Urol 151(5):293A, 1994.
7. D Smith, W Catalona. Rate of change in serum prostate specific antigen levels as a method for prostate cancer detection. J Urol 152:1163–1167, 1994.
8. D Keetch, W Catalona, D Smith. Serial prostatic biopsies in men with persistently elevated serum prostate specific antigen values. J Urol 151:1571, 1994.
9. HB Carter, JD Pearson, DW Chan, Z Waclawiw, EJ Metter, DW Chan, HA Guess, PC Walsh. Prostate specific antigen variability in men without prostate cancer: Effect of sampling interval on prostate-specific antigen velocity. Urology 45:591, 1995.
10. C Mettlin, PJ Littrup, RA Kane, GP Murphy, F Lee, A Chesley, R Badalament, FK Mostofi. Relative sensitivity and specificity of serum prostate specific antigen level

compared with age-referenced PSA, PSA density, and PSA change. Cancer 74: 1615–1620, 1994.

11. K Komatsu, N Wehner, A Prestigiacoma, Z Chen, TA Stamey. Physiologic (intra-individual) variation of serum prostate-specific antigen in 814 men from a screening population. Urology 47:343–346, 1996.

12. R Nixon, M Wener, K Smith, RE Parson, SA Strobel, MK Brawer. Biological variation of prostate-specific antigen levels in serm: An evaluation of day-to-day physiological fluctuations in a well-defined cohort of 24 patients. J Urol 157:2183–2190, 1997.

13. M Riehmann, PR Rhodes, T Cook, GS Grosse, RC Bruskwitz. Analysis of variation in prostate-specific antigen values. Urology 42:390, 1993.

14. CM Schambeck, N Schmeller, P Stieber. Methodological and clinical comparison of the ACS PSA assay and the Tandom-E PSA assay in prostate cancer. Urology 46:195–199, 1995.

6
Age Specific PSA

Ophelia Blake, Kevin McGeeney, and John M. Fitzpatrick
Mater Misericordiae Hospital, Dublin, Ireland

I. PROSTATE SPECIFIC ANTIGEN

Prostate cancer is the most common malignancy in men and the number of cases reported exceeds that of lung and colorectal cancer cases combined [1]. The incidence of prostatic disease, both benign prostatic hyperplasia (BPH) and carcinoma, is increasing with the demographic shift to longevity. There is significant regional variation in the incidence of this disease. Certain areas of Japan and China, which in the past have reported a very low incidence, are now reporting increased incidence of prostate cancer.

In the past digital rectal examination (DRE) was the conventional method of detection of prostate cancer but the majority of cancers detected were found to have spread beyond the gland at the time of diagnosis. The use of prostate specific antigen (PSA) as a screening tool or as a marker of malignancy has had a great impact on clinical practice. PSA is the most important tumor marker available for the diagnosis and management of prostate cancer. Given the poor curative rates for advanced prostate cancer, a promising alternative is the early detection of disease.

Early detection by the use of serum PSA concentration measurement and an increased public awareness about prostatic disease may lead to earlier diagnoses and better survival. However, indiscriminate use of PSA measurements could lead to overdiagnosis and overtreatment [2]. Moreover, there is conflicting evidence that early diagnosis and treatment of prostate cancer lead to a reduction in mortality [3]. The positive predictive value (PPV) of PSA as a screening test is very low (about 30%), so it is necessary to enhance the specificity of this tumor marker [4]. Measures such as the use of age specific reference ranges (ASRRs),

PSA velocity, PSA density (PSAD), or free/total PSA ratio may enhance the specificity of PSA in the diagnosis and management of prostate cancer.

Enhancing the specificity (the probability that a negative test indicates that the patient does not have the disease) of PSA as a tumor marker would reduce the number of negative biopsies in men with false-positive increases in PSA. It is important to maintain a high sensitivity (the probability of a test being positive when the patient has the disease) to ensure that a maximum number of clinically important cases are correctly identified. Because specificity and sensitivity are inversely related, increasing the specificity would result in a reduction in sensitivity. Use of ASRRs is one method proposed to overcome this problem.

II. AGE

A. What are ASRRs?

The International Federation of Clinical Chemistry (IFCC) defines a reference value as ''a value obtained by observation or measurement of a particular type of quantity on a reference individual;'' the reference individual is ''an individual selected for comparison using defined criteria.'' In practice a patient's PSA level is compared to a corresponding reference range. This range is a condensation of the information inherent in the reference values. Reference limits describe the reference distribution, giving information about the observed variation of values in a selected set of reference individuals. Clinicians aim to use PSA measurements to aid differential diagnosis [5]. The decision limit, which is determined clinically, is distinct from the upper limit of reference range, which is determined statistically. These two limits do not need to be the same but the reference values are an important factor in determining the decision limit [6].

The characteristics of the reference individuals (such as age, race, and gender) chosen for comparison and subsequently used to establish the reference values must be clearly defined. These groups of selected individuals may have to be classified into homogeneous subgroups, with clearly defined criteria for stratification. The aim of stratification of the reference group into more homogeneous subgroups is to reduce variation in the reference values, thereby giving more sensitive reference intervals. Age specific reference intervals are an example.

B. Why Do We Need Age Specific PSA Reference Intervals?

Age-specific reference ranges are based on the concept that serum PSA concentration increases with age in an individual. They may help in indicating when cancer is present and whether to perform a prostatic biopsy.

An ideal tumor marker should be detectable only when malignancy is present, be specific for a particular type of malignancy, correlate with the tumor burden, and respond rapidly to any change in tumor size. In practice there is no ideal tumor marker for prostate cancer or any other cancer. In a screening population, an ideal tumor marker would have a sensitivity and specificity of 100%. The relationship between sensitivity and specificity is evident from the receiver operating characteristics (ROC) of the test. ROC curves are useful in the evaluation of tumor markers and for comparing different markers for a given clinical setting.

The use of serum PSA measurement as a screening test has many limitations. For example, older men with benign enlargement and inflammation of the prostate have increased serum PSA concentration but no evidence of prostate cancer [7]. Sershon et al. [8] showed that serum PSA concentration has only a modest ability to differentiate men with BPH from patients with organ-confined prostate cancer. They found the area under the ROC curve to be only 0.66 (95% confidence interval = 0.60–0.72) for serum PSA to discriminate between these two groups. Age specific PSA reference ranges represent an attempt to improve the sensitivity and specificity of serum PSA concentration as a marker for prostate cancer.

C. Physiology of Aging and the Prostate

The prostate gland serves a role in sexual, reproductive, and lower urinary tract function. The glandular secretory component of the prostate gland is involved in the sexual and reproductive function while the fibromuscular component is involved in bladder function. The prostate plays a major role in aging by its ability to ''grow'' with age, causing direct and indirect effects on organ function. The gland is in a state of continuous development from its formative phase in utero to its ultimate state in the elderly. At birth the prostate gland has normal adult contours and anatomical relationships but its composition is predominantly muscular rather than glandular. After the third decade of life, glandular activity of the peripheral and central zones declines gradually with age.

D. Establishment of ASRRs

The combined use of digital rectal examination (DRE) and serum PSA measurement to facilitate early detection of prostate cancer is clinically very attractive. However, it is now recognized that some cases of prostate cancer are not being detected using this combination of diagnostic tests. To address this problem, investigators examine the relationship between serum PSA concentration and both prostate gland volume and patient age. Studies have shown a significant association between serum PSA concentration and both prostate gland volume and patient age [9–11]. Babaian et al. [10] showed that serum PSA concentration increases 26% per decade of age and 32% for each 10 ml increase in prostate volume. Collins et al. [11] found that prostate volume increases with age and that age and volume both influenced serum PSA concentration independently.

In another study, Babaian et al. [12] showed that PSA testing alone missed 11% of patients who had prostate cancer with a normal serum PSA concentration (<4ng/ml). Modified analytical techniques have been proposed to improve the sensitivity and specificity of PSA testing, and one such technique is ASRRs [13].

E. PSA Testing in Older Men

Serum PSA concentration has been shown to be dependent on patient age and, as a result, reference ranges wider than the standard PSA reference range of 0–4.0 ng/ml have been suggested for men of 60 years or older. Oesterling et al. [14], using age specific reference ranges, found that the sensitivity of PSA measurement for detecting early prostate cancer decreased by 9%, while the specificity and PPV increased by 11% and 5%, respectively. Some cancers that would have been detected by the standard reference range for PSA (0–4.0 ng/ml) were not detected by using the age specific PSA cutoff limits. Of the cancers missed, 95% had a favorable histopathological status.

A system to identify those men who are likely to benefit from further PSA testing following an initial baseline measurement could markedly reduce the health care cost and treatment-associated morbidity of prostate cancer. The upper age limit above which PSA testing is not cost-effective has not been established. It is generally accepted that men with less than a 10 year life expectancy are unlikely to benefit from early detection of prostate cancer because of the long natural history of untreated localized prostate cancer and other competing causes of death [15]. Gann et al. [16] showed that the increased risk of prostate cancer was doubled with serum PSA concentrations of 1.01–1.50 ng/ml and fivefold with serum PSA concentrations of 2.02–3.00 ng/ml. Thus baseline serum PSA concentrations could reflect a future risk of prostate cancer diagnosis and could be used to identify older men at lower risk for developing prostate cancer who may not benefit from intensive screening. Carter et al. [17] demonstrated that, by age 65 years, men with very low PSA concentrations (≤1.0 ng/ml) are not likely to be diagnosed with prostate cancer over the next decade. In addition the detection rate of prostate cancer would be minimally affected by less intensive PSA testing. Since an early diagnosis of prostate cancer is not likely to extend life when made after age 75 years, the target population for PSA screening is men below this age. Recommendations have been made for annual PSA testing of men starting at the age of 50 years and who have more than a 10 year life expectancy [18].

F.   Age and Serum PSA Concentration

Several researchers have established the role of age specific reference ranges for serum PSA in the screening and early detection of prostate cancer. PSA occurs in high concentrations in seminal fluid (1×10^6 ng/ml). In normal males, only a small proportion of this PSA enters the circulation; the exact mechanism by which this occurs remains unknown. Factors most likely to be responsible for the increase in serum PSA concentration with advancing age include an increase in prostate volume, inflammation in larger and older prostates, and the presence of undetectable microscopic but clinically insignificant cancer. In addition, older prostates may be more "leaky" with regard to PSA.

Several workers [7,11,13,19] found that serum PSA concentration correlated with patient age. Oesterling et al. [11] found that serum PSA concentration correlated with patient age (r = 0.43, p < 0.0001) and in this population serum PSA concentration increased by 3.2% (0.04 ng/ml) per year. DeAntoni et al. [13] reported a correlation between patient age and serum PSA concentration (r = 0.33). Uygur et al. [20] showed that serum PSA concentration correlated directly with age (r = 0.45, p < 0.00001) and the mean PSA concentration of men in each decade of age differed significantly (p < 0.0001) from the other decades of age. A study in Japanese men showed that serum PSA concentration directly correlated with patient age (r = 0.33, p < 0.001) and prostatic volume (r = 0.57, p < 0.001) [21]. If the study group is taken as a whole, the median serum PSA concentration increased with each decade of age. Use of regression analysis demonstrated that the serum PSA concentration increases by approximately 2.6% per year.

G.   Overview of ASRR Studies

It is hoped that ASRRs would have the potential of increasing the sensitivity (by detecting more cases of organ-confined prostate cancer in younger men) and specificity of serum PSA (by reducing the number of unnecessary prostate biopsies in older men). Several studies have established their own ASRRs for serum PSA in men without any evidence of detectable prostate cancer [11,13,22] (Table 1).

DeAntoni et al. [13] showed that serum PSA concentration and its variation within each decade of age differed significantly between the decades. Since previous studies did not adequately account for this greater variation in serum PSA concentration with advancing age, Anderson et al. [23] hypothesized that the

Table 1 Age Specific Upper Reference Limits for Serum Total PSA (ng/ml) Concentration in Normal Men of Different Races

	n	Race	\- Age (years) - 21–30	31–40	40–49	50–59	60–69	70–79	80–89
Oesterling [24]	471	White			2.5	3.5	4.5	6.5	
Anderson [23]	1,716				1.5	2.5	4.5	7.5	
DeAntoni [13]	71,172				2.3	3.8	5.6	6.9	
Oesterling [70]	422				2.0	3.0	4.0	5.5	
Lein [78]	1,160		1.16	1.78	1.75	2.27	3.48	4.26	2.64
Chautard [79]	1,274		1.07	1.37	1.33	2.07	2.82		
Espana [71]	237				2.9	4.7	7.2	9.0	11.4
Kalish [19]	983					2.84	5.87	9.03	
Wolff [74]	697		0.93	1.10	1.15	2.35	3.55	3.95	
Gustafsson [27]	1,708					5.2[a]	5.8/6.7[b]		
Morgan [59]	1,802				2.1	3.6	4.3	5.8	
Oesterling [21]	286	Asian			2.0	3.0	4.0	5.0	
Imai [66]	2,823				2.1	2.9	4.0	5.2	5.9
DeAntoni [13]	900				2.0	4.5	5.5	6.8	
Lin [64][c]	1,008		1.92	1.85	2.59	3.31	5.03	5.73	
Kao [65]	414			1.50[d]	1.88	2.37	4.82	5.86[e]	
Morgan [59]	1,673	African-American			2.4	6.5	11.3	12.5	
DeAntoni [13]	4,485				2.7	4.4	6.7	7.7	
DeAntoni [13]	1,543	Hispanic			2.1	4.3	6.0	6.6	

[a] Age group, 53–59 years.
[b] Age group, 60–64/65–70 years.
[c] Age group, 21–30; 31–40; 41–50; 51–60; 61–70; 71–80 years.
[d] Age group, <40.
[e] Age group, ≥70.

upper reference limits were too high for younger men (<60 years old) and poten-tially too low for older men (>70 years). They established ASRRs for normal men so that the specificity remained constant (95%) throughout all the age groups (Table 1). Oesterling et al. [24] modified their ASRRs according to each year of life to improve the diagnostic value of serum PSA concentration.

H.   Clinical Significance of ASRRs

The use of ASRRs compared with a standard reference range (0–4 ng/ml) for serum PSA resulted in a threefold increase in the probability of having an abnor-mal serum PSA concentration for men under the age of 60 years [24]. In men over 60 years only 9% instead of 15% of the patients would have been subjected to transrectal ultrasound (TRUS) studies and a prostate biopsy when ASRRs were employed. Catalona et al. [25] found, by using ASRRs for serum PSA in men aged 50–59 years, that there was a 45% increase in the number of biopsies per-formed and a projected 15% increase in the detection rate of prostate cancer. However, in older men (>70 years), fewer biopsies (44%) were performed and consequently 47% of organ-confined cancers were missed. They recommended use of the standard reference PSA range in older men. Oesterling et al. [14] concluded that by using ASRRs for serum PSA in older men, the sensitivity decreased by 9%, the specificity increased by 11%, and the positive predictive value increased by 5%. El-Galley et al. [26] observed a similar increase in speci-ficity in older men and an increase in sensitivity in younger men.

Gustafsson et al. [27] found an increase in the PPV (27% compared to 17%) of serum PSA for prostate cancer using ASRRs instead of the standard PSA cutoff value of >4.0 ng/ml. In addition, using the ASRRs, they found the cancer detection rate inadequate for screening prostate cancer. Bangma et al. [28] showed, using age specific PSA cutoff values to alert further investigations, that almost 39% of cancers would have been missed. Crawford et al. [29] reported higher but not significant (all p > 0.05) PPVs for PSA, DRE, and combined PSA and DRE when using ASRRs compared to those obtained using the 4.0 ng/ml cutoff value. They recommend the continued use of the combined tests of serum PSA and DRE with the PSA cutoff value of 4.0 ng/ml in prostate cancer screen-ing. Partin et al. [30] were in favor of the use of ASRRs in men <60 years, since 81% of the additional cancers detected had a favorable histological appearance compared to 76% in the older group of men. In addition, of the missed T1c tumors in the older men, 95% of them had a favorable histological appearance and were unlikely to be clinically significant. They concluded that the use of ASRRs in older men remained controversial but recommended their use in men aged under 60 years. In contrast, Borer et al. found in older men that 60% of the undetected cancers had unfavorable histological characteristics. They recom-mended the use of a serum PSA level > 4.0 ng/ml as the cut-off value for prostate biopsy in men with a negative DRE [31].

There is disagreement as to the optimal serum PSA cut-off value that should indicate the need for further examination to detect cancer. A lower serum PSA cut-off value may be more appropriate for younger men who are likely to benefit from treatment if cancer is detected [32]. Changing the serum PSA cut-off value from 4.0 to 2.5 ng/ml would more than double the number of men requiring further investigations: 8% of a screened population have a serum PSA concentration between 4.0 and 10.0 ng/ml and 12% of men have a serum PSA concentration between 2.6 and 4.0 ng/ml [33]. There are no data to suggest that the detection of prostate cancer at lower PSA concentrations would result in improved outcomes for younger men. The use of serum PSA measurements helps detect early prostate cancer an average of 4–6 years earlier than DRE [34]. Catalona et al. [35] found that about 30% of men with serum PSA concentrations between 4.0 and 10.0 ng/ml had cancers that had extended beyond the prostatic capsule at the time of diagnosis. Detecting these cancers earlier should enable more men to seek treatment while their cancer is still treatable. This could lead to virtual elimination of metastatic disease [36]. Despite the potential for early detection of curable prostate disease, Carter et al. [37] question the validity of a serum PSA cut-off value below 4.0 ng/ml to improve significantly the clinical outcome. Catalona et al. [35], using ASRRs, found that approximately 80% of the cancers detected were pathologically organ-confined compared to about 70% of organ-confined cancers in men with PSA concentrations greater than 4.0 ng/ml.

Gustafsson et al. [27] found that although the PPV of serum PSA increased when ASRRs were used, the problems of differentiating malignancy from benign conditions (such as BPH) and the reduction in cancer detection rate still existed. Etzioni et al. [38] looked at expected survival benefits using ASRRs relative to the standard PSA cut-off value of 4.0 ng/ml. They found that the average years of life saved per cancer case appeared to be greater for the standard PSA cut-off value (>4.0 ng/ml) than for the age specific cut-off value of 6.5 ng/ml. This should be borne in mind when trading off the merits of standard cut-off value against the apparently greater specificity of age specific PSA.

I.   Age as a Prognostic Factor

Age is an important factor in the management of organ-confined carcinoma of the prostate. There is an impression that prostate cancer is more aggressive in younger men [39], but others have found either improved survival [40] or no significant correlation between age and survival [41]. The optimal management of organ-confined carcinoma of the prostate is yet to be defined. Treatment is based on factors such as patient age, clinical stage of the disease, serum PSA concentration, and Gleason score. The estimated remaining life span of a patient decreases with increasing age because of a higher risk of death from other causes. Radical treatment is usually reserved for patients with at least a 10 year life expectancy. Obek et al. [42] found that older patients (>70 years) are approximately twice as likely to have biochemical recurrence than those under 70 years of age. Carter et al. [37] reported that older men had a greater likelihood of having more extensive disease than younger men with the same preoperative serum PSA concentration. Pienta et al. [43] found that survival for men after radical prostatectomy for organ-confined cancer decreased dramatically with increasing age.

The use of ASRRs is based on the correlation, which is assumed to be uniform across all the age groups, between age and serum PSA concentrations. Kirollos [44] found that the value of this correlation is sufficiently high to allow for its application in patients up to the age of 60 years. Above 60 years, the correlation is so low that its use becomes statistically flawed.

III. PROSTATE VOLUME

The most likely cause of the increase in serum PSA concentration with advancing age is the simultaneous increase in prostate volume. Stamey et al. [9] found that each gram of resected tissue following TURP in BPH patients accounted for 0.3 ng/ml of PSA. Collins et al. [45] showed that prostate gland volume increases with age ($r = 0.56$) and estimated an increase of 1 ml in prostate volume would result in a 4% increase in serum PSA concentration.

The concept of prostate specific antigen density (PSAD) was introduced by Benson et al. [46] and is defined as the serum PSA concentration divided by the volume of the prostate gland as determined by TRUS. It is reviewed in Chapter 4. A PSAD of less than 0.15 is normal. The use of PSAD was limited due to individual variations in epithelial/stromal ratios and to significant errors in the measurement of gland volume using TRUS [11]. Oesterling et al. [11] reported that use of ASRRs for serum PSA concentrations removed the need for PSAD as a diagnostic parameter for the detection of prostate cancer.

A. Age and Prostate Volume

Both Oesterling et al. [11] and Gustafsson et al. [27] have shown that the prostate volume increases by 1.6% per year. For a 60-year-old man, this would correspond to an annual increase of 0.5 ml. Oesterling et al. [11] showed that over the entire range of prostate sizes, serum PSA concentration directly correlated with prostate volume ($r = 0.55$; $p < 0.0001$). This means that the serum PSA concentration would increase by 4% per ml increase in prostate tissue. For a 30 ml prostate gland, this corresponds to an increase of 0.04 ng/ml for each ml enlargement in size. The amount of PSA produced depends on the quantity of prostate cells. This would explain the age-dependent increase in serum PSA concentrations seen in men with no evidence of prostate carcinoma as the prostate volume increases with age. However, continuous growth of the prostate gland does not occur in all men and the resultant variability in serum PSA concentration has an impact on the use of age specific reference ranges. DeAntoni et al. [13] have shown that the degree of variation in serum PSA concentrations increases among older men. In contrast, men in the 40 year age group have the least variability, because benign prostatic enlargement and prostate cancer are not common in this age group. With increasing age, prostate growth rates differ due to changes in circulating androgen concentrations and other prostatic insults such as inflammation.

In summary, it is clear that both the serum PSA concentration and prostate volume are dependent upon the patient's age. The concentration of PSA in serum correlates with the volume of prostatic epithelium. Normal prostatic tissue contributes an average of 0.1 ng/ml PSA per gram of tissue to the serum concentration of PSA. The corresponding PSA contribution for BPH tissue is 0.3 ng/ml, and for cancerous tissue it is 3.5 ng/ml [9].

B.   Age and BPH

BPH is the most common benign tumor in men aged over 60 years and appears to be a normal aging phenomenon. Age and normal androgenic function are the main factors causing BPH.

In patients with BPH, serum PSA concentration and prostate volume increase with increasing age, suggesting that in older men more PSA is released into the serum. This could be due to unrecognized subclinical prostate cancer in older men or to pathophysiological alterations within the prostate gland, such as changes in membrane permeability, microscopic infarctions, and others. The finding that prostate gland volume in men is a strong predictor of acute urinary retention [47] and the documented inaccuracies in determining prostate size by DRE [48] makes using serum PSA concentration as a proxy to estimate prostate volume very appealing to both clinicians and patients. This estimate of prostate enlargement may be useful in the therapeutic management of men with BPH.

C.   Age and Prostate Cancer

Aging is the most significant risk factor for prostate carcinoma, which is not surprising given the many similarities between the molecular changes that occur with aging and those that occur with cancer [49]. The prevalence of prostate carcinoma markedly increases with increasing age. Doubling times of 2–4 years indicate the unusually slow development of prostate cancer. Changes in release rate of PSA into the circulation may occur during tumor development. This may be due to a decrease in PSA production with loss of differentiation [50], and a simultaneous increase in secretion of PSA into the circulation with loss of tumor cell architecture. Therefore, the increase in serum PSA may reflect tumor growth

Table 2 Age Specific Values for Serum Total PSA ng/ml in Patients with BPH and Prostate Cancer

Age	Djavan [76]		Chen [73]		Uygur [20]
	Prostate Ca	BPH	BPH	Prostate Ca	BPH
50–59	11.2*	9.3	13.4	16.4	3.80
60–69	11.0*	10.0	13.5	15.0	5.40
70–79	10.9†	10.1	17.6	14.9	6.90
≥80	10.4‡	9.9			8.80

Comparison between BPH and prostate Ca groups in the Djavan [76] study.
* p < 0.001.
† p < 0.05.
‡ p > 0.05 (not significant).

only for a limited period of time [51]. Some studies have established ASRRs for patients with prostate cancer and patients with BPH (Tables 2 and 3).

IV. RACE

The incidence of prostate cancer varies markedly among ethnic groups [52]. The highest incidence and mortality rate is found in the African-American population, while the incidence in Asian men may be 50-fold lower [52]. Studies have suggested that nutrition, genetic factors, and patients' androgenic status may be responsible for some of the striking racial differences in the incidence and clinical

Table 3 Age Specific Values for Serum Free/Total PSA% in Patients with BPH and Prostate Cancer

Age (years)	Djavan [76]		Chen [73]	
	BPH	Prostate Ca	BPH	Prostate Ca
50–59	75.0	33.3*	19	20
60–69	63.8	36.9*	26	15
70–79	69.0	39.8†	36	16
≥80	68.8	24.2†		

Comparison between BPH and prostate Ca groups in the Djavan [76] study.
* p < 0.001.
† p < 0.05.

behavior of prostate cancer [53–55]. Further investigations are necessary to determine the reasons for the racial differences in serum PSA concentrations.

Whittemore et al. [56] found that a strong family history was associated with a much higher relative risk (RR) of developing prostate cancer in African-American men (RR = 9.7) than in white men (RR = 3.9) or in Asian men (RR = 1.6). Between the ages of 60 and 69 years, Borer et al. [31] found that the interracial cancer detection rates were 45.3%, 28.2%, 26.1% and 25% for African-American, white, Hispanic, and Asian men, respectively.

A.   Race and Prostate Gland Size

Oesterling et al. [21] and other researchers [45,57] found that Japanese men had smaller prostate glands than white men ($p < 0.001$). The prostate volume in this study group correlated directly with age ($r = 0.19$, $p < 0.01$). Berry et al. [57] hypothesized that as large prostate glands have more epithelial cells and have a potential for a higher degree of inflammation, this would account for the increase in serum PSA seen in men with large prostates. However, the difference in serum PSA concentration between Japanese men and white men remains significant ($p < 0.001$), even after adjusting for both prostate size and patient age.

1.   African-American

African-Americans have the highest incidence of prostate carcinoma of any racial group [58]. Morgan et al. [59] found that serum PSA concentration correlated directly with advancing age ($r = 0.40$, $p < 0.001$) in a large cohort of African-American men. Using the ASRRs established by Oesterling et al. [11] in this group would result in missing 41% of the cancers. Morgan et al. [59] therefore established ASRRs for this population and recommended a higher serum PSA cut-off for biopsy in African-American men younger than 50 years of age, and a lower serum PSA cut-off for biopsy in African-American men 40–49 years of age. The greater variance in serum PSA among African-American men leads to a higher upper limit of normal, thus making the assay less sensitive to detection of prostate cancer in the racial group with the highest incidence of the disease. However, Powell et al. [60] questioned the use of a higher PSA cut-off value for African-American than for white men and recommended a lower PSA cut-off value for biopsy in African-American men at any age group to maximize detection of prostate cancer in this high-risk group.

Studies have demonstrated that African-American men have higher serum PSA concentrations than white men following radical prostatectomy [61]. Furthermore, African-American men undergoing radical prostatectomy for localized prostate cancer have been shown to have poor prognosis. Smith et al. [62] have shown that being African-American was an independent predictor of prostate cancer even at serum PSA cut-off values of 2.6–4.0 ng/mL. They reported a PPV of serum PSA in a screening setting of 45% for African-American men and 35% for white men. This suggests that serum PSA measurement may be more useful for African-American than for white men. Guo et al. [63] reported a significantly higher rate of apoptosis in the tumor tissue of African-American men than in white men undergoing radical prostatectomy for localized prostate cancer. They suggested that this loss of apoptotic control may be due to downregulation of the expression of bcl-2.

2. Asian

Asians, in contrast with African-American men, have the lowest incidence rate of prostate cancer. Oesterling et al. [21] determined age specific reference ranges for serum PSA in Japanese men, which were significantly lower than for white men ($p < 0.001$). This is probably due to the small size of the prostate gland in Japanese men. However, the incidence rate of prostate cancer in Asians living in America is increasing and is higher than the incidence in men living in Asia.

Lin et al. [64] found in Chinese men that serum PSA concentration increases with age and established an upper limit for serum PSA so as to enhance cancer detection in this group. Fewer than 2% of the men studied under 60 years of age had serum PSA concentrations >4.0 ng/ml.

Kao [65] established age-related reference ranges for serum free PSA, total PSA, and free PSA/total PSA ratios in Chinese men. They observed a correlation between age and serum FPSA and serum TPSA concentrations ($r = 0.35$ and $r = 0.33$, respectively). This study found no significant correlation between age and F/T ratios ($r = 0.095$). The observed ratios were constant across all the age groups of the men studied. Imai et al. [66] established age specific reference ranges for normal Japanese men during a mass screening program for prostate cancer. The positive predictive value for serum PSA concentration in Asians is lower than in white men because of the lower prevalence of prostate cancer in the former population.

3. White

Numerous investigators have derived age-specific reference ranges for serum PSA for men (Tables 1 and 2) in a predominantly white population.

V. DISTRIBUTION OF MOLECULAR FORMS

Prostate specific antigen (PSA) exists in the serum in several molecular forms. The concentration of these molecular forms varies according to the disease state

Table 4 Age Specific Upper Reference Limits for Serum Complexed PSA ng/mL in Normal Men

Age (years)	Oesterling [70]	Espana [71]
40–49	1.0	1.8
50–59	1.5	3.3
60–69	2.0	5.9
≥70	3.0	6.4

of the prostate gland [67,68]. Specific serum measurement of these molecular forms may improve the clinical use of PSA. This concept is covered in detail in Chapters 7 and 8. Lilja et al. [69] showed that PSA complexed to α_1-antichymotrypsin is the predominant form of immunoreactive PSA in serum (~85%) and that the free (uncomplexed) form makes up the rest. Christensson et al. [68] measured the concentration of these various molecular forms of PSA in the serum of patients with BPH and prostate cancer. They reported that the proportion of free to total PSA ratio in the patients with prostate cancer was significantly lower than in the men with BPH (p < 0.0001).

Oesterling et al. [70] reported that serum concentrations of free, complexed, and total PSA correlated directly with patient age (r = 0.45, r = 0.43, and r = 0.45, respectively) and increased by approximately 2.8%, 3.3%, and 3.3% per year, respectively. They did not find any correlation between the ratios (free/total, complexed/total, and free/complexed PSA) and the patient age. This indicates that the ratio of one molecular form to another may be useful in differentiating men with BPH from those with early prostate cancer.

Espana et al. [71] found a significant positive correlation between the patient's age and both total serum PSA (r = 0.424, p < 0.0001) and complexed serum PSA (r = 0.379, p < 0.0001). The complexed to total PSA ratio showed no significant correlation with patient age (r = 0.026, p > 0.2) in this study. Their upper limit of normality (95th percentile) for the complexed to total PSA ratio was 0.8 regardless of the patient's age. Measurement of the molecular forms of PSA may be useful in refining the patient's risk assessment for developing prostate cancer.

The molecular forms of serum PSA have also been examined for a relationship with age. Kalish et al. [19] found that both total PSA and free PSA concentrations increased with age, but the percentage of free PSA did not show a strong systematic trend with age. The correlation coefficients between age and total PSA, free PSA, and percentage free PSA were 0.34 (p < 0.001), 0.33 (p < 0.001), and −0.08 (p = 0.01), respectively.

Table 5 Age Specific Upper Reference Limits for Serum Free PSA ng/mL in Normal Men

Age (years)	Kao [65]	Oesterling [70]	Lein [78]	Chautard [79]	Kalish [19]	Wolff [74]
20–29			0.20	0.42		0.21
30–39	0.63[a]		0.34	0.43		0.27
40–49	0.55	0.5	0.30	0.38		0.27
50–59	0.63	0.7	0.35	0.47	0.61	0.42
60–69	1.32	1.0	0.45	0.53	1.33	0.58
70–79	1.65	1.2	0.59		1.75	0.65
80–89			0.60			

[a]Different age groups, <40.

A. Free PSA and Free/Total Ratio

In order to interpret free and percentage free PSA (%fPSA) measurements, careful consideration must be paid to the in vitro stability of free PSA. Because the serum free PSA is less stable than total PSA, it is recommended that the blood specimen be processed within 3 hr of sample collection and frozen at −70°C if analysis is not carried out within 24 hr [72]. A summary of the studies with ASRRs for serum F/T PSA are shown in Tables 3 and 6, that for serum free PSA is shown in Table 5.

Chen et al. [73] showed that the F/T PSA ratio in serum improved the diagnostic efficiency in differentiating between patients with benign disease and those with cancer, with total serum PSA concentration in the 2.5–20 ng/ml range.

Table 6 Age Specific Values for Serum Free/Total PSA Ratio in Normal Men

Age (years)	Kao [65]	Oesterling [70]	Lein [78]	Chautard [79]	Kalish [19]	Wolff [74]
20–29			1.00	0.68		0.42
30–39	0.64*		0.47	0.65		0.40
40–49	0.68	0.25	0.46	0.62		0.33
50–59	0.68	0.23	0.46	0.61	0.21	0.28
60–69	0.59	0.25	0.42	0.49	0.23	0.28
70–79	0.51	0.22	0.43		0.19	0.32
80–89			0.47			

* Different age groups, <40.

Older patients (>70 years) with a high PSA concentration (10–20 ng/mL) have a greater probability (98%) of being diagnosed with cancer. F/T PSA ratio significantly improves the predictive power of serum PSA concentration [73].

Wolff et al. [74] found direct correlations with free PSA, total PSA, and the F/T PSA ratio in serum and age. Although the free and total PSA increase (r = 0.855, r = 0.857 respectively), the F/T PSA ratio decreases (r = −0.788) with advancing age. Studies have shown that F/T PSA ratio in serum may be useful in differentiating prostate cancer from benign disease such as BPH [69,75]. Lower F/T PSA ratios have been observed in patients with prostate carcinoma than in patients with BPH. Djavan et al. [76] found that in patients of all age groups without prostate cancer, the F/T PSA ratio significantly exceeded (p < 0.001) that of patients in all age groups with prostate cancer. The determination of the F/T PSA ratio in serum can improve the diagnostic efficiency of PSA testing.

Partin et al. [77] also showed that the F/T PSA increased with patient age; however, the correlation between prostate volume and patient age was not significant (r = 0.12, p = 0.21) in this study cohort with total PSA between 4 and 10 ng/ml. Use of F/T PSA should prevent approximately 20–30% of negative biopsies (improving specificity) while maintaining a 90–95% sensitivity of cancer detection. Lein et al. [78] found that F/T PSA ratio is an age-independent tumor marker for prostate cancer. They determined ranges for serum total PSA, free PSA, and F/T PSA ratio for the different age groups (Tables 1,5,6). Chautard et al. [79] found that there was a linear regression between age and free PSA (r = 0.12, p < 0.0001) and between age and F/T PSA ratio (r = 0.17, p < 0.0001).

In men with serum PSA concentrations in the range 2.6–4.0 ng/ml, Catalona et al. [32], using a percentage free PSA cutoff of 27% as a criterion for biopsy, would have detected 90% of the cancers and avoided 18% of unnecessary biopsies. Lowering the serum PSA cut-off concentration to 2.5 ng/ml for biopsy may be beneficial for African-American men whose incidence of prostate cancer is nearly 40% higher than that of white men [59].

B. Complexed PSA

Stenman et al. [75] found that the concentration of PSA bound to α1-antichymotrypsin in serum is higher in men with prostate cancer than in men without prostate cancer. Sokoll et al. [80] showed that complexed serum PSA had an improved specificity for cancer detection compared to total serum PSA between 4 and 10 ng/ml. At 95% sensitivity the complexed PSA concentration had a specificity of 25%, which is similar to data on F/T PSA ratio. ASRRs for serum complexed PSA in normal men is summarized in Table 4.

Table 7 Age Specific Upper Reference Limits
for Complexed/Total PSA Ratio in Normal Men

Age (years)	Espana [71]	Oesterling [70]
40–49	0.86	0.50
50–59	0.86	0.50
60–69	0.94	0.50
70–79	0.90	0.55
80–89	0.89	

VI. SUMMARY

The diagnosis of prostate cancer is improved when age specific reference ranges are used. This improvement ensures low false-positive biopsy rates but also leads to low true-positive rates (low sensitivity) in older age groups. The variation in the ASRRs seen in Tables 1–7 may be explained by the differences in the assay methods and also by the differences in the populations studied. The correlation between age and serum PSA concentration forms the basis for the use of age specific reference ranges. The low correlation between age and serum PSA concentration in men above the age of 60 restricts the potential use of age specific reference ranges. Thus they should only be employed for men under 60 years of age. Polascik et al. [81] indicate that neither the Food and Drug Administration nor the manufacturers of PSA assays recommend the use of ASRRs. They suggest that these ranges should be used in clinical practice with discretion.

REFERENCES

1. SH Landis, T Murray, S Bolden, PA Wingo. Cancer statistics, 1999. CA-Cancer J Clin 49:8–31, 1999.
2. TA Stamey, F Freiha, JE McNeal, EA Redwine, AS Whittemore, HP Schmid. Localized prostate cancer: Relationship of tumour volume to clinical significance for treatment of prostate cancer. Cancer 71:933–938, 1993.
3. S Selley, J Donovan, A Faulkner, J Coast, D Gillatt. Diagnosis, management and screening of early localized prostate cancer. Health Technol Assess 1:1997.
4. FH Schroder, CH Bangma. The European randomized study of screening for prostate cancer (ERSPC). Br J Urol 79:68–71, 1997.
5. MR Pincus. Interpreting laboratory results: Reference values and decision-making. In: JB Henry, ed. Clinical Diagnosis and Management by Laboratory Methods. Philadelphia: W.B. Saunders, 1996, pp 74–91.

6. UH Stenham, J Leinonen, W-M Zhang, P Finne. Prostate-specific antigen. Cancer Biol 9:83–93, 1999.

7. RB Nadler, PA Humphrey, DS Smith, WJ Catalona, TL Ratliff. Effect of inflammation and benign prostatic hyperplasia on elevated serum prostate specific antigen levels. J Urol 154:407–413, 1995.

8. PD Sershon, MJ Barry, JE Oesterling. Serum prostate specific antigen discriminates weakly between men with benign prostatic hyperplasia and patients with organ-confined prostate cancer. Eur Urol 25:281–287, 1994.

9. TA Stamey, N Yang, AR Hay, JE McNeal, FS Freiha, E Redwine. Prostate-specific antigen as a serum marker for adenocarcinoma of the prostate. N Engl J Med 317: 909–916, 1987.

10. RJ Babaian, H Miyashita, RB Evans, EI Ramirez. The distribution of prostate specific antigen in men without clinical or pathological evidence of prostate cancer: Relationship to gland volume and age. J Urol 147:837–840, 1992.

11. JE Oesterling, SJ Jacobsen, CG Chute, HA Guess, CJ Girman, LA Panser, MM Lieber. Serum prostate-specific antigen in a community-based population of healthy men. Establishment of age-specific reference ranges. JAMA 270:860–864, 1993.

12. RJ Babaian, CP Dinney, EI Ramirez, RB Evans. Diagnostic testing for prostate cancer detection: Less is best. Urology 41:421–425, 1993.

13. EP DeAntoni, ED Crawford, JE Oesterling, CA Ross, ER Berger, DG McLeod, F Staggers, NN Stone. Age- and race-specific reference ranges for prostate-specific antigenfrom a large community-based study. J Urol 48:234–239, 1996.

14. JE Oesterling, SJ Jacobsen, WH Cooner. The use of age-specific reference ranges for serum prostate specific antigen in men 60 years old or older. J Urol 153:1160–1163, 1995.

15. PC Albertsen, JA Hanley, DF Gleason, MJ Barry. Competing risk analysis of men aged 55 to 74 years at diagnosis managed conservatively for clinically localized prostate cancer. JAMA 280:975–980, 1998.

16. PH Gann, CH Hennekens, MJ Stampfer. A prospective evaluation of plasma prostate-specific antigen for detection of prostatic cancer. JAMA 273:289–294, 1995.

17. HB Carter, PK Landis, EJ Metter, LA Fleisher, JD Pearson. Prostate-specific antigen testing of older men. J Natl Cancer Inst 91:1733–1737, 1999.

18. A von Eschenbach, R Ho, GP Murphy, M Cunningham, N Lins. American Cancer Society guidelines for the early detection of prostate cancer: Update. Cancer 80: 1805–1807, 1997.

19. LA Kalish, JB McKinlay. Serum prostate-specific antigen levels (PSA) in men without clinical evidence of prostate cancer: Age-specific reference ranges for total PSA, free PSA and percent PSA. Urology 54:1022–1027, 1999.

20. MC Uygur, D Erol, M Cetinkaya, Y Gungen, Y Laleli, U Altug. The correlation between prostate specific antigen and age. Analysis of prostate specific antigen values from 4,846 Turkish men with symptomatic benign prostatic hyperplasia. Eur Urol 32:416–419, 1997.

21. JE Oesterling, Y Kumamoto, T Tsukamoto, CJ Girman, HA Guess, N Masumori, SJ Jacobsen, MM Lieber. Serum prostate specific antigen in a community-based

population of healthy Japanese men: Lower values than for similarly aged white men. Br J Urol 75:347–353, 1995.

22. ED Crawford, EP DeAntoni. PSA as a screening test for prostate cancer. Urol Clin North Am 20:637–646, 1993.

23. JR Anderson, D Strickland, D Corbin, JA Byrnes, E Zweiback. Age-specific reference ranges for serum prostate-specific antigen. J Urol 46:54–57, 1995.

24. JE Oesterling, WH Cooner, SJ Jacobsen, HA Guess, MM Lieber. Influence of patient age on the serum PSA concentration. An important clinical observation. Urol Clin N Am 20:671–680, 1993.

25. WJ Catalona, MA Hudson, PT Scardino, JP Richie, F Ahmann, RC Flanigan, JB deKernion, TL Ratliff, LR Kavoussi, BL Dalkin, WB Waters, MT MacFarlane, PC Southwick. Selection of optimal prostate specific antigen cutoffs for early detection of prostate cancer: Receiver operating characteristic curves. J Urol 152:2037–2042, 1994.

26. RES El-Galley, JA Petros, WH Sanders, TE Keane, NTM Galloway, WH Cooner, SD Graham. Normal range prostate-specific antigen versus age-specific prostate-specific antigen in screening prostate adenocarcinoma. Urology 46:200–204, 1995.

27. O Gustafsson, E Mansour, U Norming, A Carlsson, M Tornblom, CR Nyman. Prostate specific antigen (PSA), PSA density and age-adjusted PSA reference values in screening for prostate cancer. A study of a randomly selected population of 2,400 men. Scand J Urol Nephrol 32:373–377, 1998.

28. CH Bangma, R Kranse, BG Blijenberg, FH Schroder. The value of screening tests in the detection of prostate cancer. Part II: Retrospective analysis of free/total prostate specific analysis ratio, age-specific reference range, and PSA density. J Urol 46: 779–784, 1995.

29. ED Crawford, S Leewansangtong, S Goktas, K Holthaus, M Baier. Efficiency of prostate-specific antigen and digital rectal examination in screening, using 4.0 ng/mL and age-specific reference range as a cutoff for abnormal values. Prostate 38: 296–302, 1999.

30. AW Partin, SR Criley, ENP Subong, H Zincke, PC Walsh, JE Oesterling. Standard versus age-specific prostate specific antigen reference ranges among men with clinically localized prostate cancer: A pathological analysis. J Urol 155:1336–1339, 1996.

31. JG Borer, J Sherman, MC Solomon, MW Plawker, RJ Macchia. Age specific prostate specific antigen reference ranges: Population specific. J Urol 159:444–448, 1998.

32. WJ Catalona, DS Smith, DK Ornstein. Prostate cancer detection in men with serum PSA concentrations of 2.6 to 4.0 ng/mL and benign prostate examination. JAMA 14:1452–1455, 1997.

33. DS Smith, WJ Catalona, JD Herschman. Longitudinal screening for prostate cancer with prostate-specific antigen. JAMA 276:1309–1315, 1996.

34. HB Carter, JD Pearson. PSA and the natural course of prostate cancer. In: FH Schroder, ed. Recent Advances in Prostate Cancer and BPH. New York: Parthenon Publishing Group, 1997, pp 187–193.

35. WJ Catalona, DS Smith, TL Ratliff, JW Basler. Detection of organ-confined prostate cancer is increased through prostate-specific antigen-based screening. JAMA 270: 948–954, 1993.

36. F Labrie, B Candas, L Cusan, J-L Gomez, P Diamond, R Suburu, M Lemay. Diagnosis of advanced or non-curable prostate cancer can be practically eliminated by prostate specific antigen. Urology 47:212–217, 1996.
37. HB Carter, JL Epstein, AW Partin. Influence of age and prostate specific antigen on the chance of curable prostate cancer among men with nonpalpable disease. Urology 53:126–130, 1999.
38. R Etzioni, Y Shen, JC Petteway, MK Brawer. Age-specific prostate-specific antigen: A reassessment. Prostate Suppl 7:70–77, 1996.
39. JM Wilson, IW Kemp, Stein GJ. Cancer of the prostate. Do younger men have a poorer survival rate? Br J Urol 56:391–396, 1984.
40. HM Smedley, L Sinnott, LS Freedman. Age and survival in prostatic carcinoma. Br J Urol 55:529–533, 1983.
41. CJ Mettlin, GP Murphy, MP Cunningham, HR Menck. The national cancer data base report on race, age and region variations in prostate cancer treatment. Cancer 80:1261–1266, 1997.
42. C Obek, S Lai, S Sadek, F Civantos, MS Soloway. Age as a prognostic factor for disease recurrence after radical prostatectomy. Urology 54:533–538, 1999.
43. K Pienta, R Demers, M Hoff, TY Kau, JE Montie, RK Severson. Effect of age and race on the survival of men with prostate cancer in the metropolitan Detroit Tri-county Area, 1973 to 1987. Urology 45:93–102, 1995.
44. MM Kirollos. Statistical review and analysis of the relationship between serum prostate specific antigen and age. J Urol 158:143–145, 1997.
45. GN Collins, RJ Lee, GB McKelvie, ACN Rogers, M Hehir. Relationship between prostate specific antigen, prostate volume and age in the benign prostate. Br J Urol 71:445–450, 1993.
46. MC Benson, IS Whang, A Pantuck, K Ring, SA Kaplan, CA Olsson, WH Cooner. Prostate specific antigen density: A means of distinguishing benign prostatic hypertrophy and prostate cancer. J Urol 147:815–816, 1992.
47. SJ Jacobsen, DJ Jacobson, CJ Girman, RO Roberts, T Rhodes, HA Guess, MM Lieber. Natural history of prostatism: Risk factors for acute urinary retention. J Urol 158:481–487, 1997.
48. CG Roehrborn, CJ Girman, T Rhodes, KA Hanson, GN Collins, SM Sech, SJ Jacobsen, WM Garraway, MM Lieber. Correlation between prostate size estimated by digital rectal examination and measured by transrectal ultrasound. Urology 49:548–557, 1997.
49. WD Dunsmuir, D Hrouda, RS Kirby. Malignant changes in the prostate with ageing. Br J Urol 82:47–58, 1998.
50. PA Abrahamsson, H Lilja, S Falkmer, LB Wadstrom. Immunohistochemical distribution of the three predominant secretory proteins in the parenchyma of hyperplastic and neoplastic prostate glands. Prostate 12:39–46, 1988.
51. UH Stenham. Prostate specific antigen, clinical use and staging: an overview. Br J Urol 79:53–60, 1997.
52. DM Parkin, CA Muir, SL Whelan. Cancer Incidence in Five Continents. Lyon, France: IARC Press, 1992.
53. SA Ingles, RK Ross, MC Yu, RA Irvine, RW Haile, GA Coetzee. Association of

prostate cancer risk with genetic polymorphisms in vitamin D receptor and androgen receptor. J Natl Cancer Inst 89:166–170, 1997.

54. GD Steinberg, BS Carter, TH Beaty, B Childs, PC Walsh. Family history and the risk of prostate cancer. Prostate 17:337–347, 1990.

55. AS Whittemore, LN Kolonel, AH Wu, EM John, RP Gallagher, RS Paffenbarger, Jr. Prostate cancer in relation to diet, physical activity, and body size in blacks, whites and Asians in the United States and Canada. J Natl Cancer Inst 87:652–662, 1995.

56. AS Whittemore, AH Wu, LN Kolonel, EM John, RP Gallagher, GR Howe, DW West, CZ Teh, TA Stamey. Family history and prostate cancer risk in black, white and Asian men in the United States and Canada. Am J Epidemiol 141:732–740, 1995.

57. SJ Berry, DS Coffey, Walsh PC, LL Ewing. The development of human benign prostatic hyperplasia with age. J Urol 132:474–479, 1984.

58. RK Ross, H Shimizu, A Paganini-Hill, G Honda, BE Henderson. Case–control studies of prostate cancer in blacks and whites in southern California. J Natl Cancer Inst 78:869–874, 1987.

59. TO Morgan, SJ Jacobsen, WF McCarthy, DJ Jacobson, DG McLeod, JW Moul. Age-specific reference ranges for prostate-specific antigen in African American men. N Engl J Med 335:304–310, 1996.

60. I Powell, M Banerjee, M Novallo, W Sakr, D Grignon, DP Wood, JE Pontes. Should the age specific prostate specific antigen cutoff for prostate biopsy be higher for black than for white men older than 50 years? J Urol 163:146–149, 2000.

61. JW Moul, TH Douglas, WF McCarthy, DG McLeod. Black race is an adverse prognostic factor for prostate cancer recurrence following radical prostatectomy in an equal access health care setting. J Urol 155:1667–1673, 1996.

62. DS Smith, GF Carvalhal, DE Mager, AD Bullock, WJ Catalona. Use of lower prostate specific antigen cutoffs for prostate cancer screening in black and white men. J Urol 160:1734–1738, 1998.

63. Y Guo, DB Sigman, A Borkowski, N Kyprianou. Racial differences in prostate cancer growth: Apoptosis and cell proliferation in Caucasian and African American patients. Prostate 42:130–136, 2000.

64. WY Lin, CJ Gu, CH Kao, SP Changlai, SJ Wang. Serum prostate-specific antigen in healthy Chinese men: Establishment of age-specific reference ranges. Neoplasma 43:103–105, 1996.

65. CH Kao. Age-related free PSA, total PSA and free PSA/total PSA ratios: Establishment of reference ranges in Chinese males. Anticancer Res 17:1361–1366, 1997.

66. K Imai, Y Ichinose, Y Kubota, H Yamanaka, J Sato. Diagnostic significance of prostate specific antigen and the development of a mass screening system for prostate cancer. J Urol 154:1085–1089, 1995.

67. T Bjork, A Bjartell, P-A Abrahamsson, S Hulko, A di SantAgnese, H Lilja. Alpha-1-antichymotyrpsin production in PSA-producing cells is common in prostate cancer but rare in benign prostatic hyperplasia. Urology 43:427–434, 1994.

68. A Christensson, CB Laurell, H Lilja. Enzymatic activity of prostate-specific antigen

and its reaction with extracellular serine proteinase inhibitors. Eur J Biochem 194: 755–763, 1990.

69. H Lilja, A Christensson, U Dahlen, MT Matikainen, O Nilsson, K Pettersson, T Lovgren. Prostate-specific antigen in human serum occurs predominantly in complex with alpha-1-antichymotrypsin. Clin Chem 37:1618–1625, 1991.

70. JE Oesterling, SJ Jacobsen, GG Klee, K Pettersson, T Piironen, UH Stenham, B Dowell, T Lovgren, H Lilja. Free, complexed and total serum prostate specific antigen: The establishment of appropriate reference ranges for their concentrations and ratios. J Urol 154:1090–1095, 1995.

71. F Espana, M Martinez, M Royo, CD Vera, A Estelles, J Aznar, JF Jimenez-Cruz. Reference ranges for the concentrations of total and complexed plasma prostate-specific antigen and their ratio in patients with benign prostate hyperplasia. Eur Urol 32:268–272, 1997.

72. D Woodrum, C French, LB Shamel. Stability of free prostate-specific antigen in serum samples under a variety of sample collection and sample storage conditions. Urology 48:33–39, 1996.

73. Y-T Chen, AA Luderer, Thiel RP, G Carlson, CL Cuny, TF Soriano. Using proportions of free to total prostate-specific antigen, age, and total prostate-specific antigen to predict the probability of prostate cancer. Urology 47:518–524, 1996.

74. JM Wolff, H Borchers, D Rohde, G Jakse. Age related changes of free and total prostate-specific antigen in serum. Anticancer Res 19:2629–2632, 1999.

75. UH Stenman, J Leinonen, H Alfthan, S Rannikko, K Tuhkanen, O Alfthan. A complex between prostate-specific antigen and al-antichymotrypsin is the major form of prostate-specific antigen in serum of patients with prostatic cancer: Assay of the complex improves clinical sensitivity for cancer. Cancer Res 51:222–226, 1991.

76. B Djavan, AR Zlotta, M Remzi, K Ghawidel, B Bursa, S Hruby, R Wolfram, CC Schulman, M Marberger. Total and transition zone prostate volume and age: How do they affect the utility of PSA-based diagnostic parameters for early prostate cancer detection? Urology 54:846–852, 1999.

77. AW Partin, WJ Catalona, PC Southwick, ENP Subong, GH Gasior, DW Chan. Analysis of percent free prostate-specific antigen (PSA) for prostate cancer detection: Influence of total PSA, prostate volume and age. Urology 48:55–61, 1996.

78. M Lein, F Koenig, K Jung, FJ McGovern, SJ Skates, D Schnorr, SA Loening. The percentage of free prostate specific antigen is an age-independent tumour marker for prostate cancer: Establishment of reference ranges in a large population of healthy men. Br J Urol 82:231–236, 1998.

79. D Chautard, A Daver, B Mermod, A Tichet, V Bocquillon, J-Y Soret. Values for the free to total prostate-specific antigen ratio as a function of age: Necessity of reference range validation. Eur Urol 36:181–186, 1999.

80. LJ Sokoll, DJ Bruzek, JL Cox, AW Partin, DW Chan, DL Morris, KK Yeung, WJ Allard. Is complexed PSA alone clinically useful? J Urol 159:234, 1998.

81. TJ Polascik, JE Oesterling, AW Partin. Prostate specific antigen: A decade of discovery—what we have learned and where we are going. J Urol:293–306, 1999.

7
Free and Total PSA

Paul E. Li and Paul H. Lange
University of Washington School of Medicine, Seattle, Washington

I. SCREENING FOR PROSTATE CANCER WITH SERUM PROSTATE SPECIFIC ANTIGEN

A. Introduction

Prostate cancer is the most common noncutaneous malignancy in men in the United States, and the second most frequent cause of cancer-related deaths in men, with an estimated 37,000 deaths and 179,300 new diagnoses in 1999 [1]. It is variable in its natural history: some patients have a slowly progressive low-grade disease while others with poorly differentiated cancers have a rapidly declining course. Therefore, early detection and treatment is the objective in large-scale screening programs, and this has been revolutionized by the ability of serum prostate specific antigen (PSA) to detect and monitor the presence of prostate cancer.

PSA is a single-chain 33-kDa serine protease [2] that belongs to the kallikrein family of proteases, and is also called human kallikrein 3 (hK3) [3]. PSA is produced by epithelial cells that line the acini and ducts of the prostate [4], and its substrates include semenogelin I, semenogelin II, and fibronectin. Hydrolysis of these proteins causes the liquefaction of semen and liberation of motile spermatozoa [5]. PSA is normally secreted into the lumen of the prostatic ducts but small amounts diffuse into the serum, where it exists in several molecular forms. Approximately 70–90% of the total pool of PSA (tPSA) is covalently complexed to the protein α_1-antichymotrypsin (ACT). PSA is also complexed in much lesser quantities to members of the serine protease inhibitor (serpin) superfamily, such as α_1-antitrypsin (α_1-protease inhibitor [API]) and protein C inhibitor (PCI), but these forms are not considered clinically significant [6]. It is also complexed to another protease inhibitor similar to ACT called α_2-macroglobulin (A2M), but this form is not detectable with current immunoassays because the PSA epitopes are blocked by A2M [7]. The remainder of the serum PSA, which accounts for 10–30% of the tPSA pool, exists in an uncomplexed state and is called free PSA (fPSA) [8–10]. Clinically, the difference between the tPSA and the fPSA equals the cPSA, or:

fPSA [ng/ml] + cPSA [ng/ml] = tPSA [ng/ml].

The percentage of free PSA relative to total PSA, or the f/t PSA ratio, is calculated as:

(fPSA [ng/ml]/tPSA [ng/ml]) × 100%.

As initial screening tests for the early detection of prostate cancer, the combination of a digital rectal examination (DRE) and serum tPSA is the current standard as recommended by the American Urological Association and the American Cancer Society [11]. The range of 0–4.0 ng/ml tPSA is widely considered the reference range of normal [12], but approximately 65% of men with a tPSA greater than 4.0 ng/ml do not have prostate cancer, and 30–40% of men with organ-confined prostate cancer show tPSA levels within the reference range [13–16]. Many factors other than prostate cancer can cause the tPSA to be elevated, including prostatic manipulations from a DRE, prostate biopsy, cystoscopy, transurethral resection of the prostate (TURP), or benign conditions such as benign prostatic hyperplasia (BPH), urinary retention, and prostatitis [17–21]. The tPSA value can also be affected by a high-fiber diet [22], medications such as finasteride [23], antiandrogens [24], estrogens [25], and PC-SPES [26], hepatic dysfunction [27], and ejaculation [28], although the last is controversial [29,30]. In addition, it is now known that PSA is produced (albeit in much smaller quantities) by tissues other than the prostate. With the use of sensitive immunofluorometric assays, PSA was detected in pancreatic [31], colon, ovarian, liver, kidney, adrenal, and parotid tumors [32]; and, in women, in up to 30% of breast carcinomas [33,34]. The biological significance of these findings has not yet been elucidated. Because of this wide overlap of tPSA in prostate cancer with other conditions, especially in the so-called "intermediate" or "gray" zone of tPSA from 4.0 to 10.0 ng/ml, other derivatives of the tPSA assay were developed to enhance the specificity of tPSA and therefore reduce the number of unnecessary prostate biopsies. These tests, such as PSA density [35], PSA velocity [36], and age specific PSA ranges [37] are discussed elsewhere in this book.

B. Overview

Stenman et al. [10] first reported that a higher fraction of cPSA was found in men with prostate cancer than in men with BPH and therefore the f/t PSA ratio was lower. Since that report, multiple clinical trials have been conducted to determine the efficacy of the f/t PSA ratio as an enhancement to tPSA as a screening test. As in the tPSA assay, the reference range of normal is controversial, and there is also variability between different assays. However, a growing amount of evidence supports the utility of the f/t PSA test as a more sensitive and specific screening tool for prostate cancer. The f/t PSA test has been investigated for its utility in deciding whether or not to repeat a prostate biopsy after an initial negative biopsy result. Some groups also advocate the f/t PSA test for clinical staging of prostate cancer. However, contradictory studies conclude the f/t PSA serum test is not useful in the screening of prostate cancer. Finally, in studies now underway, fPSA is combined with novel serum markers, such as hK2, to improve further the screening strategies for prostate cancer. These issues will be discussed in this chapter.

II. fPSA BIOCHEMISTRY, ASSAYS, AND MECHANISMS IN PROSTATE CANCER

A. fPSA Metabolism

In a series of 12 men undergoing cardiac catheterization, Agha et al. [38] demonstrated that the likely site of greatest tPSA metabolism was in the liver; very little change was seen across the renal circulation. In a similar study with cardiac catheterizations in 20 men, Kilic et al. [39] also demonstrated that liver primarily metabolizes most tPSA, fPSA, and cPSA in the serum; renal clearance was responsible for some fPSA elimination but not of the complexed forms. However, Bjork et al. [40] concluded that the majority of fPSA clearance was performed by glomerular filtration when they examined serum clearance after radical retropubic prostatectomies. In the rat model, Birkenmeier et al. [41] showed that both the liver and kidney were responsible for PSA clearance. PSA-A2M was cleared solely by the liver, PSA-ACT by both the liver and kidney, and fPSA was mostly likely cleared by renal filtration, with any remaining fPSA being complexed rapidly with A2M or ACT. The disagreement in their conclusions may be a result of the nature of the study designs, since the prostatectomy group may represent a nonphysiological state in which a large amount of fPSA is suddenly liberated into the circulation.

Half-life determinations for fPSA after radical retropubic prostatectomies were also reported by Partin et al. [42] to follow a two-compartment model of clearance, with the first $t_{1/2}$ at approximately 1.2 hr, which then increases to 22 hr. Richardson et al. [43], in a similar study in patients after radical retropubic prostatectomy, reported that the $t_{1/2}$ of serum fPSA was 1.83 hr, but this group did not utilize the two-compartment model. Despite the differences in study design, it is evident that the $t_{1/2}$ of fPSA is shorter than the complexed forms and it is either rapidly eliminated or complexed in the circulation.

The storage conditions of blood after phlebotomy were reported to have a significant effect on tPSA and fPSA values. Several groups noted that fPSA is more labile than cPSA *in vitro*, but could be stabilized by acidifying the sample and freezing it immediately [44–46]. However, Leinonen et al. [47] reported that cPSA actually decreased and fPSA increased after long-term storage at $-20°C$, resulting in a net decrease in tPSA and an increase in the f/t PSA ratio. In an interesting report, Yoshida et al. [48] used an incubation treatment at 58°C to fractionate fPSA from ACT. With this treatment, they were able to enhance differentiation of benign hyperplasia and prostate carcinoma in the range of tPSA from 4.1 to 10.0 ng/ml by comparing the area under the receiver-operating characteristic (ROC) curves between tPSA (AUC; area under curve = 0.675) and the f/t PSA ratio (AUC = 0.871). This suggests that fPSA is heat stable at least in the short term (under 60 min). Further details on the biochemistry of PSA are discussed in Chapter 2.

B. Skew vs. Equimolar Assays

Depending on the particular PSA assay, there can be tremendous variability within patients and laboratories. Great care should be taken in interpreting individual PSA values when comparing results from larger clinical trials in different populations. Many factors contribute to this variability, such as the large number of manufacturers for PSA assays, the assay's specific technique and antibodies used in the immunodetection of particular PSA isoforms, the laboratory's particular calibration of standards, and even the patient's own concentration of PSA isoforms. Brawer et al. [49] described the variation in tPSA values between the IMx (Abbott Laboratories, Abbott Park, IL) and Tandem R (Hybritech Inc., San Diego, CA) assays as a function of the f/t PSA ratio. In comparing tPSA results from the two manufacturers, if both assays were in good agreement within 5%, the mean f/t PSA ratio was 18.6%. However, when the IMx tPSA result was ≤75% of the Tandem R result, the mean f/t PSA ratio was much lower at 11.8%; when the IMx assay was ≥20% or higher than the Tandem R assay, the mean f/t PSA ratio was much higher at 29.8%.

The explanation for this finding is that different antibodies have variable affinities for the fPSA or cPSA moieties. An "equimolar" assay recognizes both the free and complexed forms equivalently, and so the tPSA result is independent of the f/t PSA ratio. Conversely, the example above has "skew," meaning that the assay does not recognize the free moiety equivalently to the complexed moiety. The data thus suggest that the IMx assay is skewed toward overdetecting the free isoform of PSA, therefore giving a higher tPSA when the fPSA isoform is in high concentration. Semjonow et al. [50] reported that the tPSA could vary up to 36% depending on the assay and the amount of fPSA. This significant intertest variability highlights the need for international standardization for PSA immunoassays [51,52].

C. Why is the f/t PSA Ratio Lower in Men with Prostate Cancer?

There is currently no satisfactory explanation for why PSA is complexed in higher amounts in men with prostate cancer. ACT is normally present at a 10^4–10^5-fold molar excess in the extracellular fluid space [8]. Although there can be an increased production of ACT from the liver resulting in elevated serum levels of ACT, this does not correlate with serum levels of either cPSA or f/t PSA ratios [53].

One possible explanation is that the PSA produced by benign or BPH tissues is in another isoform. Chen et al. [54] reported that the PSA obtained from BPH tissue was mainly in a "nicked form" (PSA-ni) that had multiple internal cleavages resulting in a different three-dimensional structure than in seminal fluid PSA. This new structure may result in altered detection with standard fPSA detection antibodies but still have affinity for the protease inhibitors ACT and A2M. Furthermore, however, Leinonen et al. [55] showed that only 5–18% of PSA-ni complexed with ACT, whereas almost 54–67% reacted with A2M. This would suggest that in BPH nodules that produce more PSA-ni than PSA, most of the PSA-ni would bind to A2M, which is undetectable, and the tPSA has a correspondingly higher f/t PSA ratio because only a minority of the PSA-ni is bound as PSA-ACT.

Another possible explanation is that there is higher production of ACT in prostate cancer cells than in benign hyperplastic prostate cells. Although the majority of ACT is produced in the liver, it has been demonstrated by in situ hybridization and immunocytochemistry that there is local production of ACT in the prostate [56]. Both the ACT mRNA and expressed protein were found in most of the tumor cells in prostate cancers, and in much lesser amounts in benign prostate nodules [57]. This suggests that the PSA–ACT complex may be preformed in prostate cancer cells producing both PSA and ACT before it is released into the peripheral circulation. This concept is further supported by another study by Tanaka et al. [58], who examined benign and malignant prostate tissue immunostained with PSA and ACT antibodies. The percentage of ACT-stained cells in prostate cancer was significantly higher than that in benign prostatic hyperplasia specimens. Unfortunately, in this study the serum f/t PSA ratio did not correlate with the number of ACT stained cells. However, this theory is controversial and there is conflicting evidence: Bostwick et al. [59] reported that there was only a minimal difference in ACT-stained cells in benign vs. cancer specimens. An even more contradictory result was noted by Igawa et al. [60], who found that the cells in patients with prostate cancer actually had a lower proportion immunostaining for ACT compared to cells from patients with BPH.

On a slightly different note, Ornstein et al. [61] recently reported using the laser capture microdissection technique to isolate a pure population of prostatic epithelial cells from both benign and cancerous specimens, and demonstrated that the vast majority of intracellular PSA exists in the free form in both cases. They also showed that the intracellular fPSA isoform was still capable of binding with ACT, and concluded that binding to ACT occurs exclusively outside of the cell. Although this provides a mechanistic basis for PSA binding, the primary question of why the fPSA is decreased in patients with prostate cancer is still largely unanswered.

III. f/t PSA FOR ENHANCING THE SENSITIVITY AND SPECIFICITY OF tPSA AS A SCREENING TEST

Because of the aforementioned limitations of tPSA as a screening test for cancer, especially in the intermediate range from 4.0 to 10.0 ng/ml where there is significant overlap in men with BPH, additional tPSA-derived tests were developed to increase the specificity. These tests include measurement of PSA density, PSA velocity, age specific PSA ranges, and complexed PSA (see Chaps. 4, 5, 6, 8). Likewise, the sensitivity of the tPSA assay can be improved if more true-positive results were detected in situations in which the tPSA is normal (tPSA≤4.0 ng/ ml) and a biopsy would not be routinely performed. Among the different assays for the molecular isoforms (fPSA, cPSA, tPSA), there is evidence that the f/t PSA ratio improves both the sensitivity and the specificity compared to the tPSA value alone.

A.   Early Studies on the Utility of fPSA

Stenman et al. [10] described in 1991 that cPSA was higher in men with prostate cancer and that this test could be used to differentiate better between patients with benign and malignant disease. The correlate to this finding is that the fPSA is lower in men with cancer, as the sum of the isoforms equals the tPSA. In 1993, Christensson et al. [53] reported that the f/t PSA ratio was significantly lower in men with untreated prostate cancer than in men with benign disease. At a tPSA cutoff of 5 ng/ml, they reported a sensitivity of 90% and specificity of 55%, but when a tPSA cutoff at 10 ng/ml was combined with the f/t PSA ratio at 18%, the sensitivity remained at 90% and the specificity improved to 73%. Their study population, however, included men with an unselected tPSA level at varying levels, including some even into the thousands of ng/ml.

In 1995, Luderer et al. [62] specifically addressed the question of using fPSA for improving the specificity of the screening test within the "diagnostic gray zone" from 4.0 to 10.0 ng/ml. Within all ranges of tPSA (n = 181), both the f/t PSA ratio and tPSA could differentiate between men with prostate cancer and men with benign or normal prostate conditions; the ROC curves for both tPSA and the f/t PSA ratio were almost identical. However, in the subset of men with a tPSA between 4.0 and 10.0 ng/ml (n = 57), the tPSA showed no significant difference between the benign and malignant groups (mean tPSA for benign and cancer groups was 6.18 and 6.92 ng/mL respectively, p = 0.13, Wilcoxon test). For the f/t PSA ratio, on the other hand, the mean values for the benign and cancer groups were 22 and 13%, respectively (p = 0.0004). At a f/t PSA ratio of 25% or less, they reported a sensitivity of 100% and specificity of 31%, thereby correctly identifying almost one-third of patients with BPH. In contrast, using a tPSA cutoff of 4.0 ng/ml, in this group the sensitivity was 100% but the specificity was 0%.

   Various studies published in 1995 and 1996 were in agreement with these findings (see Table 1). Drawbacks in these earlier studies were that the range and cutpoint of tPSA in the studies varied greatly, and the assays were from different manufacturers. One of the most significant drawbacks was that most of the study sizes were all fairly small; only two reports had a sample size > 450, and one of these trials did not support the overall finding that the f/t PSA ratio could improve the specificity of tPSA. In the largest multi-institutional collaboration at that time, Thiel et al. [63] reported a study of 1081 subjects. Despite significant variations in results from the test sites, they concluded that only 4% of men with prostate cancer had an f/t PSA ratio > 25% and only 2% of men with BPH had an f/t PSA ratio < 7%, thus establishing these two numbers as valuable cutpoints. Within the selected tPSA range of 2.5–20.0 ng/ml, they reported that the f/t PSA ratio was a valuable adjunct to the tPSA test.

   Conversely, Bangma et al. [64] described a study with 1726 subjects, but it was a retrospective study with an unselected tPSA range of 0–165 ng/ml. Only 67 cancers were detected out of 308 men who underwent biopsies, and of those, only 140 men had a tPSA between 4.0 and 10 ng/ml. ROC curves of this latter group showed that the minimal improvement from the f/t PSA ratio compared to tPSA did not reach statistical significance (AUC = 0.74 and 0.67 respectively, with a standard error = 0.05). It is likely that with a larger study size within a selected tPSA range the improvement may have been able to reach statistical significance. The variability between the results of these early studies may be attributable to the low power of the studies as well as variations in study design.

B. Increasing the Specificity: tPSA 4.0–10.0 ng/ml

In 1998, Catalona et al. [65] reported findings from a multicenter prospective trial using the f/t PSA ratio to improve the specificity of the tPSA. Seven univer-

Table 1 Comparison of Free PSA Studies for the Detection of Prostate Cancer

References	PSA assay	Total PSA range (ng/ml)	No. Ca/ no. no Ca	Population	% Free PSA cut-off	% Sensitivity	% Specificity
Christenssen et al. [53]		4–20	Not applicable		18	71	95
Luderer et al. [62]	Immunocorp Sciences[a] free + TOSOH[b] total	4–10	25/32		25	100	31
Catalona et al. [83]	Hybritech[c] free prototype + Tandem total	4–10	63/50		20	88	50
Bangma et al. [64]	Delfia[d] free + total	4–10	26/48	Nonsuspicious digital rectal examination only	20	90	38
					23	90	31
Chen et al. [139]	Immunocorp Sciences free + TOSOH total	2.5–2.0	33/107		28	91	19
Prestigiacomo et al. [140]	Hybritech free + total	4–10	165/263		25	95	26
Elgamal et al. [141]	Centocor[e] free + total	3–15	20/28		23	90	32
					14	95	64
			37/48	T1c	15	95	56
			32/48		18	95	40
					18	78	40
Van Cangh et al. [142]	Hybritech free + total	2–30	154/266	T2	25	90	38
Catalona et al. [69]	Hybritech free + total	2–10	90/205	Nonsuspicious digital rectal examination only	25	90	38
		2.6–4	52/232		26	90	24
Partin et al. [79]	Hybritech free prototype + Tandem total	4–10	139/78		20	95	29

[a] Montreal, Canada.
[b] Tokyo, Japan.
[c] San Diego, California.
[d] Wallac, Oy, Finland.
[e] Malvern, Pennsylvania.
Source: Ref. 143.

Table 2 Percentage of Free PSA Cutoffs, Sensitivity, and Specificity

Free PSA cut-off (%)	Sensitivity, % (no.) of cancers detected [95% CI]	Specificity, % (No.) of unnecessary biopsies avoided [95% CI]
≤22	90 (341/379) [86–93]	29 (115–394) [25–34]
≤25	95 (358/379) [92–97]	20 (80–394) [16–24]

Source: Ref. 65.

sity medical centers in the United States participated in the study, and they enrolled a total of 773 men aged 50–75 with a benign DRE and a tPSA between 4.0 and 10.0 ng/ml. The Tandem PSA and free assays (Hybritech Inc., San Diego, CA) were used in the study, which determined that with a 25% f/t PSA ratio, 95% of prostate cancers were detected and 20% of unnecessary biopsies were avoided (see Table 2). With a 22% f/t PSA ratio, the sensitivity dropped to 90% but the specificity increased to 29%, thus avoiding almost one-third of unnecessary biopsies. In their ROC curves the AUC for the f/t PSA ratio was significantly higher (AUC = 0.72) than for tPSA (AUC = 0.53, see Fig. 1).

This group concluded that the f/t PSA ratio could be used in two ways: either as a single cutoff value at 25% (i.e., biopsy all men ≤ 25%), or to assess an individual's risk for prostate cancer along with tPSA (i.e., biopsy ≤ 25% only if an individual's risk for cancer is high). There was a statistically significant correlation with favorable pathological findings (Gleason score < 7, stage I and II, no metastases at lymph nodes, and tumor volume ≤ 10% of gland) as the f/t PSA ratio increased. The authors stated that men with higher f/t PSA ratios were likely to have less aggressive disease. Finally, they also showed that the sensitivity f/t PSA ratio correlated negatively with prostate volume; at a 25% f/t PSA cutoff, sensitivity was 99% with a gland ≤ 30 cm³, but the sensitivity decreased to 87% at a volume > 50 cm³.

This important study resulted in the approval by the Food and Drug Administration (FDA) of the f/t PSA assay for a select group of men with a tPSA between 4.0 and 10.0 ng/ml.

C. Increasing the Sensitivity: tPSA ≤ 4.0 ng/ml

Sensitivity of the tPSA test can be improved if a cancer is detected in someone who normally would not undergo a prostate biopsy, and thus reduce the false-negative rate. Most physicians do not recommend a biopsy for patients with a tPSA level under 4.0 ng/ml, unless the patient is age 40–59 years of age or has

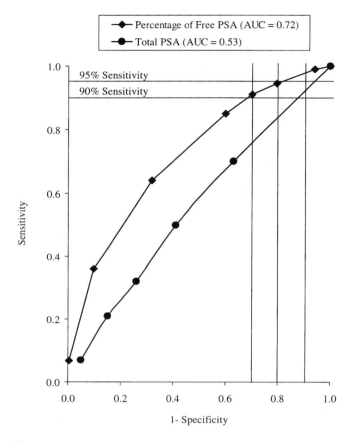

Figure 1 Percentage of free PSA and total PSA ROC curve. A cut-off of 25% or less free PSA provides 95% sensitivity and 20% specificity (i.e., it spares 20% of men with benign prostatic disease from an inappropriate biopsy). AUC indicates area under the ROC curve. (From Ref. 65.)

an abnormal DRE. However, 13–20% of men with a tPSA between 2.6 and 4.0 will have a cancer detected in 3–5 years [66,67]. In a study that evaluated the f/t PSA ratio in a range of tPSA from 1.8 to 10 ng/ml, Van Cangh et al. [68] reported that in addition to gaining an improvement in both sensitivity and specificity with the f/t PSA ratio, 29 of 92 (31.5%) patients with prostate cancer had a tPSA < 4.0 ng/ml. Earlier detection of these cancers would allow curative treatment while disease is still localized in the prostate, and there is evidence that this detection can be achieved with the f/t PSA test.

Catalona et al. [69] in 1997 reported 914 consecutive volunteers over the age of 50 with a tPSA of 2.6–4.0 ng/ml; 332 of these men underwent a biopsy of the prostate, and cancer was detected in 73 (22%). The authors determined that with a f/t PSA ratio cutoff of ≤27% for performing a prostate biopsy, they were able to obtain a sensitivity of 90% and avoid 18% of unnecessary biopsies. A majority of these cancers were "medically important tumors": only 17% of the cancers that were surgically staged were low-volume and low or moderately low-grade tumors.

Lodding et al. [70] reported on 243 men, ages 50–65 years, with tPSA levels of 3–4 ng/ml. Prostate cancer was detected in 32 of 243 men (13.2%), and in this group 30 (94%) had a f/t PSA ratio ≤ 27%. Surgical specimens were available for 14 of these men; all tumors were greater than 0.5 cc with a mean volume of 1.8 cc; 6 patients had pT3 disease; and 5 had positive margins. These results further illustrate that cancers detected with a tPSA ≤ 4.0 ng/ml are not always "harmless" or "clinically insignificant."

More recently, Tornblom et al. [71] performed a retrospective screening study of 1782 men who underwent DRE, transrectal ultrasound (TRUS), and PSA testing. An fPSA assay was performed on 1748 men, and 367 underwent a biopsy based on abnormal findings on DRE or TRUS, or a tPSA > 10.0 ng/ml. Sixty-four cases of prostate cancer were detected (3.7%), and 9 of these (14% of all prostate cancers) were in men with a tPSA ≤ 18%. The authors concluded that for screening, the combination of a tPSA ≤ 3.0 ng/ml and a f/t PSA ratio ≥ 18% selects for a population with a very low risk of cancer. These men could be spared an annual DRE and could be screened at intervals longer than every year. However, the risk of cancer is not negligible in men with tPSA ≤ 3.0 ng/ml and f/t PSA ratio ≤ 18%, and these men should undergo a biopsy of the prostate.

It is intuitive that earlier detection of these prostate cancers should be beneficial in men with tPSA ≤ 4.0 ng/ml, and certainly in those with a higher risk, such as a positive family history, African-American heritage, or age <60. Approximately 30% of men with cancer and a tPSA between 4.0 and 10.0 ng/ml already have prostatic capsule invasion at the time of diagnosis [72,73]. By decreasing the false-negative rate for men with tPSA ≤ 4.0 ng/ml, the addition of an f/t PSA test would increase the amount of cancers detected that are "clinically significant," but at a cost of increasing the number of negative biopsies. Catalona et al. [74] developed models for identifying men with cancer and a tPSA level between 2.51 and 4.0 ng/ml in a retrospective analysis of archived serum samples. In this select group, by choosing a f/t PSA ratio cut-off between 10 and 15%, a sensitivity range of 30–54% could be achieved, with only 9–36% of men in this group recommended for biopsy. It seems prudent to detect these cancers in men who otherwise would not have ordinarily undergone a biopsy and thus would have a delayed diagnosis.

D. What is the Reflex Range?

In general, despite a fair amount of variability in the above studies, most seem to concur that the f/t PSA ratio can improve the sensitivity and specificity of the tPSA assay. However, no complete agreement exists among the studies regarding the appropriate cutpoint for f/t PSA ratio, nor is there agreement on the appropriate reflex range for tPSA: the range of values of tPSA outside of which a laboratory would automatically proceed with determining the f/t PSA ratio.

Vashi et al. [75] investigated the ability of both the tPSA and the f/t PSA ratio to differentiate BPH and prostate cancer in 413 men with a tPSA range from 2 to 20 ng/ml. They generated ROC curves to determine the optimal ranges of tPSA and cutpoints for the f/t PSA ratio. They concluded that the appropriate reflex range of tPSA was 3.0–10.0 ng/ml; in this range, the f/t PSA ratio improved the tPSA ratio by 21% (AUC = 0.72 and 0.51, respectively; p < 0.001). When the tPSA was between 3.0 and 4.0 ng/ml, a cutpoint for the f/t PSA ratio of 19% resulted in 90% sensitivity, with a biopsy rate of 73% and a cancer detection rate of 44%. This means that for this select group of men, one cancer, would be found for every 1.7 biopsies performed. The authors likewise calculated that if the tPSA was between 4.1 and 10.0 ng/ml, an f/t PSA ratio cutpoint of 24% resulted in a 95% sensitivity and 13% fewer negative biopsies.

One caveat is that the study population for Vashi et al. [75] was from a tertiary-care university-based center, and the prevalence of cancer among this group may not be the same as for other populations. However, their cutpoint of 24% f/t PSA for the range 4.1–10 ng/ml tPSA with 95% sensitivity is in surprisingly good agreement with that of Catalona et al. [65] who used the same criteria to generate a 25% f/t PSA ratio cutpoint. The prevalence of cancer, different sample sizes, and different assay manufacturers may account for some of the variations with other studies. For instance, Carlson et al. [76] reported that in their series of 479 men the lowest tPSA value at which the f/t PSA ratio differed from tPSA in predicting cancer was 4.0 ng/ml, and there was no improvement in sensitivity for tPSA values below that cutpoint.

Other controversies abound. For example, although many studies have shown that tPSA is dependent on age [77–79], several studies have indicated that the f/t PSA ratio is age-independent [80–82]. Several studies showed that a similar disagreement exists for the dependence of the f/t PSA ratio on prostate volume [78,79,83–85]. A large, multi-institutional prospective trial is needed to clarify the associations between fPSA and f/t PSA ratios with age and prostate volume.

E. Recent Clinical Trials

A plethora of recent reports with similar study designs have described congruent results with the f/t PSA assay [86–96]. Despite variations with sample size, study design, assay manufacturer, as well as the f/t PSA ratio cutoff and resultant sensitivity and specificity, many of the studies generally concur that there is an improvement in specificity when the tPSA is between 4.0 and 10.0 ng/ml. The f/t PSA ratio was also shown to be useful in the African-American population for the detection of prostate cancer [97], although there were only 79 African-American and 647 white males in that study. In another study with 222 African-American and 298 white males with a serum tPSA of 2.5–9.9, Fowler et al. [98] reported that there were significant racial differences with the test. In African-Americans, there was a mild improvement in the AUC for the f/t PSA ratio (0.66) over the tPSA ratio (0.58) that did not reach statistical significance (p = 0.15), although there was a significant improvement in whites (p < 0.00001). A greater proportion of African-American men with a f/t PSA ratio ≥25% had cancer (32% vs. 13%, p = 0.005), as well for those with a f/t PSA ratio <25% (53% vs. 41%, p = 0.03). This underscores the concept that African-American men are at a higher risk for developing prostate cancer, and suggests that a different reference range may be needed for African-American men in this country.

IV. f/t PSA AFTER AN INITIAL NEGATIVE BIOPSY

Another clinical scenario useful for the f/t PSA ratio is the situation in which a man has a persistently elevated tPSA level despite a negative DRE and a previous prostate biopsy that did not show any evidence of cancer. This important clinical scenario is reviewed in Chapter 10. In an initial study with a low sample size of 67 men, Morgan et al. [99,100] reported that the median f/t PSA ratio was significantly lower in men who eventually had a biopsy positive for prostate cancer than in men without cancer (6.7% vs. 18.0%, respectively; p < 0.00005). In their ROC curve analysis, the AUC for the f/t PSA ratio was 0.93 vs. 0.51 for tPSA. They concluded that in this select population a 10% f/t PSA ratio cutpoint resulted in a sensitivity of 91%, while reducing the false biopsy rate by 86%.

Catalona et al. [101] also looked at a similar population of men who had a tPSA range from 4.1 to 10 ng/ml, benign findings on DRE, and a prior negative biopsy. Of 163 men in this series, 99 agreed to undergo another biopsy, and cancer was then detected in 20 (20%). An f/t PSA ratio cutpoint of 28% resulted in a 90% sensitivity and 13% specificity, whereas at a cutpoint of 30% the sensitivity was 95% with a 12% specificity. Letran et al. [102] came to a similar conclusion but also showed a significant difference in using assays from different manufacturers. The study used archived sera from only 51 men, and the tPSA range was 2–15 ng/ml. The fPSA was calculated with assays from both Hybritech (Hybritech, Inc, San Diego, CA) and Dianon (Dianon Systems, Stratford, CT), but only the Hybritech tPSA was used as the denominator in comparing both f/t PSA ratios (i.e., Hybritech free/Hybritech total vs. Dianon free/Hybritech total). The Hybritech f/t PSA ratio was significantly lower in men with a positive repeat biopsy; the Dianon free/Hybritech total PSA ratio and the tPSA was not significantly different between the two groups. An f/t PSA ratio cutpoint of 27% gave a 100% sensitivity and 25% specificity, while a 22% cutpoint resulted in a 95% sensitivity and a 44% specificity.

Trinkler et al. [103] investigated a similar population but also used assays from two different manufacturers (Diagnostic Products Corporation, Los Angeles, CA; and Ciba Corning, East Walpole, MA). They determined that the reflex range of tPSA should be 2.5–10.0 ng/ml, and they also noted a significant difference of as much as 197% with the tPSA results from the two assay manufacturers. They concluded that the combination of tPSA with an f/t PSA ratio cutpoint of 19% could maintain the sensitivity level of tPSA alone (82.8%) but also increase the specificity to eliminate 39.8% of unnecessary prostate biopsies.

Larger series have shown similar results; Fowler et al. [104] reported that in 298 men with a previous negative biopsy, 27% subsequently had a positive biopsy. With multiple logistic regression analyses, they concluded that the f/t PSA ratio was the most powerful predictor of cancer in these patients. Djavan examined 820 men with a previous negative biopsy [105] and found cancer in 10% of men who underwent a repeat biopsy. They showed that the f/t PSA ratio was the most accurate predictor of prostate cancer in this population; with a cutpoint of 30%, they were able to maintain a sensitivity of 90% and a specificity of 50%. The AUC for the f/t PSA ratio was 74.5% compared to 60.3% for tPSA.

Despite all the above reports that the f/t PSA ratio may be helpful to determine who should undergo a repeat prostate biopsy, Hayek et al. [106] presented some evidence that the f/t PSA ratio was of no additional benefit than just tPSA alone. The controversy is not yet resolved and a multi-institutional prospective study is needed to resolve this issue.

V. f/t PSA FOR CLINICAL STAGING

The f/t PSA ratio has also been investigated for its utility in predicting the pathological grade and stage of prostate cancer, which is further discussed in Chapter 11. Although the molecular mechanism explaining why the fPSA is lower in men with prostate cancer has not yet been elucidated, it seems initially intuitive that perhaps with a lower f/t PSA ratio the prostate cancer may be more aggressive or widespread than a cancer with a relatively higher f/t PSA ratio. Carter et al. [107] used the f/t PSA ratio assay retrospectively to analyze archival sera from men up to 18 years before the diagnosis of cancer. Although tPSA was not statistically different, the f/t PSA ratio was significantly different ($p < 0.008$) between men who had aggressive disease (stage T3, presence of bone or nodal metastases, positive surgical margins, or Gleason score 7 or greater) and those with nonaggressive disease (none of the above). The men with aggressive disease were more likely to have a low f/t PSA ratio, which suggested that the f/t PSA ratio might predict the clinical course of the tumor before tPSA. Several other studies [108–110] also showed that the f/t PSA ratio has a positive correlation with predicting pathological stage. In predicting the histological characteristics of the biopsy, some groups report [104,111,112] that the f/t PSA ratio was useful for differentiating cancer from BPH, but was not able to differentiate cancer from prostatic intraepithelial neoplasia (PIN).

However, some results contradict the above findings. Bjork et al. [113] reported that although f/t PSA provided prognostic information in a multivariate analysis, there was a tendency for a high f/t PSA ratio to be associated with a poor prognosis. They reported that patients who died from poorly differentiated prostate cancer had a mean f/t PSA ratio of 21.2%; those with moderately differentiated tumors had a lower mean f/t PSA ratio of 14.5%; and those with well differentiated tumors had even lower ratios, although this value did not reach statistical significance. Furthermore, in a histological analysis, Jung et al. [114] showed that the tissue concentration of tPSA in cancer and benign prostate tissue had no correlation with serum values of tPSA and f/t PSA, although they did confirm that a lower f/tPSA was seen in prostate cancer tissue than in benign tissue. Other studies [115–117] reported that there was no differentiation of the f/t PSA ratio between organ-confined disease and extraprostatic spread. Lin et al. [118] examined a population of patients with biochemical recurrence after radical prostatectomy and reported no significant relationship between the f/t PSA ratio with the patient's grade, stage, or severity of the disease. They also noted that the f/t PSA ratio was actually higher in patients who received treatment for their metastatic disease (hormonal, radiation, or both) than in those who did not receive treatment. Wojno et al. [119] studied a similar population of patients after prostatectomy and found that although most cancers that recur have a low f/t PSA ratio, there is a significant proportion in whom the ratio is high (9% of patients had a ratio of 15–19%, and 9% had a ratio ≥20), and, paradoxically, the patients with high ratios had more aggressive disease.

Pannek and Partin [120] recently reviewed this controversial topic and discussed the many variables between the studies, such as pathological classification, sample handling, assay manufacturer, prostate volume, patients' age, and study design. Given the current conflicting data, correlation of a low serum f/t PSA ratio with a more aggressive prostate cancer still remains to be confirmed, and the f/t PSA ratio should not be used routinely to stage or prognosticate clinical outcomes until a larger multi-institutional trial is completed.

VI. CONTRADICTORY STUDIES SHOWING THAT f/t PSA MAY NOT BE HELPFUL

Despite the enlarging body of literature demonstrating the utility of f/t PSA ratio in improving the sensitivity and specificity of tPSA, many reports also conclude that the assay has significant flaws and does not improve substantially over the tPSA test. Different groups state that there is a significant amount of variation with the f/t PSA ratio within individuals [121,122] as well as between assays from different manufacturers [123–126]. Several studies [127–129] used ROC curves to show that the f/t PSA ratio adds no additional benefit to tPSA. One group used a nested case–control study [130] on archived sera from four different institutions to show that there was only an insignificant advantage over tPSA. Jung et al. [131] reported that the f/t PSA ratio could not reliably differentiate between cancer and chronic prostatitis.

These contradictory studies emphasize the point that all of the studies are different with respect to multiple variables, such as sample size, study design, cancer prevalence, assay manufacturer, serum storage conditions, and many other factors. In order to apply conclusions from a report it is necessary to control for these variables as much as possible, as well as to remember that the study populations are never exactly identical.

VII. NEW DEVELOPMENTS WITH THE f/t PSA RATIO

Further modifications are always being introduced to increase the sensitivity and specificity of the assays to screen for prostate cancer. Permutations of fPSA with the other molecular forms of PSA, such as the f/c PSA ratio [132] and the prostate malignancy index [133], are currently under investigation. One especially promising area of future research is with human glandular kallikrein 2 (hK2). This serine protease shares a very high sequence homology with PSA and serum levels correlate well with PSA; furthermore, several groups [134–138] have shown the utility of the hk2/fPSA ratio in differentiating cancer from BPH. Larger studies need to be completed in order to confirm the utility of these new assays in mainstream clinical practices.

VIII. CONCLUSION

Reports from multiple institutions continue to accrue that describe the utility of the f/t PSA assay. However, there is always the problem of translating those results to an individual patient for whom the result of a biopsy is not a percentage risk of cancer but rather binary; and for whom the pain, hematuria, irritative symptoms, and risk of infection from a negative prostate biopsy are the result of a low sensitivity rate from the assay. It appears that currently the data support three clinical scenarios for using the f/t PSA ratio in clinical practice:

1. Benign DRE, and tPSA 4.0–10.0 ng/ml

2. Benign DRE, tPSA 4.0–10.0 ng/ml, and a previous negative biopsy
3. Benign DRE, tPSA 2.5–4.0 ng/ml, and a high risk of prostate cancer (positive family history, age 45–59, or African-American heritage)

Our approach at the University of Washington is to biopsy the prostate in patients with tPSA between 4.0 and 10.0 ng/dl without regard to the f/t PSA ratio, because the positive predictive value for tPSA at those levels is still worrisome enough for cancer, even with a high f/t PSA ratio. However, if no cancer is found on the first biopsy, the ratio becomes more helpful, but it is not the exclusive determinant for another biopsy. Family history, patient anxiety and/or life expectancy, PSA velocity, and results of the digital rectal exam all must be factored into this admittedly subjective decision until further research gives us more certain guidelines. If the patient's tPSA is between 2.5 and 4.0 ng/ml, the f/t PSA ratio likewise becomes only one of several factors that can be considered when making a decision about the initial biopsy. In general, if the patient is under 65 years old and in good health, we will recommend an initial biopsy when the f/t PSA ratio is less than 20%. If that biopsy is negative, we will watch the patient for changes in status unless the f/t PSA ratio is alarmingly low (e.g., <10%). In short, there is still so very much yet unknown in making decisions about a biopsy that an "Art of Medicine" approach is required, especially in coming to an understanding with an educated patient, including the use of the positive predictive value nomograms currently available.

The other potentially applicable scenarios for the f/t PSA ratio are still under investigation and should still be considered experimental at this point. However, in the last few years since the introduction of this assay, the f/t PSA ratio has shown great promise in its ability to supplement the tPSA test in improving both the sensitivity and specificity, and will therefore have a significant role in the early detection and treatment of prostate cancer in the new millennium.

REFERENCES

1. SH Landis, T Murray, S Bolden, PA Wingo. Cancer statistics, 1999. CA Cancer J Clin 49(1):8–31, 1999.
2. MC Wang, LA Valenzuela, GP Murphy, TM Chu. Purification of a human prostate specific antigen. Invest Urol 17(2):159–163, 1979.
3. P Henttu, P Vihko. cDNA coding for the entire prostate specific antigen shows high homologies to the human tissue kallikrein genes. Biochem Biophys Res Commun 160(2):903–910, 1989.
4. HJ Lilja. A kallikrein-like serine protease in prostatic fluid cleaves the predominant seminal vesicle protein. J Clin Invest 76(5):1899–1903, 1985.
5. HJ Lilja. Structure, function, and regulation of the enzyme activity of prostate-specific antigen. World J Urol 11(4):188–191, 1993.

6. A Christensson, H Lilja. Complex formation between protein C inhibitor and prostate-specific antigen in vitro and in human semen. Eur J Biochem 220(1):45–53, 1994.

7. RL Vessella, PH Lange. Issues in the assessment of prostate-specific antigen immunoassays. An update. Urol Clin North Am 24(2):261–268, 1997.

8. A Christensson, CB Laurell, H Lilja. Enzymatic activity of prostate-specific antigen and its reactions with extracellular serine proteinase inhibitors. Eur J Biochem 194(3):755–763, 1990.

9. H Lilja, A Christensson, U Dahlen, MT Matikainen, O Nilsson, K Pettersson, T Lovgren. Prostate-specific antigen in serum occurs predominantly in complex with alpha-1 antichymotrypsin. Clin Chem 37(9):1618–1625, 1991.

10. UH Stenman, J Leinonen, H Alfthan, S Rannikko, K Tuhkanen, O Alfthan. A complex between prostate-specific antigen and alpha 1-antichymotrypsin is the major form of prostate-specific antigen in serum of patients with prostate cancer: Assay of the complex improves clinical sensitivity for cancer. Cancer Res 51(1):222–226, 1991.

11. BS Kramer, ML Brown, PC Prolok, AL Potosky, JK Gohagan: Prostate cancer screening: What we know and what we need to know. Ann Intern Med 119:914–923, 1993.

12. JE Oesterling, SJ Jacobsen, CG Chute, HA Guess, CJ Girman, LA Panser, MM Lieber. Serum prostate-specific antigen in a community-based population of healthy men. Establishment of age-specific reference ranges. JAMA 270(7):860–864, 1993.

13. PH Lange, CJ Ercole, DJ Lightner, EE Fraley, R Vessella. The value of serum prostate specific antigen determinations before and after radical prostatectomy. J Urol 141(4):873–879, 1989.

14. JE Oesterling: Prostate specific antigen: A critical assessment of the most useful tumor marker for adenocarcinoma of the prostate. J Urol 145(5):907–923, 1991.

15. MK Brawer, MP Chetner, J Beattie, DM Buchner, RL Vessella, PH Lange. Screening for prostatic carcinoma with prostate specific antigen. J Urol 147 (3 Pt 2):841–845, 1992.

16. WJ Catalona, JP Richie, FR Ahmann, MA Hudson, PT Scardino, RC Flanigan, JB deKernion, TL Ratliff, LR Kavoussi, BL Dalkin, WB Waters, MT MacFarlane, PC Southwick. Comparison of digital rectal examination and serum prostate specific antigen in the early detection of prostate cancer: Results of a multicenter clinical trial of 6,630 men. J Urol 151(5):1283–1290, 1994.

17. JE Oesterling, DC Rice, WJ Glenski, EJ Bergstralh. Effect of cystoscopy, prostate biopsy and transurethral resection of prostate on serum prostate specific antigen concentration. Urology 42(3):276–282, 1993.

18. JJ Yuan, DE Coplen, JA Petros, RS Figenshau, TL Ratliff, DS Smith, WJ Catalona. Effects of rectal examination, prostatic massage, ultrasonography and needle biopsy on serum prostate specific antigen levels. J Urol 147(3 Pt 2):810–814, 1992.

19. TA Stamey, N Yang, AR Hay, JE McNeal, FS Freiha, E Redwine. Prostate specific antigen as a serum marker for adenocarcinoma of the prostate. N Engl J Med 317(15):909–916, 1987.

20. RB Nadler, PA Humphrey, DS Smith, WJ Catalona, TL Ratliff. Effect of inflammation and benign prostatic hyperplasia on elevated serum prostate specific antigen levels. J Urol 154(2 Pt 1):407–413, 1995.
21. E Lechevallier, C Eghazarian, JC Ortega, F Roux, C Coulange. Effect of digital rectal examination on serum complexed and free prostate-specific antigen and percentage of free prostate-specific antigen. Urology 54(5):857–861, 1999.
22. N Tariq, DJ Jenkins, E Vidgen, N Fleshner, CW Kendall, JA Story, W Singer, M D'Costa, N Struthers. Effect of soluble and insoluble fiber diets on serum prostate specific antigen in men. J Urol 163(1):114–118, 2000.
23. HA Guess, GJ Gormley, E Stoner, JE Oesterling. The effect of finasteride on prostate specific antigen: Review of available data. J Urol 155(1):3–9, 1996.
24. JP Richie. Anti-androgens and other hormonal therapies for prostate cancer. Urology 54(6A Suppl):15–18, 1999.
25. MA Ferro, D Gillatt, MO Symes, PJ Smith. High-dose intravenous estrogen therapy in advanced prostatic carcinoma. Use of serum prostate-specific antigen to monitor response. Urology 34(3):134–138, 1989.
26. RS DiPaola, H Zhang, GH Lambert, R Meeker, E Licitra, MM Rafi, BT Zhu, H Spaulding, S Goodin, MB Toledano, WN Hait, MA Gallo. Clinical and biologic activity of an estrogenic herbal combination (PC-SPES) in prostate cancer. N Engl J Med 339(12):785–791, 1998.
27. Y Kubota, I Sasagawa, H Sinzawa, T Kunii, K Itoh, H Miura, K Imai, T Nakada. Serum levels of free and total prostate-specific antigen in males with liver cirrhosis. Eur Urol 36(5):409–412, 1999.
28. JD Herschman, DS Smith, WJ Catalona. Effect of ejaculation on serum total and free prostate-specific antigen concentrations. Urology 50(2):239–243, 1997.
29. R Simak, S Madersbacher, ZF Zhang, U Maier. The impact of ejaculation on serum prostate specific antigen. J Urol 150(3):895–897, 1993.
30. A Heidenreich, R Vorreuther, S Neubauer, J Westphal, UH Engelmann, JW Moul. The influence of ejaculation on serum levels of prostate specific antigen. J Urol 157(1):209–211, 1997.
31. R Pezzilli, A Bertaccini, P Billi, L Zanarini, F Miglio, G Martorana. Serum prostate-specific antigen in pancreatic disease. Ital J Gastroenterol Hepatol 31(7):580–583, 1999.
32. M Levesque, H Hu, M D'Costa, EP Diamandis. Prostate-specific antigen expression by various tumors. J Clin Lab Anal 9(2):123–128, 1995.
33. H Yu, EP Diamandis, M Levesque, M Giai, R Roagna, R Ponzone, P Sismondi, M Monne, CM Croce. Prostate specific antigen in breast cancer, benign breast disease and normal breast tissue. Breast Cancer Res Treat 40(2):171–178, 1996.
34. JA Foekens, EP Diamandis, H Yu, MP Look, ME Meijer-van Gelder, WL van Putten, JG Klijn. Expression of prostate-specific antigen (PSA) correlates with poor response to tamoxifen therapy in recurrent breast cancer. Br J Cancer 79(5–6): 888–894, 1999.
35. MC Benson, IS Whang, A Pantuck, K Ring, SA Kaplan, CA Olsson, WH Cooner. Prostate specific antigen density: A means of distinguishing benign prostatic hypertrophy and prostate cancer. J Urol 147:815–816, 1992.

36. HD Carter, JD Pearson. PSA velocity for the diagnosis of early prostate cancer: A new concept. Urol Clin North Am 20:665–670, 1993.

37. JE Oesterling, WH Cooner, SJ Jacobsen, HA Guess, MM Liebner. Influence of patient age on the serum PSA concentration: An important clinical observation. Urol Clin North Am 20:671–680, 1993.

38. AH Agha, E Schechter, JB Roy, DJ Culkin. Prostate specific antigen is metabolized in the liver. J Urol 155(4):1332–5, 1996.

39. S Kilic, S Yalcinkaya, E Guntekin, E Kukul, N Deger, M Sevuk. Determination of the site of metabolism of total, free, and complexed prostate-specific antigen. Urology 52(3):470–473, 1998.

40. T Bjork, B Ljungberg, T Piironen, PA Abrahamsson, K Pettersson, AT Cockett, H Lilja. Rapid exponential elimination of free prostate-specific antigen contrasts the slow, capacity-limited elimination of PSA complexed to alpha-1 antichymotrypsin from serum. Urology 51(1):57–62, 1998.

41. G Birkenmeier, F Struck, R Gebhardt. Clearance mechanism of prostate specific antigen and its complexes with alpha-2 macroglobulin and alpha-1 antichymotrypsin. J Urol 162 (3 Pt 1):897–901, 1999.

42. AW Partin, S Piantadosi, EN Subong, CA Kelly, S Hortopan, DW Chan, RL Wolfert, HG Rittenhouse, HB Carter. Clearance rate of serum-free and total PSA following radical retropubic prostatectomy. Prostate Suppl 7:35–39, 1996.

43. TD Richardson, KJ Wojno, LW Liang, DA Giacherio, BG England, WH Henricks, A Schork, JE Oesterling. Half-life determination of serum free prostate-specific antigen following radical retropubic prostatectomy. Urology 48(6A Suppl):40–44, 1996.

44. D Woodrum, C French, LB Shamel. Stability of free prostate-specific antigen in serum samples under a variety of sample collection and sample storage conditions. Urology 48(6A Suppl):33–39, 1996.

45. T Piironen, K Pettersson, M Suonpaa, UH Stenman, JE Oesterling, T Lovgren, H Lilja. In vitro stability of free prostate-specific antigen (PSA) and prostate-specific antigen (PSA) complexed to alpha 1-antichymotrypsin in blood samples. Urology 48(6A Suppl):81–87, 1996.

46. E Paus, O Nilsson, OP Bormer, SD Fossa, B Otnes, E Skovlund. Stability of free and total prostate specific antigen in serum from patients with prostate carcinoma and benign hyperplasia. J Urol 159(5):1599–1605, 1998.

47. J Leinonen, UH Stenman. Reduced stability of prostate-specific antigen after long-term storage of serum at −20 degrees C. Tumour Biol 21(1):46–53, 2000.

48. K Yoshida, M Honda, S Sumi, K Arai, S Suzuki, S Kitahara. Levels of free prostate-specific antigen (PSA) can be selectively measured by heat treatment of serum: free/total-PSA ratios improve detection of prostate carcinoma. Clin Chim Acta 280(1–2):195–203, 1999.

49. MK Brawer, MH Wener, HG Rittenhouse, RL Wolfert. Proportion of free form of PSA explains the majority of bias between the IMx (Abbott) and Tandem (Hybritech) PSA assays. J Urol 155(Suppl):416A, 1996.

50. A Semjonow, F Oberpenning, B Brandt, L Hertle. Influence of the free PSA fraction on the measurement of 7 different assays for total PSA. J Urol 155(Suppl):420A, 1996.

51. Z Chen, A Prestigiacomo, TA Stamey. Purification and characterization of prostate-specific antigen (PSA) complexed to alpha 1-antichymotrypsin: Potential reference material for international standardization of PSA immunoassays. Clin Chem 41(9): 1273–1282, 1995.

52. AF Prestigiacomo, Z Chen, TA Stamey. A universal calibrator for prostate specific antigen (PSA). Scand J Clin Lab Invest Suppl 221:57–59, 1995.

53. A Christensson, T Bjork, O Nilsson, U Dahlen, MT Matikainen, AT Cockett, PA Abrahamsson, H Lilja. Serum prostate specific antigen complexed to alpha 1-antichymotrypsin as an indicator of prostate cancer. J Urol 150(1):100–105, 1993.

54. Z Chen, H Chen, TA Stamey. Prostate specific antigen in benign prostatic hyperplasia: Purification and characterization. J Urol 157(6):2166–2170, 1997.

55. J Leinonen, WM Zhang, UH Stenman. Complex formation between PSA isoenzymes and protease inhibitors. J Urol 155(3):1099–1103, 1996.

56. A Bjartell, T Bjork, MT Matikainen, PA Abrahamsson, A di Sant'Agnese, H Lilja. Production of alpha-1-antichymotrypsin by PSA-containing cells of human prostate epithelium. Urology 42(5):502–510, 1993.

57. T Bjork, A Bjartell, PA Abrahamsson, S Hulkko, A di Sant'Agnese, H Lilja. Alpha 1-antichymotrypsin production in PSA-producing cells is common in prostate cancer but rare in benign prostatic hyperplasia. Urology 43(4):427–434, 1994.

58. M Tanaka, Y Suzuki, K Takaoka, S Murakami, N Suzuki, J Shimazaki. Immunohistochemical finding of alpha-1-antichymotrypsin in tissues of benign prostatic hyperplasia and prostate cancer. Int J Urol 6(12):600–606, 1999.

59. DG Bostwick, JE Oesterling, G MacLennan, A Pacelli, PA Abrahammson, H Lilja: PSA and alpha-1-antichymotrypsin expression in prostatic intraepithelial neoplasia and adenocarcinoma. J Urol 155 (Suppl):625A, 1996.

60. M Igawa, S Urakami, H Shiina, T Ishibe, T Shirane, T Usui, GW Chodak. Immunohistochemical evaluation of proliferating cell nuclear antigen, prostate-specific antigen and alpha 1-antichymotrypsin in human prostate cancer. Br J Urol 77(1):107–12, 1996.

61. DK Ornstein, C Englert, JW Gillespie, CP Paweletz, WM Linehan, MR Emmert-Buck, Petricoin EF 3rd. Characterization of intracellular prostate-specific antigen from laser capture microdissected benign and malignant prostatic epithelium. Clin Cancer Res 6(2):353–356, 2000.

62. AA Luderer, YT Chen, TF Soriano, WJ Kramp, G Carlson, C Cuny, T Sharp, W Smith, J Petteway, MK Brawer, R Thiel. Measurement of the proportion of free to total prostate-specific antigen improves diagnostic performance of prostate-specific antigen in the diagnostic gray zone of total prostate-specific antigen. Urology 46(2):187–194, 1995.

63. RP Thiel, JE Oesterling, KJ Wojno, AW Partin, DW Chan, HB Carter, TA Stamey, AR Prestigiacomo, MK Brawer, JC Petteway, G Carlson, AA Luderer. Multicenter comparison of the diagnostic performance of free prostate-specific antigen. Urology 48(6A):45–50, 1996.

64. CH Bangma, R Kranse, BG Blijenberg, FH Schroder. The value of screening tests in the detection of prostate cancer. Part 1: Results of a retrospective evaluation of 1726 men. Urology 46(6):773–778, 1995.

65. WJ Catalona, AW Partin, KM Slawin, MK Brawer, RC Flanigan, A Patel, JP Ri-

chie, JB deKernion, PC Walsh, PT Scardino, PH Lange, EN Subong, RE Parson, GH Gasior, KG Loveland, PC Southwick. Use of the percentage of free prostate-specific antigen to enhance differentiation of prostate cancer from benign prostatic disease: a prospective multicenter clinical trial. JAMA 279(19):1542–1547, 1998.

66. DS Smith, WJ Catalona, JD Herschman. Longitudinal screening for prostate cancer with prostate-specific antigen. JAMA 276:1309–1315, 1996.

67. PH Gann, CH Hennekens, MJ Stampfer. A prospective evaluation of plasma prostate-specific antigen for detection of prostatic cancer. JAMA 273:289–294, 1995.

68. PJ Van Cangh, P De Nayer, L De Vischer, P Sauvage, B Tombal, F Lorge, FX Wese, R Opsomer. Free to total prostate-specific antigen (PSA) ratio improves the discrimination between prostate cancer and benign prostatic hyperplasia (BPH) in the diagnostic gray zone of 1.8 to 10 ng/mL total PSA. Urology 48(6A Suppl): 67–70, 1996.

69. WJ Catalona, DS Smith, DK Ornstein. Prostate cancer detection in men with serum PSA concentrations of 2.6 to 4.0 ng/mL and benign prostate examination. Enhancement of specificity with free-PSA measurements. JAMA 277(18):1452–1455, 1997.

70. P Lodding, G Aus, S Bergdahl, R Frosing, H Lilja, CG Pihl, J Hugosson. Characteristics of screening detected prostate cancer in men 50 to 66 years old with 3 to 4 ng/mL prostate-specific antigen. J Urol 159(3):899–903, 1998.

71. M Tornblom, U Norming, J Adolfsson, C Becker, PA Abrahamsson, H Lilja, O Gustafsson. Diagnostic value of percent free prostate-specific antigen: Retrospective analysis of a population-based screening study with emphasis on men with PSA levels less than 3.0 ng/mL. Urology 53(5):945–950, 1999.

72. WJ Catalona, DS Smith, TL Ratliff, KM Dodds, DE Coplen, JJ Yuan, JA Petros, GL Andriole. Measurement of prostate-specific antigen in serum as a screening test for prostate cancer. N Engl J Med 324(17):1156–116, 1991.

73. WJ Catalona, DS Smith, TL Ratliff, JW Basler. Detection of organ-confined prostate cancer is increased through prostate-specific antigen-based screening. JAMA 270(8):948–954, 1993.

74. WJ Catalona, AW Partin, JA Finlay, DW Chan, HG Rittenhouse, RL Wolfert, DL Woodrum. Use of percentage of free prostate-specific antigen to identify men at high risk of prostate cancer when PSA levels are 2.51 to 4 ng/mL and digital rectal examination is not suspicious for prostate cancer: An alternative model. Urology 154(2):220–224, 1999.

75. AR Vashi, KJ Wojno, W Henricks, BA England, RL Vessella, PH Lange, GL Wright Jr, PF Schellhammer, RA Weigand, RM Olson, BL Dowell, KK Borden, JE Oesterling. Determination of the "reflex range" and appropriate cutpoints for percent free prostate-specific antigen in 413 men referred for prostatic evaluation using the AxSYM system. Urology 49(1):19–27, 1997.

76. GD Carlson, CB Calvanese, SJ Childs. The appropriate lower limit for the percent free prostate-specific antigen reflex range. Urology 52(3):450–454, 1998.

77. GD Carlson, CB Calvanese, AW Partin. An algorithm combining age, total prostate-specific antigen (PSA), and percent free PSA to predict prostate cancer: Result on 4298 cases. Urology 52(3):455–461, 1998.

78. DK Ornstein, DS Smith, PA Humphrey, WJ Catalona. The effect of prostate vol-

ume, age, total prostate specific antigen level and acute inflammation on the percentage of free serum prostate specific antigen levels in men without clinically detectable prostate cancer. J Urol 159(4):1234–1237, 1998.

79. AW Partin, WJ Catalona, PC Southwick, EN Subong, GH Gasior, DW Chan. Analysis of percent free prostate-specific antigen (PSA) for prostate cancer detection: Influence of total PSA, prostate volume, and age. Urology 48(6A Suppl):55–61, 1996.

80. JE Oesterling, SJ Jacobsen, GG Klee, K Pettersson, T Piironen, PA Abrahamsson, UH Stenman, B Dowell, T Lovgren, H Lilja. Free, complexed and total serum prostate specific antigen: The establishment of appropriate reference ranges for their concentrations and ratios. J Urol 154(3):1090–1095, 1995.

81. CH Kao. Age-related free PSA, total PSA and free PSA/total PSA ratios: Establishment of reference ranges in Chinese males. Anticancer Res 17(2B):1361–1365, 1997.

82. M Lein, F Koenig, K Jung, FJ McGovern, SJ Skates, D Schnorr, SA Loening. The percentage of free prostate specific antigen is an age-independent tumour marker for prostate cancer: Establishment of reference ranges in a large population of healthy men. Br J Urol 82(2):231–236, 1998.

83. WJ Catalona, DS Smith, RL Wolfert, TJ Wang, HG Rittenhouse, TL Ratliff, RB Nadler. Evaluation of percentage of free serum prostate-specific antigen to improve specificity of prostate cancer screening. JAMA 274(15):1214–1220, 1995.

84. CM Yemoto, R Nolley, AF Prestigiacomo. Free (f) and total (t) PSA density in patients with prostate cancer (CaP) and benign prostatic hypertrophy (BPH). J Urol 155(Suppl):374A, 1996.

85. M Kuriyama, H Uno, H Watanabe, H Yamanaka, Y Saito, K Shida. Determination of reference values for total PSA, F/T and PSAD according to prostatic volume in Japanese prostate cancer patients with slightly elevated serum PSA levels. Jpn J Clin Oncol 29(12):617–622, 1999.

86. M Kuriyama, Y Kawada, Y Arai, H Maeda, S Egawa, K Koshiba, K Imai, H Yamanaka. Significance of free to total PSA ratio in men with slightly elevated serum PSA levels: A cooperative study. Jpn J Clin Oncol 28(11):661–665, 1998.

87. JT Wu, GH Liu, P Zhang, RA Stephenson. Monitoring percent free PSA in serial specimens: Improvement of test specificity, early detection, and identification of occult tumors. J Clin Lab Anal 12(1):26–31, 1998.

88. R Mione, P Barioli, M Barichello, F Zattoni, T Prayer-Galetti, M Plebani, G Aimo, C Terrone, F Manferrari, G Madeddu, L Caberlotto, A Fandella, C Pianon, L Vianello, M Gion. Prostate cancer probability after total PSA and percent free PSA determination. Int J Biol Markers 13(2):77–86, 1998.

89. M Gion, R Mione, P Barioli, M Barichello, F Zattoni, T Prayer-Galetti, M Plebani, G Aimo, C Terrone, F Manferrari, G Madeddu, L Caberlotto, A Fandella, C Pianon, L Vianello. Percent free prostate-specific antigen in assessing the probability of prostate cancer under optimal analytical conditions. Clin Chem 44(12):2462–2470, 1998.

90. D Weckermann, C Maassen, F Wawroschek, R Harzmann. Improved discrimination of prostate cancer and benign prostatic hyperplasia by means of the quotient of free and total PSA. Int Urol Nephrol 31(3):351–359, 1999.

91. J Morote, G Encabo, MA Lopez, IM De Torres. The free-to-total serum prostatic

specific antigen ratio as a predictor of the pathological features of prostate cancer. Br J Urol 83(9):1003–1006, 1999.

92. GN Collins, K Alexandrou, A Wynn-Davies, S Mobley, PH O'Reilly. Free prostate-specific antigen 'in the field': A useful adjunct to standard clinical practice. Br J Urol Int 83(9):1000–1002, 1999.

93. RW Veltri, MC Miller. Free/total PSA ratio improves differentiation of benign and malignant disease of the prostate: Critical analysis of two different test populations. Urology 53(4):736–745, 1999.

94. C Dincel, T Caskurlu, AI Tasci, M Cek, G Sevin, A Fazlioglu. Prospective evaluation of prostate specific antigen (PSA), PSA density, free-to-total PSA ratio and a new formula (prostate malignancy index) for detecting prostate cancer and preventing negative biopsies in patients with normal rectal examinations and intermediate PSA levels. Int Urol Nephrol 31(4):497–509, 1999.

95. C Mettlin, AE Chesley, GP Murphy, G Bartsch, A Toi, R Bahnson, P Church. Association of free PSA percent, total PSA, age, and gland volume in the detection of prostate cancer. Prostate 39(3):153–158, 1999.

96. K Jung, U Elgeti, M Lein, B Brux, P Sinha, B Rudolph, S Hauptmann, D Schnorr, SA Loening. Ratio of free or complexed prostate-specific antigen (PSA) to total PSA: Which ratio improves differentiation between benign prostatic hyperplasia and prostate cancer? Clin Chem 46(1):55–62, 2000.

97. WJ Catalona, AW Partin, KM Slawin, CK Naughton, MK Brawer, RC Flanigan, JP Richie, A Patel, PC Walsh, PT Scardino, PH Lange, JB deKernion, PC Southwick, KG Loveland, RE Parson, GH Gasior. Percentage of free PSA in black versus white men for detection and staging of prostate cancer: A prospective multicenter clinical trial. Urology 55(3):372–376, 2000.

98. JE Fowler JR, J Sanders, SA Bigler, J Rigdon, NK Kilambi, SA Land. Percent free prostate specific antigen and cancer detection in black and white men with total prostate specific antigen 2.5 to 9.9 ng/mL. J Urol 163(5):1467–1470, 2000.

99. TO Morgan, DG McLeod, ES Leifer, JW Moul, GP Murphy. Prospective use of free PSA to avoid repeat prostate biopsies in men with elevated total PSA. Prostate Suppl 7:58–63, 1996.

100. TO Morgan, DG McLeod, ES Leifer, GP Murphy, JW Moul. Prospective use of free prostate-specific antigen to avoid repeat prostate biopsies in men with elevated total prostate-specific antigen. Urology 48(6A Suppl):76–80, 1996.

101. WJ Catalona, JA Beiser, DS Smith. Serum free prostate specific antigen and prostate specific antigen density measurements for predicting cancer in men with prior negative prostatic biopsies. J Urol 158(6):2162–2167, 1997.

102. JL Letran, AB Blase, FR Loberiza, GE Meyer, SD Ransom, MK Brawer. Repeat ultrasound guided prostate needle biopsy: Use of free-to-total prostate specific antigen ratio in predicting prostatic carcinoma. J Urol 160(2):426–429, 1998.

103. FB Trinkler, DM Schmid, D Hauri, P Pei, FE Maly, T Sulser. Free/total prostate-specific antigen ratio can prevent unnecessary prostate biopsies. Urology 52(3): 479–486, 1998.

104. JE Fowler Jr, SA Bigler, D Miles, DA Yalkut. Predictors of first repeat biopsy cancer detection with suspected local stage prostate cancer. J Urol 163(3):813–818, 2000.

105. B Djavan, A Zlotta, M Remzi, K Ghawidel, A Basharkhah, CC Schulman, M Marb-

erger. Optimal predictors of prostate cancer on repeat prostate biopsy: A prospective study of 1051 men. J Urol 163(4):1144–1148, 2000.

106. OR Hayek, CB Noble, A de la Taille, E Bagiella, MC Benson. The necessity of a second prostate biopsy cannot be predicted by PSA or PSA derivatives (density or free: total ratio) in men with prior negative prostatic biopsies. Curr Opin Urol 9(5):371–375, 1999.

107. HB Carter, AW Partin, AA Luderer, EJ Metter, P Landis, DW Chan, JL Fozard, JD Pearson. Percentage of free prostate-specific antigen in sera predicts aggressiveness of prostate cancer a decade before diagnosis. Urology 49(3):379–384, 1997.

108. J Pannek, HG Rittenhouse, DW Chan, JI Epstein, PC Walsh, AW Partin. The use of percent free prostate specific antigen for staging clinically localized prostate cancer. J Urol 159(4):1238–1242, 1998.

109. JI Epstein, DW Chan, LJ Sokoll, PC Walsh, JL Cox, H Rittenhouse, R Wolfert, HB Carter. Nonpalpable stage T1c prostate cancer: Prediction of insignificant disease using free/total prostate specific antigen levels and needle biopsy findings. J Urol 160(6 Pt 2):2407–2411, 1998.

110. PC Southwick, WJ Catalona, AW Partin, KM Slawin, MK Brawer, RC Flanigan, A Patel, JP Richie, PC Walsh, PT Scardino, PH Lange, GH Gasior, RE Parson, KG Loveland. Prediction of post-radical prostatectomy pathological outcome for stage T1c prostate cancer with percent free prostate specific antigen: A prospective multicenter clinical trial. J Urol 162(4):1346–1351, 1999.

111. S Kilic, E Kukul, A Danisman, E Guntekin, M Sevuk. Ratio of free to total prostate-specific antigen in patients with prostatic intraepithelial neoplasia. Eur Urol 34(3): 176–180, 1998.

112. CG Ramos, GF Carvahal, DE Mager, B Haberer, WJ Catalona. The effect of high grade prostatic intraepithelial neoplasia on serum total and percentage of free prostate specific antigen levels. J Urol 162(5):1587–1590, 1999.

113. T Bjork, H Lilja, A Christensson. The prognostic value of different forms of prostate specific antigen and their ratios in patients with prostate cancer. Br J Urol Int 84(9):1021–1027, 1999.

114. K Jung, B Brux, M Lein, B Rudolph, G Kristiansen, S Hauptmann, D Schnorr, SA Loening, P Sinha. Molecular forms of prostate-specific antigen in malignant and benign prostatic tissue: Biochemical and diagnostic implications. Clin Chem 46(1): 47–54, 2000.

115. WH Henricks, BG England, DA Giacherio, JE Oesterling, KJ Wojno. Serum percent-free PSA does not predict extraprostatic spread of prostate cancer. Am J Clin Pathol 109(5):533–539, 1998.

116. J Noldus, M Graefen, E Huland, C Busch, P Hammerer, H Huland. The value of the ratio of free-to-total prostate specific antigen for staging purposes in previously untreated prostate cancer. J Urol 159(6):2004–2007, 1998.

117. H Maeda, Y Arai, S Ishitoya, K Okubo, Y Aoki, T Okada, S Maekawa. Free-to-total prostate specific antigen ratio in clinical staging of prostate cancer. Hinyokika Kiyo 44(5):307–311, 1998.

118. DW Lin, JL Noteboom, BA Blumenstein, WJ Ellis, PH Lange, RL Vessella. Serum percent free prostate-specific antigen in metastatic prostate cancer. Urology 52(3): 366–371, 1998.

119. KJ Wojno, AR Vashi, PF Schellhammer, GL Wright Jr, JE Montie. Percent free prostate-specific antigen values in men with recurrent prostate cancer after radical prostatectomy. Urology 52(3):474–478, 1998.

120. J Pannek, AW Partin. The role of PSA and percent free PSA for staging and prognosis prediction in clinically localized prostate cancer. Semin Urol Oncol 16(3):100–105, 1998.

121. J Morote, G Encabo, M Lopez, IM De Torres. Individual variations of total and percent free serum prostatic specific antigen: Could they change the indication of prostatic biopsy? Oncol Rep 6(4):887–890, 1999.

122. J Morote, CX Raventos, JA Lorente, G Enbabo, M Lopez, I de Torres. Intraindividual variations of total and percent free serum prostatic-specific antigen levels in patients with normal digital rectal examination. Eur Urol 36(2):111–115, 1999.

123. . A Semjonow, F Oberpenning, B Brandt, C Zechel, W Brandau, L Hertle. Impact of free prostate-specific antigen on discordant measurement results of assays for total prostate-specific antigen. Urology 48(6A Suppl):10–15, 1996.

124. JM Wolff, G Stocker, H Borchers, H Haubeck, H Greiling, G Jakse. Critical aspects related to the interpretation of the free-to-total PSA-ratio. Anticancer Res 19(4A): 2633–2636, 1999.

125. MP Fox, AA Reilly, E Schneider. Effect of the ratio of free to total prostate-specific antigen on interassay variability in proficiency test samples. Clin Chem 45(8 Pt 1): 1181–1189, 1999.

126. D Chautard, A Daver, B Mermod, A Tichet, V Bocquillon, J Soret. Values for the free to total prostate-specific antigen ratio as a function of age: Necessity of reference range validation. Eur Urol 36(3):181–186, 1999.

127. GP Murphy, RJ Barren, SJ Erickson, VA Bowes, RL Wolfert, G Bartsch, H Klocker, J Pointner, A Reissigl, DG McLeod, T Douglas, T Morgan, GM Kenny, H Ragde, AL Boynton, EH Holmes. Evaluation and comparison of two new prostate carcinoma markers. Free-prostate specific antigen and prostate specific membrane antigen. Cancer 78(4):809–818, 1996.

128. JG Masters, PE Keegan, AJ Hildreth, DR Greene. Free/total serum prostate-specific antigen ratio: How helpful is it in detecting prostate cancer? Br J Urol 81(3):419–423, 1998.

129. HC Klingler, H Woo, D Rosario, PE Cutinha, J Anderson, AM Ward, CR Chapple. The value of prostate specific antigen (PSA) density and free: Total PSA ratio in selecting patients with a normal digital rectal examination and intermediate total PSA levels for further investigation. Br J Urol 82(3):393–397, 1998.

130. NJ Wald, HC Watt, L George, P Knekt, KJ Helzlsouer, J Tuomilehto. Adding free to total prostate-specific antigen levels in trials of prostate cancer screening. Br J Cancer 82(3):731–736, 2000.

131. K Jung, A Meyer, M Lein, B Rudolph, D Schnorr, SA Loening. Ratio of free-to-total prostate specific antigen in serum cannot distinguish patients with prostate cancer from those with chronic inflammation of the prostate. J Urol 159(5):1595–1598, 1998.

132. T Okegawa, M Kinjo, K Watanabe, H Noda, M Kato, A Miyata, A Murata, M Yoshii, K Nutahara, E Higashihara. The significance of the free-to-complexed

prostate-specific antigen (PSA) ratio in prostate cancer detection in patients with a PSA level of 4.1–10.0 ng/mL. Br J Urol Int 85(6):708–714, 2000.

133. C Dincel, T Caskurlu, AI Tasci, M Cek, G Sevin, A Fazlioglu. Prospective evaluation of prostate specific antigen (PSA), PSA density, free-to-total PSA ratio and a new formula (prostate malignancy index) for detecting prostate cancer and preventing negative biopsies in patients with normal rectal examinations and intermediate PSA levels. Int Urol Nephrol 31(4):497–509, 1999.

134. MK Kwiatkowski, F Recker, T Piironen, K Pettersson, T Otto, M Wernli, R Tscholl. In prostatism patients the ratio of human glandular kallikrein to free PSA improves the discrimination between prostate cancer and benign hyperplasia within the diagnostic "gray zone" of total PSA 4 to 10 ng/mL. Urology 52(3): 360–365, 1998.

135. AW Partin, WJ Catalona, JA Finlay, C Darte, DJ Tindall, CY Young, GG Klee, DW Chan, HG Rittenhouse, RL Wolfert, DL Woodrum. Use of human glandular kallikrein 2 for the detection of prostate cancer: Preliminary analysis. Urology 54(5):839–845, 1999.

136. A Magklara, A Scorilas, WJ Catalona, EP Diamandis. The combination of human glandular kallikrein and free prostate-specific antigen (PSA) enhances discrimination between prostate cancer and benign prostatic hyperplasia in patients with moderately increased total PSA. Clin Chem 45(11):1960–1966, 1999.

137. C Becker, T Piironen, K Pettersson, T Bjork, KJ Wojno, JE Oesterling, H Lilja. Discrimination of men with prostate cancer from those with benign disease by measurements of human glandular kallikrein 2 (HK2) in serum. J Urol 163(1):311–316, 2000.

138. A Haese, C Becker, J Noldus, M Graefen, E Huland, H Huland, H Lilja. Human glandular kallikrein 2: A potential serum marker for predicting the organ confined versus non-organ confined growth of prostate cancer. J Urol 163(5):1491–1497, 2000.

139. Y Chen, AA Luderer, RP Thiel, G Carlson, CL Cuny, TF Soriano. Using proportions of free to total prostate-specific antigen, age, and total prostate-specific antigen to predict the probability of cancer. Urology 47(4):518–524, 1996.

140. AF Prestigiacomo, H Lilja, K Pettersson, RL Wolfert, TA Stamey. A comparison of the free fraction of serum prostate specific antigen in men with benign and cancerous prostates: the best case scenario. J Urol 156(2 Pt 1):350–354, 1996.

141. AA Elgamal, FJ Cornillie, HP Van Poppel, WM Van de Voorde, R McCabe, LV Baert. Free-to-total prostate specific antigen ratio as a single test for detection of significant stage T1c prostate cancer. J Urol 156(3):1042–1047, 1996.

142. PJ Van Cangh, P De Nayer, P Sauvage, B Tombal, M Elsen, F Lorge, R Opsomer, FX Wese. Free to total prostate-specific antigen (PSA) ratio is superior to total-PSA in differentiating benign prostate hypertrophy from prostate cancer. Prostate Suppl 7:30–34, 1996.

143. DL Woodrum, MK Brawer, AW Partin, WJ Catalona, PC Southwick. Interpretation of free prostate specific antigen clinical research studies for the detection of prostate cancer. J Urol 159(1):5–12, 1998.

8

Alpha-1-Antichymotrypsin Complexed Prostate Specific Antigen

Michael K. Brawer
Northwest Prostate Institute, Seattle, Washington

Prostate specific antigen (PSA) is the most important tumor marker in human oncology. Indeed, those who deal with other cancers would welcome the availability of such a marker. The fact that those of us who treat patients with prostate cancer have such a beneficial tool in our armamentarium has stimulated a number of us to try and improve on its performance. As reviewed in previous chapters, these efforts have primarily been associated with enhancement in test specificity, at least in early detection and screening applications. This results from the observation that a false-negative test (low sensitivity) is less important if repeat testing is available. Conversely, false-positive tests (low specificity) are expensive. This is obvious in economic terms, since all of the cost of biopsy is incurred. However, false-positive results are expensive psychologically due to their associated stress. Efforts to enhance specificity have resulted in the utilization of so-called PSA derivatives, including age specific PSA, PSA velocity, and PSA density as well as the measurement of PSA isoforms.

The biochemistry of PSA forms in the bloodstream and the decreased ratio of free to total PSA in men with malignancy relative to those without has been well reviewed in Chapter 2 To reiterate briefly, once PSA gains access to the systemic circulation, the majority becomes complexed to protease inhibitors including alpha-1-antichymotrypsin (ACT) and alpha-2-macroglobulin. The former actually occurs to a greater proportion in men with malignancy. This latter observation has been recognized for a number of years.

Considerable effort has been expended in creating a specific assay for the ACT-complexed form of PSA (CPSA). Only recently have specific assays for the ACT-complexed form been realized [1–3]. The benefits of a specific assay

Table 1 Diagnosis Performance at Set Levels of Sensitivity

% Sensitivity	Hybritech Free/total PSA		Dianon Free PSA/Hybritech Total PSA		Chiron Free PSA/Hybritech Total PSA	
	% Free/total cut-off	Specificity	% Free/total cut-off	Specificity	% Free/total cut-off	Specificity
2.0–20 ng/ml range (25 with Ca, 100 with no evidence of malignancy)						
90	20	44	33	22	34	33
95	22	38	34	19	35	32
100	29	16	42	13	43	16
2.0–10 ng/ml, range (18 with Ca, 87 with no evidence of malignancy)						
90	20	45	33	23	33	38
95	22	38	34	19	35	36
100	29	15	40	15	42	21

Table 2 Comparison of the Sensitivity and Specificity of Total PSA and the Free to Total PSA Ratio

Assay	Sensitivity (%)	Specificity (%) total PSA	Specificity (%) F/T PSA	Cut-point total PSA (ng/ml)	Cut-point F/T PSA (%)
ACS: 180 PSA 2 and free PSA	100	0	0	0.02	90
	95	10	17	1.7	25
	90	25	54	3.3	15
Enzymum PSA and free PSA	100	0	0	0.02	100
	95	5	7	1.1	43
	90	24	32	3.0	23
Tandem-R PSA and free PSA	100	1	1	0.4	52
	95	7	22	2.1	25
	90	17	31	3.4	21

Data from all patients in the BPH and prostate cancer groups are included.

for the complexed form of PSA are numerous. One would expect that such an assay would provide the same specificity enhancement realized with the free to total PSA but would require only the measurement of a single analyte. In addition to the economic advantage of only a single test over measuring both the free and the total form of PSA, several other benefits accrue. One is avoiding the variability of different manufacturers' assays, which leads to the lack of uniformity in total PSA or free PSA measured by different manufacturers. This important issue is discussed in detail in Chapter 3.

Although effort has been expended to create an international standard for PSA testing, particularly led by the efforts of Thomas Stamey [4–6] at Stanford, no consensus, has been reached. This creates obvious problems when one is comparing literature values, for example, a cutoff of the free to total PSA with the clinically determined level on an individual patient. Unless the same assay by the same manufacturer is used, different results may accrue.

For example, we have investigated three different free forms of PSA and kept the total form constant [7]. Significant differences were observed in the free to total PSA ratio. This resulted in large differences in the degree of specificity enhancement realized by different manufacturers' free PSA (Table 1).

In a subsequent investigation, we used the same manufacturer's products for both the free and total PSA determinations [8]. Even with this constraint, which may not be realized in the clinical laboratory, we observed considerable differences in the value for the free to total PSA obtained as well as its utility as evidenced by enhanced specificity (Table 2). Thus, in our opinion the measurement of free to total PSA ratio is fraught with problems.

I. INITIAL STUDIES WITH cPSA

We were encouraged by the development of assays purported to be specific for the complex form of PSA [1–3]. We set out to evaluate the diagnostic utility of the Bayer Immuno-One assay in a series of men undergoing ultrasound-guided prostate needle biopsy [9]. We selected patients for this investigation from our archival serum bank; the only constraint given was to provide a 25% prostate cancer yield. This reflects the overall experience in our ultrasound-guided biopsy series.

Sera were processed soon after collection and stored at $-80°$. There was no freeze–thaw. We measured each sample with the Bayer complex PSA and the Hybritech free and total PSA methods according to manufacturers' specifications. All assays were performed by a single technician during a 24 hr period without a freeze–thaw cycle.

All men had undergone an ultrasound-guided systematic sector biopsy with a minimum of six cores obtained. They range in aged from 43 to 93 years, with a mean age of 67.7 ± 7.72 years. There was no difference in the age of men with and without malignancy.

To access the capture of the complex form of PSA we performed a regression analysis comparing the Hybritech total PSA and the sum of the complex PSA by Bayer with the Hybritech free level (Fig. 1). While there is a close approximation to a slope of one, there is a slight positive bias, perhaps indicating measurement of some complex PSA with the free assay or, conversely, some free PSA with the complex assay method.

In Table 3 the values for total, complex, and free to total PSA values are noted. As expected, higher total and complex PSA levels were measured in men with malignancy and higher free to total PSA ratios in men without. These findings were echoed in the more truncated range of a total PSA between 4 and 10 ng/ml (the so-called gray zone) (Table 4).

A number of ways of depicting the observation from different testing approaches have been used in the literature. Many authorities have utilized the receiver operator characteristic curve analysis. We have found this clinically irrelevant because, except for the upper right hand corner of such a graphic display, the data are clinically unimportant. With sensitivities less than about 90%, the test result is inadequate for clinical cancer detection. Thus, the so-called area under the curve comparisons of different methods of PSA enhancement may

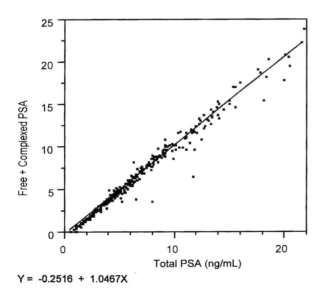

Y = -0.2516 + 1.0467X

Figure 1   Regression between the complexed PSA and total PSA (a lone outlier was removed from the analysis).

Table 3 Total PSA, Complexed PSA, and % Free/Total PSA Values for the Entire Study Population: Men with Prostate Cancer and Men with Benign Histological Findings

	All (n = 300)	CAP (n = 75)	NEM (n = 225)	p value
Total PSA (ng/ml)				
Mean	7.06	10.0	6.08	
Median	5.69	8.02	5.05	<0.0001
S.D.	6.85	11.42	3.96	
Range	0.51–99.16	1.25–99.16	0.16–6.18	
95% CI	6.28–7.84	7.38–12.62	5.56–6.60	
Complex PSA (ng/ml)				
Mean	5.93	8.85	4.95	
Median	4.61	7.56	3.94	<0.0001
S.D.	5.98	9.61	3.67	
Range	0.08–83.1	0.91–83.1	0.08–19.73	
95% CI	5.25–6.61	6.64–11.06	4.47–5.43	
Free/total PSA (%)				
Mean	0.18	0.15	0.2	
Median	0.17	0.17	0.18	<0.0001
S.D.	0.09	0.09	0.09	
Range	0.0–0.67	0.0–0.67	0.0–0.55	
95% CI	0.17–0.19	0.13–0.17	0.19–0.21	

CAP, prostate cancer; NEM, no evidence of malignancy; CI, confidence interval.

show a benefit of one approach that is only realized at low level of sensitivity that most clinicians would find inadequate for clinical testing. We prefer to report our results at given sensitivity cutoffs. We believe that in general at least a 95% sensitivity (i.e., willingness to allow missing the diagnosis of carcinoma in only 5% of men) is required.

Table 5 shows the sensitivity analysis for our initial study of complex PSA. As noted, at the 95% sensitivity level, the specificity for total PSA is 22%. Complex PSA with a cutoff of 2.52 would provide 95% sensitivity with an increased specificity of 26.7%. In this study, the free to total PSA ratio required for 95% sensitivity was 28%. This afforded only a 15.6% specificity.

The decreased performance of free to total PSA in this series may reflect the not well recognized instability of the free form of PSA with long-term storage. Degradation of the free form would result in decrease in specificity. We have shown that the ACT-complex is exceedingly stable in specimens stored for 18 months (Fig. 2) [10].

Table 4 Total PSA, Complexed PSA, and % Free/Total PSA Values for the Entire Study Population: Men with Prostate Cancer and Men with Benign Histological Findings

	All (n = 153)	CAP (n = 36)	NEM (n = 117)	p value
Total PSA (ng/ml)				
Mean	6.40	7.11	6.19	0.0038
Median	6.13	7.01	5.88	0.0045
S.D.	1.69	1.70	1.63	
Range	4.01–9.9	4.01–9.9	4.01–9.82	
95% CI	5.70–6.47	6.57–7.65	5.98–6.40	
Complex PSA (ng/ml)				
Mean	5.49	6.61	5.14	<0.0001
Median	5.22	6.6	4.69	<0.0001
S.D.	1.84	1.78	1.72	
Range	2.52–9.95	2.52–9.95	3.36–9.62	
95% CI	5.20–5.78	6.00–7.21	4.89–5.39	
Free/total PSA (%)				
Mean	0.17	0.15	0.18	0.0152
Median	0.17	0.14	0.17	0.0137
S.D.	0.07	0.06	0.07	
Range	0.04–0.43	0.04–0.32	0.05–0.43	
95% CI	0.16–0.18	0.13–0.17	0.16–0.20	

Findings are based on total PSA range at 4–10 ng/ml. Abbreviations as in Table 3.

Table 5 Specificity of Cut-Off Values of Different PSA Assays at Selected Sensitivities: Entire Total PSA Range

% Sensitivity	Total PSA		Complexed PSA		Free/Total PSA	
	Cut-off (ng/ml)	% Specificity	Cut-off (ng/ml)	% Specificity	Cut-off (%)	% Specificity
80	4.11	35.6	3.98	51.6	19	46.2
85	3.86	31.1	3.34	38.7	22	32.4
90	3.4	25.3	2.94	33.8	24	26.2
95	3.06	21.8	2.52	26.7	28	15.6
97.5	2.28	12.9	1.67	14.7	32	8.9
100	1.0	3.1	0.89	6.2	67	0

18 mo. CPSA STABILITY

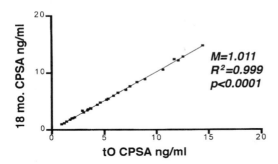

Figure 2   CPSA stability at 18 months. (From Ref. 10.)

In the more truncated range of a total PSA of 4–10 ng/ml we again showed significant enhancement and specificity with the complexed form of PSA. These data are shown in Table 6. At the 95% sensitivity there was a reduction of the specificity of complex PSA. However, it was higher than the free to total PSA at the 90 and 100% sensitivity levels. This suggests an artifact due to low numbers at this high sensitivity level.

These findings are depicted graphically in Figure 3. Lines have been drawn at the 4.0 ng/ml cut-off for PSA and 3.75 for the complexed PSA. Note the 35 men in the lower right hand quadrant (of whom only 1 had carcinoma) who have a total PSA greater than 4 ng/ml but a complex PSA less than 3.75 ng/ml. With the use of complexed PSA and a threshold for biopsy of 7.5, all of these latter men could potentially have avoided undergoing a biopsy.

Table 6   Specificity of Cut-Off Values of Different PSA Assays at Selected Sensitivities: Total PSA Range of 4.0–10.0 ng/ml

	Total PSA		Complexed PSA		Free/Total PSA	
% Sensitivity	Cut-off (ng/ml)	% Specificity	Cut-off (ng/ml)	% Specificity	Cut-off (%)	% Specificity
80	5.27	38.1	4.55	43.9	20	29.8
85	4.66	22.9	4.21	34.2	22	25.4
90	4.01	0.8	3.92	25.4	24	19.3
95	4.0	0	3.36	7.9	29	11.4
100	4.0	0	3.26	7	34	4.4

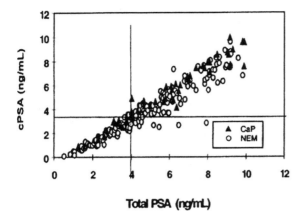

Figure 3 Regression analysis compares different cut-offs for complexed PSA (cPSA) and total PSA. CaP, prostate cancer; NEM, no evidence of malignancy. (From Ref. 9.)

Recently, Stamey and associates [11] compared the Bayer complexed PSA assay with three manufacturers' free and total PSA measurements. In their investigation, the complex PSA was only slightly better than the total PSA and free to total PSA provided much greater improvement. Although these findings are certainly at odds with our study, several differences in patient selection between the two sites may explain these results.

The Stanford series was comprised of 160 men, 90 of whom who had benign findings. To be considered without malignancy men had to have two sets of six negative systematic sector biopsies. We applaud the Stanford group in utilizing such a criteria for absence of carcinoma, but this may introduce a bias relative to what is observed in general clinical practice. Furthermore, men with cancer were selected to have a minimum of 5 mm of cancer in the biopsy, which is a constraint that we did employ.

Perhaps of greater importance was the observation in the Stanford study of no difference in total serum PSA between men with and without malignancy. In our series, as shown in Tables 3 and 4, the total PSA was significantly greater in men with malignancy. For reasons that are obscure, in the Stanford group there was no difference in total PSA despite the use of three different manufacturers' assays (Bayer, Hybritech, and DPC) in the total PSA. Since most clinicians observe higher PSA levels in men with cancer, this may provide an additional reason for the discrepancy in the utility of complex PSA observed by the Stanford group. Another discrepancy in their series is the exceedingly low specificity observed with total PSA (Table 7).

Table 7 CPSA in Biopsy Series

Author	No. men	No. cap	Analyte	Specificity @ 90% sensitivity	Specificity @ 95% sensitivity
Brawer [9]	225	75	TPSA	25	22
			F/T PSA	26	16
			CPSA	34	27
Brawer [12]	385[a]	237[b]	TPSA	28	18
			F/T PSA	31	23
			CPSA	32	24
Croal [15]	58	21	TPSA	52	43
			F/T PSA	54	52
			CPSA	60	57
Jung [16]	40[c]	40[d]	TPSA	18	—
			F/T PSA	55	—
			CPSA	25	—
Maeda [17][e]	114	23	TPSA	24	13
			F/T PSA	18	18
			CPSA	27	15
Mitchell [18]	109	51	TPSA	33[g], 24[h]	17[g], 16[h]
			F/T PSA	32[g], 32[h]	16[g], 19[h]
			CPSA	47	25
Sokoll [19][f]	60	76	TPSA	40	35
			F/T PSA	—	—
			CPSA	42	37
Stamey [11]	90	70	TPSA	12	4
			F/T PSA	47	29
			CPSA	14	10

[a] Includes 225 cases from Brawer [9].
[b] Includes 75 cases from Brawer [9].
[c] Selected from 89 patients to simulate overlapping TPSA values.
[d] Selected from 144 patients to simulate overlapping TPSA values.
[e] 91% specificity reported.
[f] 96% specificity reported.
[g] Bayer assays.
[h] Abbott assays.

II. COMPLEX PSA MULTICENTER TRIAL

In an effort to understand further the utility of the complex form of PSA, we have expanded our Seattle series by incorporating patients evaluated at the Johns Hopkins University by Dr. Alan Partin as well as a small cohort derived from a multicenter screening trial that is underway [12]. In this investigation, 272 men with carcinoma detected on ultrasound-guided biopsy were contrasted with 385 men with benign findings [12]. The Bayer complex PSA was compared with the Hybritech total and free assays according to manufacturers' specifications. Table 8 demonstrates the distribution of PSA levels in men with and without malignancy. The medium, free, complex, and total PSA as well as the free-to-total PSA ratio along with the interquartile range may be found in Table 9. As in our prior series, a significantly higher total, complex, and lower free to total PSA ratio was found in those in men with malignancy (p < 0.0001).

Sensitivity analysis for this investigation is shown in Tables 10 and 11. For the overall series, at the 95% sensitivity level, total PSA provided 18% specificity at a cutoff of 3.06. The complex PSA afforded a 24% specificity at a cutoff value of 2.75 ng/ml. The free to total PSA ratio at the 95% sensitivity level with a cutoff of 23.9% afforded a 23% specificity.

In Table 11 the sensitivity analysis over the more truncated range of total PSA between 4 and 10 ng/ml is demonstrated. At the 95% sensitivity level a cutoff of 4.24 afforded only a 7% specificity for total PSA. Complex PSA with a cut-off of 3.70 resulted in an 18% specificity, which is very similar to the 17% shown with the free to total ratio of 23.9%.

The optimum cut-off for complex PSA has not been established. Table 12 indicates the performance of total PSA, complex PSA, and free to total PSA ratio at commonly utilized cut-offs of 4.0, 3.75, and 25% respectively. When these cut-offs are used, the complex PSA affords approximately equal sensitivity to the free-to-total PSA ratio over various total PSA ranges but with enhanced specificity. As shown in Table 12, the sensitivity of complex PSA and the free to total PSA ratio are fairly similar, although they are lower than achieved with total PSA. In contrast, while the free-to-total PSA ratio provides 8% improvement in specificity in all samples and 13% improvement in samples in the range of 4–10 ng/ml of total PSA, the complex PSA assay had a 13% improved specificity in all samples and a 21% improvement in the gray zone of 4–10 ng/ml. An intriguing finding is that in the range of 4–6 ng/ml for total PSA, the complex PSA assay provides an even greater increase in specificity of 37% compared to only 13% with the free to total PSA ratio.

This latter finding intrigued us and we carried out an analysis of the specificity enhancement with complex PSA over various total PSA ranges. These data are shown in Figure 4. In this analysis we contrasted the chance of identifying a negative biopsy correctly utilizing a complex PSA cutoff of 3.75 ng/ml in

Table 8 Distribution of Men With and Without Malignancy at Each Site Stratified by Total PSA

Site	No. Pts. No Evidence of Malignancy			No. Pts. Prostate Ca		
	Total	4–10 ng/ml PSA	4–6 ng/ml PSA	Total	4–10 ng/ml PSA	4–6 ng/ml PSA
Seattle	225	117	64	75	36	9
Baltimore	104	86	46	143	133	54
Bayer multisite	56	34	17	54	33	11
Totals	385	237	127	272	202	74

Table 9 Median Values of Free, Complexed, and Total PSA, and the Free to Total PSA Ratio in 385 Patients with No Evidence of Malignancy and 272 with Prostate Cancer

	Median ng/ml (interquartile range)		
PSA Test	No evidence of malignancy	Prostate Ca	p Value
Free	0.89 (0.71)	0.83 (0.63)	0.30
Complexed	4.34 (3.38)	5.93 (3.56)	0.001
Total	5.4 (3.81)	6.66 (3.63)	0.001
Free-to-total	17.18 (10.21)	12.02 (8.11)	0.001

contrast to a free to total PSA ratio of 25%. As was observed, the benefit of the complexed to total PSA ratio is greater primarily in the lower range of total PSA: between 4.0 and 6.0 ng/ml. At higher levels, the free to total PSA offers greater enhancement.

These findings need to be put into the context of what is observed in early detection programs. For example, in Figure 5 we have demonstrated the total PSA in men recruited through media in an ongoing early detection program at Northwest Hospital in Seattle. As is readily apparent, far more men have a total PSA between 4 and 6 than greater than 6 in an early detection cohort. These data would suggest that the complex PSA will provide a greater benefit in early detection than the free to total ratio, since higher percentage of patients' results will fall into the range of total PSA where complex PSA affords the best stratification.

Table 10 Specificity of Total and Complexed PSA, and the Free to Total PSA Ratio for All Samples within the Sensitivity Range of 80–95%

	Total PSA		Complexed PSA		Free-to-Total PSA Ratio	
% Sensitivity	Cut-off (ng/ml)	% Specificity	Cut-off (ng/ml)	% Specificity	Cut-off (ng/ml)	% Specificity
80	4.64	41	4.09	46	17.1	52[a,b]
85	4.33	33	3.79	41[a]	18.9	42[a]
90	3.99	28	3.40	32	20.9	31
95	3.06	18	2.75	24[a]	23.9	23[a]

[a] Significantly different from total PSA.
[b] Significantly different from complexed PSA.

Table 11 Specificity of Total and Complexed PSA, and the Free to Total PSA Ratio within the Sensitivity Range of 80–95% for Samples in the Total PSA Range 4–10 ng/ml

% Sensitivity	Total PSA		Complexed PSA		Free to Total PSA Ratio	
	Cut-off (ng/ml)	% Specificity	Cut-off (ng/ml)	% Specificity	Cut-off (ng/ml)	% Specificity
80	5.06	30	4.37	37	17.10	48[a,b]
85	4.67	21	4.19	31[a]	18.90	34[a]
90	4.42	11	3.94	25	20.50	25[a]
95	4.24	7	3.70	18[a]	23.30	17[a]

[a] Significantly different from total PSA.
[b] Significantly different from complexed PSA.

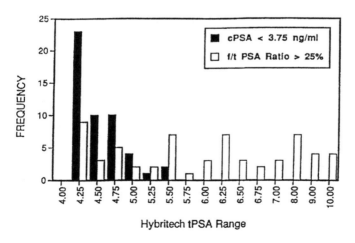

Figure 4 Incidence of patients with no evidence of malignancy and total (t) PSA in 4–10 ng/ml range with complexed PSA less than 3.75 ng/ml and free to total (f/t) PSA ratio greater than 25%. (From Ref. 12.)

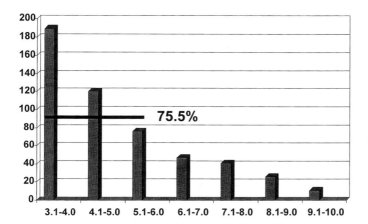

Figure 5 Total PSA 3.0–10.0 ng/ml in a contemporary screening cohort (n = 2375, 510 between 3.0–10.0 ng/ml).

III. cPSA ADDITIONAL STUDIES

Table 7 summarizes the literature of cPSA in populations who have undergone biopsy. As noted, all series demonstrate, at clinically relevant sensitivity levels, enhanced performance of cPSA compared with TPSA. Most rival that afforded by the free/total PSA ratio. The discrepancy noted in the Stamey paper [11] has been discussed above. The Jung Study [11] is difficult to evaluate for two reasons. This represents the highly select cohort. For example, the median PSA in men with cancer was 8.30 ng/ml compared with only 1.88 ng/ml for men without. For the sensitivity analysis the authors chose to "match" total PSA in the benign and malignant subjects, resulting in a subset of only 40 of 89 men with benign findings compared with 40 of 144 men with prostate cancer. The ability to extrapolate these data to routine clinical practice is doubtful.

IV. CPSA IN MEN WITH TOTAL PSA < 4.0 NG/ML

We have evaluated the utility of cPSA in men with TPSA < 4.0 ng/ml.) [13]. Ninety-eight men were studied and 12 had carcinoma. Table 13 shows the significant findings. Both free/total and cPSA provide specificity enhancement. For example, at the 83% sensitivity level (not unreasonable given the lower prevalence

Table 12 Sensitivity and Specificity of the Various PSA Assays at Published Cut-Off Values

		Sensitivity					Specificity		
Total PSA range	No. pts.	Total PSA	Complexed PSA	Free to total PSA ratio	No. pts.	Total PSA	Complexed PSA	Free to total PSA ratio
Cut-off (ng/ml)		4.0	3.75	25% when total PSA greater than 4 and less than 10		4.0	3.75	25% When total PSA greater than 4 and less than 10
All concentrations	272	90	85	86	385	28	41	36
4–10 ng/ml	201	100	93	96	237	0	21	13
4–6 ng/ml	74	100	81	100	127	0	37	13

Table 13 Utility of cPSA and % FPSA in Men Undergoing Biopsy with TPSA <4.0 ng/ml

Sensitivity	cPSA Cut-off (ng/ml)	cPSA Spec (%)	% FPSA Cutoff	% FPSA Spec
62	2.5	62	22	48
83	1.5	51	24	45
100	0.9	30	25	44

of cancer in the cohort) complex PSA would allow one to avoid 51% of negative biopsies, and the % free 45% at cut-offs of 1.5 ng/ml and 24%, respectively.

V. CONCLUSION

The complex form of PSA has been approved for the monitoring of men with prostatic carcinoma. In a multicenter investigation of the clinical utility of complexed PSA compared to total PSA for monitoring patients with established malignancy, no difference was observed [14]. These findings would suggest that the complex form of PSA may serve as a substitute for total PSA in all current applications.

REFERENCES

1. WJ Allard, Z Zhou, KK Yeung. Novel immunoassay for the measurement of complexed prostate-specific antigen in serum. Clin Chem 44(6):1216–1223, 1998.
2. K Chichibu, K Kuroe, C Hashimoto, et al. Specific quantification of gamma-seminoprotein-alpha 1 antichymotrypsin complex in serum by monoclonal antibody-based enzyme immunoassay. Jpn J Clin Pathol (Rinsho Byori) 43:1153–1158, 1995.
3. M Kuriyama, K Euno, et al. Clinical evaluation of serum prostate-specific antigen-alpha$_1$-antichymotrypsin complex values in diagnosis of prostate cancer: A cooperative study. Int J Urol 5:48–54, 1998.
4. TA Stamey. Progress in standardization of immunoassays for prostate-specific antigen. Urol Clin North Am 24(2):269–273, 1997.
5. Z Chen, A Prestigiacomo, TA Stamey. Purification and characterization of prostate-specific antigen (PSA) complex alpha 1-antichymotrypsin: potential reference material for international standardization of PSA immunoassays. Clin Chem 41(9):1273–1282, 1995.
6. TA Stamey. Second Stanford conference on international standardization of PSA immunoassays: September 1 and 2, 1994. Urology 45(2):173–184, 1995.

7. RG Nixon, MH Gold, AB Blase, GE Meyer, MK Brawer. Comparison of three investigative assays for the free form of prostate-specific antigen. J Urol 160:420–425, 1998.

8. HJ Roth, S Christensen-Stewart, MK Brawer. A comparison of three free and total PSA assays. PCPD 1(6):326–331, 1998.

9. MK Brawer, GE Meyer, JL Letran, et al. Measurement of complexed PSA improves specificity for early detection of prostate cancer. Urology 52(3):372–378, 1998.

10. LF Ferreri, DD Bankson, MK Brawer. Long-term stability of complex prostate specific antigen (PSA) in frozen serum. J Urol (suppl) 161:318, 1999.

11. TA Stamey, CE Yemoto. Examination of the 3 molecular forms of serum prostate specific antigen for distinguishing negative from positive biopsy: Relationship to transition zone volume. J Urol 163(1):119–126, 2000.

12. MK Brawer, CD Cheli, IE Neaman, et al. Complexed prostate specific antigen provides significant enhancement of specificity compared with total prostate specific antigen for detecting prostate cancer. J Urol 163:1476–1480, 2000.

13. E Yu, S McNight, LF Ferreri, MK Brawer. Prostate needle biopsy in men with total prostate specific antigen (PSA) less than 4.0 ng/ml: the role of complex PSA (cPSA). J Urol (Suppl) 159:321, 1998.

14. WJ Allard, CD Cheli, DL Morris, et al. Multicenter evaluation of the performance and clinical utility in longitudinal monitoring of the Bayer Immuno 1 complexed PSA assay. Int J Biol Markers 14:73–83, 1999.

15. BL Croal, IDC Mitchell, A Dickie, et al. Complexed PSA and complexed PSA/prostatic volume ratio in the diagnosis of prostatic carcinoma. Clin Chem (Suppl) 45:A108, 1999.

16. K Jung, U Elgeti, M Lein, et al. Ratio of free or complexed prostate-specific antigen (PSA) to total PSA: Which ratio improves differentiation between benign prostatic hyperplasia and prostate cancer? Clin Chem 46(1):55–62, 2000.

17. H Maeda, Y Arai, Y Aoki, K Okubo, T Okada, S Maekawa. Complexed prostate-specific antigen and its volume indexes in the detection of prostate cancer. Urology 54(2):225–228, 1999.

18. I Mitchell, B Croal, A Dickie, N Cohen, I Ross. A prospective study to evaluate the role of complexed prostate specific antigen and free to total prostate specifici ratio in the diagnosis of prostate cancer. J Urol 2000 (submitted).

19. LI Sokoll, JL Cox, DJ Bruzek, et al. Clinical utility of complexed PSA. Clin Chem (Suppl) 44:A46, 1998.

9
PSA and Early Detection

David K. Ornstein
University of North Carolina, Chapel Hill, North Carolina

Alfredo Velasco
Catholic University Hospital, Santiago, Chile

Gerald L. Andriole
Washington University, St. Louis, Missouri

Symptoms related to prostate cancer usually do not manifest themselves until spread beyond the prostate has occurred, at which point curative therapy is not possible. Therefore, the opportunity to cure prostate cancer depends on detection prior to the onset of symptoms. Physicians have historically relied on the digital rectal examination for early prostate cancer detection. Unfortunately, digital rectal examination alone is not adequate, and results in metastatic or locally advanced disease in 70–80% of patients at the time of diagnosis.

Researchers in the early 1980s demonstrated that serum prostate specific antigen (PSA) was a sensitive test for advanced prostate cancer and was a useful biomarker to monitor prostate cancer progression. In the late 1980s it was shown that PSA was also a sensitive biomarker for localized prostate cancer and that serum measurements could aid in early detection of prostate cancer [1,2]. Since that time, the implementation of PSA-based prostate cancer screening has become widespread, and it is estimated that today more that 75% of prostate cancers are detected based on an ''abnormal'' PSA test result [3,4]. Despite the apparent widespread acceptance of PSA testing, the appropriateness of prostate cancer screening is a topic of great debate. Some cite that, to date, no randomized controlled study has demonstrated PSA screening to be an effective means of reducing prostate cancer morbidity/mortality, and that widespread testing should not be encouraged. Others point to substantial inferential evidence suggesting that

PSA-based prostate cancer screening is responsible for the recently observed reductions in prostate cancer mortality. This controversy is exemplified by the disparate recommendations propounded by different medical organizations. For example, both the American Urologic and the American Cancer Associations recommend annual PSA testing, while other organizations such as the American Academy of Family Physicians do not [5–7].

This chapter will review evidence supporting the value of PSA testing, and then discuss some strategies to improve the efficacy and efficiency of prostate cancer screening. There are several important criteria required for a test to be considered a useful cancer screening tool. The prevalence of the disease must be sufficiently common within the general population or within selected cohorts of at-risk subjects to warrant systematic screening. An effective management strategy (either a more definitive diagnostic test or a therapeutic intervention) for positive results of screening must be clearly defined and the cost and morbidity of false-positive screening must be acceptable. An effective screening test must be sensitive enough that it has a reasonable chance of detecting the disease, but should not detect "clinically irrelevant" cancers that would not otherwise have been discovered. In other words, implementation of an effective screening test should not result in a long-term increase in disease incidence. An effective test should detect cancers at an earlier stage than previously used detection methods, and should primarily detect curable cancers. An effective and minimally morbid treatment for the cancer must be available, and the effectiveness of the therapy should be enhanced by early detection. A useful screening test should possess sufficient specificity and the cost and morbidity of false-positive results should be relatively minimal. The screening test's eventual result should be to reduce morbidity and mortality for affected and at-risk patients.

I. PROSTATE CANCER PREVALENCE

Prostate cancer is the most common noncutaneous malignancy in American men, and is the leading cause of death due to cancer among men in the United States [8]. The incidence of prostate cancer-related death is similar to or greater than other cancers for which widespread screening programs have already been accepted (Table 1). It is estimated in the year 2000 that 31,900 men will die from prostate cancer, 40,800 women from breast cancer, and 22,100 men from colon cancer [8]. The lifetime risk of prostate cancer is now 1:8 and the disease has no racial or hereditary barriers. Therefore, all men are at risk for prostate cancer and could potentially benefit from early detection. The effectiveness of systematic PSA-based prostate cancer screening is exemplified by results of several large screening trials. These trials have demonstrated that 10–15% of American men

Table 1 Incidence, Mortality, and Lifetime Risk for the Four Most Common Solid Tumors in the United States

Cancer	New cases per year	Deaths per year	Lifetime risk
Breast (female)	182,800	40,800	1:8
Prostate	180,400	31,900	1:6
Lung (male)	89,500	89,300	1:12
Colon/rectal (male)	63,600	27,800	1:18

Source: Ref. 8.

will have an "abnormal" PSA test (> 4 ng/ml), and 2–3% will have prostate cancer detected [9].

II. SAFETY AND EFFICACY OF PROSTATE BIOPSY

The diagnosis of prostate cancer is always made histologically. The ability to obtain prostate tissue samples safely and efficiently from men is a critical factor in the success of PSA-based detection strategies. Ultrasound-guided transrectal biopsy of the prostate was pioneered in the 1980s and is currently used to facilitate a systematic sampling of the prostate. This outpatient procedure can be performed in less than 10 min and results in minimal morbidity. In fact, in a series of more than 1,500 men undergoing transrectal ultrasound-guided sextant biopsies of the prostate, low-grade fever was reported in 4.2% and sepsis in only 0.4% [10].

Random systematic sextant biopsy is a common technique practiced by most urologists today; however, this strategy may not be optimal for all men. Studies have shown that nearly 25% of men undergoing radical prostatectomy for clinically localized prostate cancer required at least two biopsy sessions before prostate cancer was diagnosed [11]. The histological characteristics of cancers detected by more than one set of biopsies are not more likely to be indolent than cancers detected by a single set of biopsies suggesting that clinically important prostate cancers are missed by current biopsy strategies [12,13]. Furthermore, computer simulation [14] and mathematical modeling [15] have determined that more than six cores are needed for some men in order to minimize the chance of missing a clinically significant cancer. Several researchers have shown, in nonrandomized, retrospective studies, that obtaining additional tissue cores (i.e., more than the standard six) may reduce that number of missed cancers. Escew et al. reported that adding four laterally and three medially directed biopsies improved cancer detection by 35% compared to standard sextant biopsies [16]. Levine et al. confirmed these general findings using a somewhat different biopsy protocol. They showed that performing 2 sets of sextant biopsies (i.e., 12 laterally directed cores) improved overall cancer detection by 30% [17]. Men with prostates larger than 50 g experienced a 63% improvement in cancer detection compared to 21% for men with prostates smaller than 30 g. However, a large randomized trial comparing the efficacy of 6 and 12 biopsy cores failed to detect a difference in cancer detection, and the optimal number of biopsy cores remains to be determined [18]. Performance of six additional biopsy cores did not increase morbidity. The authors concluded that further study of this issue was warranted.

Approximately 20% of clinically relevant prostate cancers arise from the transition zone [19] but a majority are associated with additional peripheral zone cancers [20]. Standard sextant biopsies generally do not sample the transition zone. Several studies have shown that routine transition zone biopsies in men undergoing their initial prostate biopsy are not beneficial [21–23]. However, studies have shown that additional transition zone biopsies may improve cancer detection when repeat biopsies are taken of men with persistently elevated PSA levels. Fleshner et al. showed that adding transition zone biopsies in this setting improved cancer detection by 16% in 156 men with a mean PSA of 11.4 ng/ml [23]. Lui et al. showed a 53% improvement in cancer detection among 47 men with a previously negative biopsy and a mean PSA of 34.6 ng/ml [24]. Collectively these studies suggest that transition zone biopsies are only indicated among men who have previously shown negative results on a sextant biopsy and have a persistently elevated PSA level.

III. IMPACT OF PROSTATE CANCER SCREENING

A. Impact on Prostate Cancer Incidence

The introduction of PSA-based prostate cancer screening to clinical practice has indeed had a profound impact on prostate cancer incidence. Between 1987 and 1992, PSA-based prostate cancer became widely accepted and prostate cancer incidence rose by 85% [25]. Subsequently, incidence rates began to fall and are now only slightly higher than in the ''pre-PSA'' era [26]. These trends are not unexpected: it is anticipated that the introduction of any effective screening program will result in an increased incidence of the disease. If the test does not detect insignificant disease, incidence rates should eventually return toward baseline levels. If, however, the test detects insignificant disease, then incidence rates will continue to be higher than they were prior to the introduction of the screening test. The rise and subsequent fall of prostate cancer incidence, coincident with the introduction of PSA-based prostate cancer screening, is evidence used by many to support the efficacy of PSA testing. Additional supporting evidence can be found by comparing age- and race-related trends in prostate cancer incidence. That is, prostate cancer incidence has risen faster and fallen more rapidly in older men who have been more heavily screened than younger men who are less likely to have undergone screening [27]. Among African-American men, the peak incidence rates and the subsequent decline are similar but have lagged behind that of white men. This is consistent with apparent delays in the availability and acceptance of prostate cancer screening among African-American men [28].

B. Sensitivity

It is well established that serum PSA is a highly sensitive biomarker and that measurement of serum PSA is a useful test that aids in early detection of prostate cancer [29–31]. In fact, when PSA measurement is added to digital rectal examination, cancer detection is enhanced three- to fivefold [32]. Retrospective studies suggest that PSA testing detects clinically significant prostate cancer an average of 6.2 years prior to the development of an abnormal digital rectal examination [33]. It is estimated that PSA measurement will miss fewer than 20% of prostate cancers [32]. The sensitivity of PSA testing compares favorably with that of other accepted cancer screening modalities such as mammography and fecal occult blood testing [1,33–36].

C. Impact on Detection of "Insignificant" Cancers

Prostate cancer is commonly detected when autopsies are performed on men of all ages [37]. The significant prevalence of "incidental" prostate cancer suggest that many prostate cancers remain clinically indolent during patients' lifetimes. This factor has caused some people to question the importance of early prostate cancer detection and to suggest that PSA-based screening programs detect cancers that would not otherwise have been detected. A comparison of histological features of prostate cancer detected through PSA screening with those detected on autopsy demonstrate that PSA does not commonly detect "clinically irrelevant" cancers [27,38,39]. Pathological examination of surgically removed prostates from men with PSA-detected cancers show that fewer than 10% of these tumors are low volume (< 0.5 cc) and low-grade (Gleason sum < 4) (Table 2), characteristics found in approximately 90% of "autopsy" cancers [36,38–42].

D. Impact on Stage

Over the past decade there has been a dramatic stage migration for newly diagnosed prostate cancer. Today 70–80% of men are diagnosed with prostate cancer while it is pathologically organ confined (Table 2), compared to only 20–30% in the "pre-PSA era" [42]. In the SEER program, the rate of distant disease fell

Table 2 Pathological Results of Radical Prostatectomy in Men with Prostate Cancer Detected by PSA-Based Screening

Author	Number	Indication for biopsy	% Low-volume/grade	% Organ-confined
Catalona et al. [32]	160	PSA > 4.0 ng/ml and/or suspicious DRE	8	71
Ohori et al. [41]	306	PSA > 4.0 ng/ml and/or suspicious DRE	9	71
Smith et al. [38]	816	PSA > 4.0 ng/ml and/or suspicious DRE	3	71
Scaletsky et al. [40]	142	PSA > 4.0 ng/ml	6	73
Lodding et al. [64]	14	PSA 3.0–4.0 ng/ml and/or suspicious DRE	0	64
Catalona et al. [62]	52	PSA 2.6–4.0 ng/ml	17	81
Schroder et al. [63]	75	PSA 2.0–3.9 ng/ml	NA	84
	238	PSA 4.0–9.9 ng/ml	NA	62

by 52% between 1990 and 1994 [27]. This stage migration can almost certainly be attributed to the widespread acceptance of PSA-based cancer screening. Several studies have clearly demonstrated that cancers detected because of a PSA elevation are more likely to be organ confined than those detected because of an abnormal digital rectal examination [27,38–43].

There is strong inferential evidence that screening will lead to improved survival; untreated men with a life expectancy of 10–15 years have a 60–80% chance of dying from prostate cancer. Radical prostatectomy cures up to 80% of men with organ-confined prostate cancer [44–47].

E. Impact on Grade

It is well established that a man's risk of dying from prostate cancer is directly related to the tumor's Gleason grade [46,48]. Low-grade prostate cancers may remain indolent for more than 15 years [46], and some high-grade tumors may not be curable with any form of therapy [47]. Therefore, early detection and aggressive local therapy will likely have the greatest impact on men with moderate-grade tumors. Serum PSA measurement appears to be a good screening test for prostate cancer since its major impact has been on the detection of moderate-grade prostate cancers. In the pre-PSA era, low-grade cancers accounted for 24%, moderate-grade for 35%, and high-grade for 33% of cases. In contrast, in 1999,

58% of cancers diagnoses were moderate-grade and 17% were considered high-grade [49].

F. Impact on Mortality

Population-based reductions in prostate cancer mortality rates may be the only way to assess the impact of prostate cancer screening. Since we currently do not have an effective treatment for advanced disease, any reduction in mortality is likely attributable to early detection programs. In 1994, shortly after the widespread acceptance of PSA-based prostate cancer screening, annual prostate cancer deaths increased to 34,902, but have fallen an average of 1.6% per year since that time [29]. In the past decade, prostate cancer mortality has fallen by more than 14% [50,51]. The initial increase in prostate cancer deaths is most likely the result of heightened prostate cancer awareness; the subsequent persistent decline may be the result of early detection.

IV. RANDOMIZED SCREENING TRIALS

Many critics claim that recommendations in support of routine PSA testing should be withheld until the benefits of screening and early detection have been demonstrated in a randomized trial. Prospective randomized trials in both Europe and North America have been initiated in an attempt to determine if PSA-based screening reduces prostate cancer mortality in a cost-effective manner without reducing the quality of life for participants [52–54]. The European Randomized Study of Screening for Prostate Cancer (ESPRC) has already enrolled 80,000 men [54]. The National Cancer Institute's Prostate, Lung, Colorectal, Ovarian (PLCO) screening program has already enrolled 50,000 men [53]. It will likely be at least 10 years until the results of these trials can be interpreted. Unfortunately, benefits of screening may be missed by this trial because the widespread use of PSA testing may result in contamination (i.e., men undergoing PSA testing by their personal physician) in the control arm.

A large prospective randomized screening trial involving more than 46,000 Canadian men was conducted in Quebec and the results recently published. Using an "intent-to-treat" analysis, the authors found a 6% reduction in deaths among the screened population after 8 years of follow-up [55]. Unfortunately, these results are not definitive because of methodological flaws such as a high drop-out rate among the men in the screening arm and poor follow-up for unscreened men. Many believe that 8 years is premature for early detection to have an impact on mortality, and that the observed reduction in mortality may be attributed to improvements in medical care for patients with advanced prostate cancer detected in the screened population.

V. OPTIMAL SCREENING INTERVAL

One potential strategy to reduce the cost associated with widespread PSA-based prostate cancer screening is to increase the intervals between screening visits. The American Cancer Society and the American Urological Association recommend annual prostate cancer screening [56], but data suggest that it may be safe to screen some men less frequently. It appears that the serum PSA level and the age of the patient may be useful factors in determining the optimal screening interval. Longitudinal screening studies have shown that a man's PSA level at time of entry into a study is a strong predictor of his risk of eventually being diagnosed with prostate cancer [57]. For example, men with a total PSA < 2.5 ng/ml had a 1.0% chance of being diagnosed with prostate cancer within 4 years, compared to 12.7% for men with PSA levels between 2.6 and 4.0 ng/ml and 38.4% for men with PSA levels between 4.1 and 10.0 ng/ml. Data from the Baltimore Longitudinal Study of Aging showed that men with an initial PSA level less than 2.0 ng/ml had a 4% chance of converting to a PSA of 4.1–5.0 ng/ml during 4 years of follow-up, but that men with a PSA level of 2.1–4.0 ng/ml had a 27–36% chance of converting to a PSA level of 4.0–5.0 ng/ml [58]. Very similar findings (i.e., PSA became elevated in < 5% and cancer was detected in < 1% of men with initial PSA < 2.0 ng/ml) have been reported in 8187 men serially screened as part of Prostate Cancer Awareness Week [59]. Collectively these studies suggest that men with an initial PSA level at or below 2.0 ng/ml and a normal digital rectal examination may safely be screened on a biannual basis, but that men with PSA levels above 2.0 ng/ml should be screened annually.

Although the American Cancer Society recommends that prostate cancer screening should begin at age 50 for white men without a family history of prostate cancer, no recommendation regarding the age at which screening should end has been made. Preliminary results from the Baltimore Longitudinal Study of Aging suggest that prostate cancer screening could safely be stopped in 65-year-old men with a PSA level of 1.0 ng/ml or less [60]. Implementation of this could result in great cost savings; this issue should be studied further.

VI. OPTIMAL PSA CUT-OFF POINTS

Although 4.0 ng/ml has traditionally been used as the upper limit of normal for PSA in testing protocols [1,61] 20% of men with diagnosed prostate cancer have a PSA level less than 4.0 ng/ml [61]. Recent studies by Catalona et al. have demonstrated that 22% of men with a benign rectal examination and a PSA level of 2.6–4.0 ng/ml will have cancer detected on prostate biopsy, and that 81% of these cancers will be pathologically organ-confined [62]. Results from the ERSPC demonstrated a 19% cancer detection rate for men with PSA between 2.0 and 3.9 ng/ml [63]. Eighty-four percent of the cancers detected in men with PSA levels of 2.0–3.9 ng/ml were organ-confined compared to only 62% of those in men with PSA levels 4.0–10.0 ng/ml. Based on these data, the authors recommended biopsy for patients with PSA levels greater than 3.0 ng/ml. Lodding et al. reported that lowering the PSA cut-off point from 4.0 to 3.0 ng/ml improved cancer detection by 30%, but that only 9 of the 14 men who were surgically staged had organ-confined disease [64]. Differences in surgical technique may account for this apparent discrepancy in pathological stage. It appears that 2.5 ng/ml is an appropriate PSA cut-off point for younger men in whom early prostate cancer detection and aggressive treatment would be most beneficial. More study is needed to determine whether this will improve long-term survival and to determine the additional cost of using a lower PSA cut-off.

VII. OPTIMAL AGE TO BEGIN SCREENING

Current recommendations are to begin prostate cancer screening at age 50, except for African-American men or those men with a family history [5]. However, there is data to suggest that initiating screening before the age of 50 may enhance the chance of detecting "curable" prostate cancer. Carter et al. showed that for any given PSA stratum, 40–50-year-old men were more likely to be diagnosed with organ-confined prostate cancer (Table 3) [65]. For example, among men with PSA levels of 4–6 ng/ml, those 40–50 years of age had an 87% chance of

Table 3 Pathological Results of Men Undergoing Radical Prostatectomy for Clinically Localized Prostate Cancer Stratified by Total PSA (TPSA) Level and Age in Years

TPSA (ng/ml)	40–50[a] (%)	51–60[a] (%)	61–73[a] (%)
2.5–4.0	89 (87–90)	83 (82–84)	78 (77–79)
4.1–6.0	87 (85–88)	81 (80–82)	74 (73–75)
6.1–8.0	84 (83–85)	78 (77–79)	71 (70–72)
8.1–10.0	83 (82–83)	75 (74–75)	67 (66–68)
>10.0	73 (65–80)	57 (52–62)	49 (45–53)

[a] Probability of organ-confined disease.
Source: From Ref. 65.

having organ-confined disease compared to 81% for men aged 51–60 and 74% for men older than 60.

VIII. SCREENING MEN WITH A FAMILY HISTORY OF PROSTATE CANCER

One important risk factor for prostate cancer development is a positive family history. Prostate cancer can be inherited and it is estimated that hereditary cases account for 9% of prostate cancers but 40% of cancers diagnosed in men younger than 55 years of age [66,67]. In addition to true ''hereditary'' prostate cancer cases there is also a strong familial association. Studies have shown that a man's relative prostate cancer risk is increased two- to threefold if he has a first-degree relative with prostate cancer. It is estimated that 34% of men diagnosed with prostate cancer have a positive family history [68–70]. Linkage analyses of families with hereditary prostate cancer have identified at least four separate prostate cancer susceptibility loci suggesting that multiple genes can be responsible for the development of hereditary prostate cancer (HPC1 on 1q24–25, PCAP on 1q42–43, CAPB on 1p36, and HPC on Xq27–28) [71–75]. Efforts to identify specific genes, and to determine their role in the development of hereditary, familial, and sporadic prostate cancer, are underway. In the future, genetic markers to predict prostate cancer risk will be available, and their use will enhance prostate cancer screening strategies.

Prostate cancer patients with a family history present at a younger age than men without a family history [69,75]. Most reports suggest that a positive family history is not an adverse prognostic factor. Population-based studies have shown similar survival rates for men with hereditary, familial, and sporadic prostate cancer [76], and surgical series have shown similar outcomes among men undergoing radical prostatectomy [77,78]. Better characterization of the genetic defects responsible for carcinoma of the prostate will almost certainly help us determine who would most likely benefit from early and aggressive screening.

Knowledge regarding hereditary and familial prostate cancer supports early and aggressive screening for this cohort of men. Matikainen et al. identified 209 asymptomatic men from 302 families with 2 or more affected cases, and detected elevated serum PSA levels in 10% and prostate cancer in 3.3% [79]. Among the cancer families with an average age of diagnosis less than 60 years, 29% had elevated PSA levels and 14% had prostate cancer. The optimal strategy to screen men with a positive family history has yet to be determined, but for now the recommendations to begin screening men with a family history of prostate cancer at age 40 seem justified.

IX. SCREENING AFRICAN-AMERICAN MEN

Another important risk factor for prostate cancer development is race. Population studies have shown that African-American men have a substantially higher incidence of prostate cancer than age-matched Caucasian men [80,81]. In addition, African-American men tend to present with higher-grade and -stage tumors, and ultimately suffer a substantially higher mortality [82]. The underlying reason for these differences is multifactorial. Some studies suggest that differences are the result of inequalities in access to health care and that race is not an independent risk factor of poor prognosis [83,84]. Others, however, have demonstrated that African-American men develop biologically more aggressive cancers than Caucasian men. Several reports from equal-access health care systems have demonstrated differences in prostate cancer detection rates, pathological features, and survival. A large cohort study demonstrated that among men who belong to an equal-access health maintenance organization, African-American men had poorer prostate cancer survival [85]. Moul et al. studied 541 men (133 African-American and 408 white) with prostate cancer diagnosed in the military health system and found that, despite equal access to cancer screening and early treatment, African-American men had tumors that on average were 2.6 times larger than those found in whites. In addition, the average age at time of diagnosis was younger (64.9 vs. 66.8 years) for African-American men [86]. Others have shown that differences in Gleason score and recurrence rate between African-American and white men occur exclusively in men younger than 69, suggesting that clinically aggressive prostate cancer develops at a younger age in African-American men [86,87].

It has been shown that PSA-based screening can have an impact on prostate cancer diagnosis in African-American men. Powell et al. reported a profound reduction in advanced disease as the result of PSA screening [88]. They reported that 65% of African-American men undergoing radical prostatectomy for cancer detected through the Detroit Education and Early Detection program had organ-confined disease compared to only 35% men in the clinic population at Wayne State [89]. Furthermore, a study from the Veterans Administration demonstrated similar rates of distant disease (6 vs. 4%) among African-American and white prostate cancer patients diagnosed in the "PSA era" [90]. Collectively these data support the American Cancer Society's recommendation to begin screening African-American men at age 40.

Studies have shown that PSA appears to behave differently among races. Eastham et al. concluded that African-American men without prostate cancer had significantly higher PSA and PSA density levels than aged-matched white men [91]. However, these results should be regarded with some caution since men in this study were assumed to be free of cancer if their PSA level was less than 4.0 ng/ml or they otherwise had undergone a negative biopsy. Since the criteria used to exclude cancer were not very strict, it is possible that the higher PSA levels seen in African-American men may be the result of increased prevalence of undetected cancer compared to white men. In the study by Moul et al., African-American men with prostate cancer had a significantly higher PSA level at the time of diagnosis than white men (14 ng/ml vs. 8 ng/ml) [86]. Smith et al. reported that the positive predictive value of PSA level >4.0 ng/ml was 38–48% for African-American men and 22–34% for white men [87]. Powell et al. recently reported that for any PSA stratum, African-American men undergoing radical prostatectomy had higher postoperative biochemical failure rates, suggesting that race-adjusted references ranges that delay prostate biopsy for African-American men would compromise cure [92]. Collectively, these studies suggest that the most appropriate PSA cut-off point for African-American men is probably 2.5 ng/ml. Several studies have shown that percentage free PSA can be used to improve the specificity of total PSA measurement for white men [93], and a recent study has shown that it may also be useful for African-American men [94]. A lower PSA cut-off point (2.5 ng/ml) and the use of percentage free PSA should be evaluated in a large prospective screening trial.

X. EFFECT OF FINASTERIDE ON PSA

Finasteride, a 5-alpha reductase inhibitor, reduces the risk of urinary retention and the need for surgical treatment of benign prostatic hyperplasia (BPH) [95]. Studies have shown that, on average, serum total PSA levels are lowered by 50% among men without prostate cancer who have received finasteride for more than 6 months [96]. Results from 3040 men who were studied as part of the 4-year randomized controlled PLESS trial demonstrate that multiplying the PSA value by 2 among men receiving finasteride preserves the usefulness of PSA for prostate cancer detection [97]. Reports of a randomized trial comparing men receiving finasteride to untreated men have shown that while total PSA levels were reduced by 50% percentage free PSA levels were not affected [98,99]. These studies suggest that percentage free PSA measurements remain valid among men receiving finasteride, but these findings should be confirmed in a larger study.

XI. EFFECT OF EJACULATION ON PSA

Studies evaluating the effect of ejaculation on serum PSA levels have yielded conflicting results. Tchetgen et al. reported that ejaculation causes a statistically significant yet small increase in total PSA level that can persist for up to 48 hr [100]. They studied 64 men aged 49–79 years and found that, following ejaculation, PSA levels increased in 87% of the men. The mean increase was 0.8 ng/ ml at 1 hr, 0.3 ng/ml at 6 hr, 0.2 ng/ml at 24 hr, and 0.4 ng/ml at 48 hr. Herschman et al. studied 20 men aged 51–67 and showed that 24 hr after ejaculation 40% of men had elevations in total PSA and 35% of men had reductions in percentage free PSA [101]. The mean differences in total PSA level were 0.3 ng/ml at 1 hr and 0.1 ng/ml at 6 hr. Percentage free PSA rose by a mean of 9.9% at 1 hr, but was on average 2.2% below baseline at 24 hr. Stenner et al. failed to detect an impact of ejaculation on total PSA measurements determined within 12 hr [102]. The reason for these conflicting results is not clear. We can conclude from these studies that ejaculation has only a minimal effect on PSA levels and that 6 hr after ejaculation there is unlikely to be a clinically significant effect on either total or percentage free PSA measurements.

XII. EFFECT OF DIGITAL RECTAL EXAMINATION ON PSA

There have been multiple conflicting reports regarding the impact of digital rectal examination (DRE) on PSA. We reported on 93 men who were evaluated as part of a large PSA-based prostate cancer screening program. One hour following DRE, 31% of men had total PSA and 48% had percentage free PSA levels that rose above baseline levels by more than expected biological variation [103]. Both total and percentage free PSA levels returned to baseline levels by 24 hr. It seems prudent to wait 24 hr after DRE before measuring PSA. However, since the total and percentage free PSA increases were small (mean total PSA increase was 0.2 ng/ml; mean percent free PSA increase was 4.2%) PSA measurements made within 24 hr of a DRE are probably reliable unless the value is close to the desired cut-off point.

XIII. SUMMARY

Although, to date, it has not been proven in a prospective randomized trial, there is strong inferential evidence that PSA-based prostate cancer screening is beneficial since measurement of serum PSA is relatively inexpensive, with relatively robust sensitivity to identify men with early-stage prostate cancer. The availability of a safe and relatively reliable methods to biopsy the prostate enables PSA testing to be useful in clinical practice. The widespread implementation of PSA-based prostate screening has had a profound impact on prostate cancer incidence. The unprecedented increase in prostate cancer incidence coincident with introduction of PSA testing and the subsequent decline is consistent with an effective screening test. Independent of changes in incidence there has been a dramatic downward stage migration and an increase in the percentage of men diagnosed with moderate-grade tumors (for which local therapy is most likely to have the greatest impact). Furthermore, PSA testing has not resulted in detection of a significant number of "clinically indolent" prostate cancers. These facts, along with the reduction in prostate cancer mortality observed for the past 3 years, support the widespread use of PSA-based prostate cancer screening.

The optimal screening strategy remains to be determined. There are significant data to suggest that a cut-off of 4.0 ng/ml may not be appropriate for all men and that lower cut-off may be needed to maximize detection of "curable" prostate cancers. Family history and race are the most important risk factors for prostate cancer, and screening strategies (age to begin and PSA cut-off) should be adjusted accordingly. In the future genetic polymorphism and molecular markers will be used to further modify the assessment of prostate cancer risk. The common practice of screening high-risk patients beginning at the age of 40 appears justified, and there is now evidence that this recommendation (to begin screening at age 40 rather than 50) may be appropriate for all men.

The last decade has witnessed a dramatic and unprecedented improvement in the ability to diagnose and effectively treat prostate cancer. The development of serum PSA measurement as a tool for early diagnosis is primarily responsible. In the next decade,vast improvements in imaging and molecular profiling technologies will almost certainly refine prostate cancer diagnoses by complementing an already powerful test: PSA.

REFERENCES

1. WJ Catalona, DS Smith, TL Ratliff, KM Dodds, DE Coplen, JJ Yuan, JA Petros, GL Andriole. Measurement of prostate-specific antigen in serum as a screening test for prostate cancer. N Engl J Med 324:1156–1161, 1991.
2. TA Stamey, N Yang, AR Hay, JE McNeal, FS Freiha, E Redwine. Prostate-specific antigen as a serum marker for adenocarcinoma of the prostate. N Engl J Med 317: 909–916, 1987.
3. K Ito, Y Kubota, K Suzuki, N Shimizu, Y Fukabori, K Kurokawa, K Imai, H Yamanaka. Correlation of prostate-specific antigen before prostate cancer detection and clinicopathologic features: Evaluation of mass screening populations. Urology 55(5):705–709, 2000.
4. MW Plawker, JM Fleisher, EM Vapnek, RJ Macchia. Current trends in prostate cancer diagnosis and staging among United States urologists. J Urol 158(5):1859–1860, 1997.
5. RA Smith, CJ Mettlin, KJ Davis, H Eyre. American Cancer Society guidelines for the early detection of cancer. CA Cancer J Clin 50(1):34–49, 2000.
6. DK Ornstein, G Andriole. AUA Update series. Screening for prostate cancer in 1999. AVA Update Series, Lesson 1 Volume XVIII, pages 1–7.

7. American Urological Association. Prostate-specific antigen (PSA) best practice policy. Oncology 14(2):267, 2000.

8. RT Greenlee, T Murray, S Bolden, PA Wingo. Cancer statistics, 2000. CA Cancer J Clin 50(1):7–33, 2000.

9. CM Coley, MJ Barry, C Fleming, AG Mulley. Early detection of prostate cancer. Part I: Prior probability and effectiveness of tests. Ann Intern Med 126(5):394–406, 1997.

10. JB Rietbergen, AE Kruger, R Kranse, FH Schroder. Complications of transrectal ultrasound-guided systematic sextant biopsies of the prostate: Evaluation of complication rates and risk factors within a population-based screening program. Urology 49(6):875–880, 1997.

11. DW Keetch, WJ Catalona, DS Smith. Serial prostatic biopsies in men with persistently elevated serum prostate specific antigen values. J Urol 151:1571–1574, 1998.

12. JI Epstein, PC Walsh, G Akingba, HB Carter. The significance of prior benign needle biopsies in men subsequently diagnosed with prostate cancer. J Urol 162(5): 1649–1652, 1999.

13. CK Naughton, DS Smith, PA Humphrey, WJ Catalona, DW Keetch. Clinical and pathologic tumor characteristics of prostate cancer as a function of the number of biopsy cores: A retrospective study. Urology 52(5):808–813, 1998.

14. F Daneshgari, GD Taylor, GJ Miller, ED Crawford. Computer simulation of the probability of detecting low volume carcinoma of the prostate with six random systematic core biopsies. Urology 45:604–609, 1995.

15. AR Vashi, KJ Wojno, B Gillespie, JE Oesterling. A model for the number of cores per prostate biopsy based on the patient age and prostate gland volume. J Urol 159: 920–923, 1998.

16. LA Escew, RL Bare, DL McCullough. Systematic five region prostate biopsy is superior to sextant method for diagnosing carcinoma of the prostate. J Urol 157: 199–203, 1997.

17. MA Levine, M Ittman, J Melamed, H Lepor. Two consecutive sets of transrectal ultrasound guided sextant biopsies of the prostate for the detection of prostate cancer. J Urol 159:471–476, 1998.

18. CK Naughton, DK Ornstein, DS Smith, WJ Catalona. Pain and morbidity of transrectal ultrasound guided prostate biopsy: A prospective randomized trial of 6 versus 12 cores. J Urol 163(1):168–71, 2000.

19. JE McNeal, EA Rewine, FS Freiha, TA Stamey. Zonal distribution of prostatic adenocarcinoma, correlation with histologic pattern and direction of spread. Am J Surg Pathol 12:897–906, 1988.

20. DR Greene, TM Wheeler, S Egawa, JK Dunn, PT Scardino. A comparison of the morphological features of cancer arising in the transition zone and in the peripheral zone of the prostate. J Urol 146:1069–1076, 1991.

21. DW Keetch, WJ Catalona. Prostatic transition zone biopsies in men with previous negative biopsies and persistently elevated serum prostate specific antigen values. J Urol 154:1795–1797, 1995.

22. M Bazinet, PI Karakiewicz, AG Aprikan, C Trudel, S Aronson, M Nachabe, F Peloquin, J Dessureault, M Goyal, W Zheng, LR Begin, MM Elhilali. Value of

systematic transition zone biopsies in the early detection of prostate cancer. J Urol 155:605–606, 1996.

23. NE Fleshner, WR Fair. Indications for transition zone biopsy in the detection of prostatic carcinoma. J Urol 158:556–558, 1997.

24. PD Lui, MK Terris, JE McNeal, TA Stamey. Indications for ultrasound guided transition zone biopsies in the detection of prostate cancer. J Urol 153:1000–1003, 1995.

25. AL Polotsky, BA Miller, PC Albertsen, BS Kramer. The role of increasing detection in the rising incidence of prostate cancer. JAMA 273:548–552, 1995.

26. PA Wingo, S Landis, LAG Ries. An adjustment to the 1997 estimate for new prostate cancer cases. Cancer 80:1810–1813, 1997.

27. RA Stephenson. Population-based prostate cancar trends in the PSA era: data from the surveillance, epidemiology, and end results (SEER) program. Monogr Urol 19: 3–19, 1998.

28. JD Taylor, TM Holmes, GM Swanson. Descriptive epidemiology of prostate cancer in metropolitan Detroit. Cancer 73:1704–1707, 1994.

29. LK Dennis, MI Resnick. Analysis of recent trends in prostate cancer incidence and mortality. Prostate. 42(4):247–252, 2000.

30. JM Legler, EJ Feuer, AL Potosky, RM Merrill, BS Kramer. The role of prostate-specific antigen (PSA) testing patterns in the recent prostate cancer incidence decline in the United States. Cancer Causes Control 9(5):519–527, 1998.

31. CG Arcangeli, DK Ornstein, DW Keetch, GL Andriole. Prostate-specific antigen as a screening test for prostate cancer. The United States experience. Urol Clin N Am 24(2):299–306, 1997.

32. WJ Catalona, JP Richie, FR Ahmann, MA Hudson, PT Scardino, RC Flanigan, JB deKernion, TL Ratliff, LR Kavoussi, BL Dalkin, WB Waters, MT MacFarlane, PC Southwick. Comparison of digital rectal examination and serum prostate specific antigen in the early detection of prostate cancer: Results of a multicenter clinical trial of 6,630 men. J Urol 151:1283–1290, 1994.

33. PH Gann, CH Hennekens, MJ Stampfer. A prospective evaluation of plasma prostate-specific antigen for detection of prostatic cancer. JAMA 273:289–294, 1995.

34. SH Taplin, CM Rutter, JG Elmore, D Seger, D White, RJ Brenner. Accuracy of screening mammography using single versus independent double interpretation. AJR 174(5):1257–1262, 2000.

35. JD Lurie, HG Welch. Diagnostic testing following fecal occult blood screening in the elderly. J Natl Cancer Inst 6(19):1641–1646, 1991.

36. C Mettlin, GP Murphy, F Lee, PJ Littrup, A Chesley, R Babaian, R Badalament, RA Kane, FK Mostofi. Characteristics of prostate cancer detected in the American Cancer Society–National Prostate Cancer Detection Project. J Urol 152(5 Pt 2): 1737–1740, 1994.

37. WD Belville. Are T1c tumors different from incidental tumors found at autopsy? The risk and reality of overdetection. Semin Urol Oncol 13(3):181–186, 1995.

38. DS Smith, WJ Catalona. The nature of prostate cancer detected through prostate specific antigen based screening. J Urol 152:1732–1736, 1994.

39. C Mettlin, GP Murphy, F Lee, PJ Littrup, A Chesley, R Babaian, R Badalament,

RA Kane, FK Mostofi. Characteristics of prostate cancers detected in a multi-modality early detection program. Cancer 72:1701–1708, 1993.

40. R Scaletscky, MO Koch, CW Eckstein, SL Bicknell, GF Gray Jr., JA Smith Jr. Tumor volume and stage in carcinoma of the prostate detected by elevations in prostate specific antigen. J Urol 152:129–131, 1994.

41. M Ohori, TM Wheeler, JK Dunn, TA Stamey, PT Scardino. The pathological features and prognosis of prostate cancer detected with current diagnostic tests. J Urol 152:1714–1720, 1994.

42. WJ Catalona, DS Smith, TL Ratliff, JW Basler. Detection of organ-confined prostate cancer is increased through prostate-specific antigen based screening. JAMA 270:948–954, 1993.

43. GS Gerber, IM Thompson, R Thisted, GW Chodak. Disease-specific survival following routine prostate cancer screening by digital rectal examination. JAMA 269:61–64, 1993.

44. G Aus, J Hugosson. Fifteen-year survival with prostate cancer in Sweden. JAMA 278:205–206, 1997.

45. J Johansson, L Holmberg, S Johansson, R Bergstrom, H Adavi. Fifteen-year survival in prostate cancer. JAMA 277:467–471, 1997.

46. PC Albertsen, JA Hanley, DF Gleason, MJ Barry. Competing risk analysis of men aged 55 to 74 years at diagnosis managed conservatively for clinically localized prostate cancer. JAMA 280(11):975–980, 1998.

47. GS Gerber, RA Thisted, PT Scardino, HG Frohmuller, FH Schroeder, DF Paulson, AW Middleton Jr, DB Rukstalis, JA Smith Jr, PF Schellhammer, M Ohori, GW Chodak. Results of radical prostatectomy in men with clinically localized prostate cancer. JAMA 276(8):615–619, 1996.

48. S Vesalainen, S Nordling, P Lipponen, M Talja, K Syrjanen. Progression and survival in prostatic adenocarcinoma: a comparison of clinical stage, Gleason grade, S-phase fraction and DNA ploidy. Br J Cancer 70(2):309–314, 1994.

49. M Perrotti, F Rabbanni, A Farkas, WS Ward, KB Cummings. Trends in poorly differentiated prostate cancer 1973 to 1994: observation from the Surveillance, Epidemiology and End Results database. J Urol 16:811–815, 1998.

50. BF Hankey, EJ Feuer, LX Clegg, RB Hayes, JM Legler, PC Prorok, LA Ries, RM Merrill, RS Kaplan. Cancer surveillance series: Interpreting trends in prostate cancer—part I: Evidence of the effects of screening in recent prostate cancer incidence, mortality, and survival rates. J Natl Cancer Inst 91(12):1017–1024, 1999.

51. RM Merrill, RA Stephenson. Trends in mortality rates in patients with prostate cancer during the era of prostate specific antigen screening. J Urol 163(2):503–510, 2000.

52. B Standaert, L Denis. The European randomized study of screening for prostate cancer: An update. Cancer 80:1830–1834, 1997.

53. C Vanchieri. Prostate cancer screening trials: Fending off critics to recruit men. J Natl Cancer Inst 90:10–12, 1998.

54. FH Schroder, CH Bangma. The European randomized study of screening for prostate cancer (ERSPC): An update. Eur Urol 35(5–6):539–543, 1999.

55. F Labrie, A Dupont, B Candas, L Cusan, JL Gomez, P Diamond, A Belanger, G

Brousseau, J Levesque. Decrease of prostate cancer death by screening: First data from the Quebec prospective and randomized study. Proc ASCO 17:2a, 1998.

56. B Stein, JM Lindenmayer. Proposed prostate cancer screening recommendations. Med Health/RI 80:343–345, 1997.

57. DS Smith, WJ Catalona, JD Herschman. Longitudinal screening for prostate cancer with prostate-specific antigen. JAMA 276:1309–1315, 1996.

58. HB Carter, JI Epstein, DW Chan. Recommended prostate-specific antigen testing intervals for the detection of curable prostate cancer. JAMA 277:1456–1460, 1997.

59. S Leewansangtong, ED Crawford, SG Gordon, G Serdar, K Holthaus, M Baier, NN Stone, M Eisenberger, F Staggers, D McLoed. Longitudinal follow up for Prostate Cancer Awareness Week (PCAW): Screening intervals. J Urol 159:177–180, 1998.

60. JD Pearson, B Bell, P Landis, JL Fozard, HB Carter. When is PSA testing no longer necessary? J Urol 159:178–180, 1998.

61. GL Andriole, WJ Catalona. Using PSA to screen for prostate cancer: The Washington University experience. Urol Clin North Am 20:647–651, 1993.

62. WJ Catalona, DS Smith, DK Ornstein. Prostate cancer detection in men with serum PSA concentrations of 2.6 to 4.0 ng/ml and benign prostate examination: Enhancement of specificity with free PSA measurements. JAMA 277:1452–1455, 1997.

63. FH Schroder, I van der Cruijsen-Koeter, HJ de Koning, AN Vis, RF Hoedemaeker, R Kranse. Prostate cancer detection at low prostate specific antigen. J Urol 163(3): 806–812, 2000.

64. P Lodding, G Aus, S Bergdahl, R Frosing, H Lilja, C Pihl, J Hugosson. Characteristics of screening detected prostate cancer in men 50 to 66 years old with 3 to 4 ng/mL prostate specific antigen. J Urol 159:899–903, 1998.

65. HB Carter, JI Epstein, AW Partin. Influence of age and prostate-specific antigen on the chance of curable prostate cancer among men with nonpalpable disease. Urology 53(1):126–130, 1999.

66. BS Carter, TH Beaty, GD Steinberg, B Childs, PC Walsh. Mendelian inheritance of familial prostate cancer. Proc Natl Acad Sci USA 89(8):3367–3371, 1992.

67. H Gronberg, SD Isaacs, JR Smith, JD Carpten, GS Bova, D Freije, J Xu, DA Meyers, FS Collins, JM Trent, PC Walsh, WB Isaacs. Characteristics of prostate cancer in families potentially linked to the hereditary prostate cancer 1 (HPC1) locus. JAMA 278:1251–1255, 1997.

68. DW Keetch, JP Rice, BK Suarez, WJ Catalona. Familial aspects of prostate cancer: A case control study. J Urol 154:2100–2101, 1995.

69. PC Walsh, AW Partin. Family history facilitates the early diagnosis of prostatic carcinoma. Cancer 80:1871–1874, 1997.

70. SM Lesko, L Rosenberg, S Shapiro. Family history and prostate cancer risk. Am J Epidemiol 144:1041–1047, 1996.

71. J Xu, D Meyers, D Freije, S Isaacs, K Wiley, D Nusskern, C Ewing, E Wilkens, P Bujnovszky, GS Bova, P Walsh, W Isaacs, J Schleutker, M Matikainen, T Tammela, T Visakorpi, OP Kallioniemi, R Berry, D Schaid, A French, S McDonnell, J Schroeder, M Blute, S Thibodeau, J Trent. Evidence for a prostate cancer susceptibility locus on the X chromosome. Nat Genet 20(2):175–179, 1998.

72. P Berthon, A Valeri, A Cohen-Akenine, E Drelon, T Paiss, G Wohr, A Latil, P

Millasseau, I Mellah, N Cohen, H Blanche, C Bellane-Chantelot, F Demenais, P Teillac, A Le Duc, R de Petriconi, R Hautmann, I Chumakov, L Bachner, NJ Maitland, R Lidereau, W Vogel, G Fournier, P Mangin, O Cussenot, et al. Predisposing gene for early-onset prostate cancer, localized on chromosome 1q42.2–43. Am J Hum Genet 62(6):1416–1424, 1998.

73. M Gibbs, L Chakrabarti, JL Stanford, EL Goode, S Kolb, EF Schuster, VA Buckley, M Shook, L Hood, GP Jarvik, EA Ostrander. Analysis of chromosome 1q42.2-43 in 152 families with high risk of prostate cancer. Am J Hum Genet 64(4):1087–1095, 1999.

74. S Narod. Genetic epidemiology of prostate cancer. Biochim Biophys Acta 1423(1): F1–13, 1999.

75. JR Smith, D Freije, JD Carpten, H Gronberg, J Xu, SD Isaacs, MJ Brownstein, GS Bova, H Guo, P Bujnovsky, DR Nusskern, JE Damber, A Bergh, M Emanuelsson, OP Kallioniemi, J Walker-Daniels, JE Bailey-Wilson, TH Beaty, DA Meyers, PC Walsh, FS Collins, JM Trent, WB Isaacs. Major susceptibility locus for prostate cancer on chromosome 1 suggested by a genome-wide search. Science 274(5291):1371–1374, 1996.

76. H Gronberg, L Damber, B Tavelin, JE Damber. No difference in survival between sporadic, familial and hereditary prostate cancer. Br J Urol 82(4):564–567, 1998.

77. GS Bova, AW Partin, SD Isaacs, BS Carter, TL Beaty, WB Isaacs, PC Walsh. Biological aggressiveness of hereditary prostate cancer: long-term evaluation following radical prostatectomy. J Urol 160(3 Pt 1):660–663, 1998.

78. JJ Bauer, S Srivastava, RR Connelly, IA Sesterhenn, DM Preston, DG McLeod, JW Moul. Significance of familial history of prostate cancer to traditional prognostic variables, genetic biomarkers, and recurrence after radical prostatectomy. Urology 51(6):970–976, 1998.

79. MP Matikainen, J Schleutker, P Morsky, OP Kallioniemi, TL Tammela. Detection of subclinical cancers by prostate-specific antigen screening in asymptomatic men from high-risk prostate cancer families. Clin Cancer Res 5(6):1275–1279, 1999.

80. CR Baquet, JW Horm, T Gibbs, P Greenwald. Socioeconomic factors and cancer incidence among blacks and whites. J Natl Cancer Inst 83:223–230, 1991.

81. RA Morton. Racial differences in adenocarcinoma of the prostate in North American men. Urology 44:637–645, 1994.

82. AP Polednak, JT Flannery. Black versus white racial differences in clinical stage at diagnosis and treatment of prostatic cancer in Connecticut. Cancer 70:2152–2155, 1992.

83. JA Eastham, MW Kattan. Disease recurrence in black and white men undergoing radical prostatectomy for clinical stage T1-T2 prostate cancer. J Urol 163(1):143–145, 2000.

84. MN Witte, MW Kattan, J Albani, DS Sharp, JA Eastham, RA Morton Jr. Race is not an independent predictor of positive surgical margins after radical prostatectomy. Urology 54(5):869–874, 1999.

85. AS Robbins, AS Whittemore, SK Van Den Eeden. Race, prostate cancer survival, and membership in a large health maintenance organization. J Natl Cancer Inst 90(13):986–990, 1998.

86. JW Moul, IA Sesterhenn, RR Connelly, T Douglas, S Srivastava, FK Mostofi, DG McLeod. Prostate-specific antigen values at the time of prostate cancer diagnosis in African-American men. JAMA 274:1277–1281, 1995.
87. DS Smith, AD Bullock, WJ Catalona, JD Herschman. Racial differences in a prostate cancer screening study. J Urol 156(4):1366–1369, 1996.
88. IJ Powell, M Banerjee, W Sakr, D Grignon, DP Wood Jr, M Novallo, E Pontes. Should African-American men be tested for prostate carcinoma at an earlier age than white men? Cancer 85(2):472–477, 1999.
89. KT Pienta, R Demers, M Hoff, TY Kau, JE Montie, RK Severson. Effect of age and race on the survival of men with prostate cancer in the metropolitan Detroit tri-county area, 1973 to 1987. Urology 45:93–102, 1995.
90. SJ Freedland, ME Sutter, J Naitoh, F Dorey, GS Csathy, WJ Aronson. Clinical characteristics in black and white men with prostate cancer in an equal access medical center. Urology 55(3):387–390, 2000.
91. JA Eastham, RA May, T Whatley, A Crow, DD Venable, O Sartor. Clinical characteristics and biopsy specimen features in African-American and white men without prostate cancer. J Natl Cancer Inst 90:756–760, 1998.
92. IJ Powell, M Banerjee, M Novallo, W Sakr, D Wood, JE Pontes. Should the age specific PSA cut-point for prostate biopsy be higher among African American vs. American Caucasian men above age 50 years. J Urol 159:74–76, 1998.
93. WJ Catalona, DS Smith, RL Wolfert, TJ Wang, HG Rittenhouse, TL Ratliff, RB Nadler. Evaluation of percentage of free serum prostate-specific antigen to improve specificity of prostate cancer screening. JAMA 274(15):1214–1220, 1995.
94. WJ Catalona, AW Partin, KM Slawin, CK Naughton, MK Brawer, RC Flanigan, JP Richie, A Patel, PC Walsh, PT Scardino, PH Lange, JB deKernion, PC Southwick, KG Loveland, RE Parson, GH Gasior. Percentage of free PSA in black versus white men for detection and staging of prostate cancer: A prospective multicenter clinical trial. Urology 55(3):372–376, 2000.
95. JD McConnell, R Bruskewitz, P Walsh, G Andriole, M Leber, HL Holtgrewe, P Albertson, CG Roehrborn, JC Nickel, DZ Wang, AM Taylor, J Waldstreicher. The effect of finasteride on the risk of acute urinary retention and the need for surgical treatment among men with benign prostatic hyperplasia. N Engl J Med 338:557–563, 1998.
96. HA Guess, GJ Gormley, E Stoner, JE Oesterling. The effect of finasteride on prostate specific antigen: Review of available data. J Urol 155:3–9, 1996.
97. GL Andriole, PC Walsh, JI Epstein, P Hudson, N Romas, TJ Cook, J Waldstreicher, H Guess. Treatment with finasteride preserves the usefulness of PSA in prostate cancer (CaP) detection. J Urol 159:73, 1998.
98. J Pannek, LS Marks, JD Pearson, HG Rittenhouse, DW Chan, ED Shery, GJ Gormley, ENP Subong, CA Kelley, E Stoner, AW Partin. Influence of finasteride on free and total serum prostate specific antigen levels in men with benign prostatic hyperplasia. J Urol 159:449–453, 1998.
99. DW Keetch, GL Andriole, TL Ratliff, WJ Catalona. Comparison of percent free prostate-specific antigen levels in men with benign prostatic hyperplasia treated with finasteride, terazosin, or watchful waiting. Urology 50:901–905, 1997.
100. MB Tchetgen, JT Song, M Strawderman, SJ Jacobson, JE Oesterling. Ejaculation

increases the serum prostate-specific antigen concentration. Urology 47:511–516, 1996.

101. JD Herschman, DS Smith, WJ Catalona. Effect of ejaculation on serum total and free prostate-specific antigen concentrations. Urology 50:239–243, 1997.

102. J Stenner, K Holthaus, SH Mackenzie, ED Crawford. The effect of ejaculation on prostate-specific antigen in a prostate cancer-screening population. Urology 51: 455–459, 1998.

103. DK Ornstein, GS Rao, DS Smith, TL Ratliff, JW Basler, WJ Catalona. Effect of digital rectal examination and needle biopsy on serum total and percentage of free prostate specific antigen levels. J Urol 157:195–198, 1997.

10
PSA and Repeat Biopsy

Bob Djavan
University of Vienna, Vienna, Austria

Although prostate specific antigen (PSA) is regarded as the best biochemical marker for prostate cancer (CaP) [1], an important limitation in its use in cancer detection is the considerable overlap of patients with CaP and those with benign prostatic hyperplasia (BPH) when serum PSA levels range between 4.0 and 10.0 ng/ml [2–4]. Most studies on early detection of CaP use a serum PSA level of 4.0 ng/ml as the cut-off. However, a cut-off of 4.0 ng/ml does not detect 20% of cancer cases (false-negative results) and incorrectly identifies about 65% of patients with benign disease as potentially cancerous (false-positive results) [5]. Therefore, the false-positive group will unnecessarily undergo prostatic biopsy, which is both invasive and costly.

Furthermore, in men with one or two sets of prostate biopsies that showed no cancer, persistently elevated serum PSA concentrations pose a diagnostic dilemma: What further evaluation should be performed to exclude prostate cancer adequately?

For subjects within the ''gray zone'' of a 4–10 ng/ml serum PSA level, several concepts have been introduced to improve cancer detection (sensitivity) and reduce the number of unnecessary prostatic biopsies (specificity) or even repeat biopsies [6]. These concepts include PSA density (PSAD; the ratio of the serum PSA level to the volume of the prostate gland), PSAD of the transition zone (PSA-TZ; the ratio of the serum PSA level to the prostatic transition zone volume), PSA velocity (PSAV; the rate of change of serum PSA levels over time), age-adjusted PSA reference ranges (evaluating the PSA level with regard to patient age), and measurement of different molecular forms of PSA in the serum (unbound [free] PSA vs. protein-bound forms of PSA). During the past decade, % free PSA (the ratio of free PSA to total PSA) has emerged as the most clinically useful method of improving CaP detection [7–10]. The value of the other methods is still the subject of considerable debate [2,11–19].

Urologists routinely select patients for prostate biopsy on the basis of digital rectal examination (DRE) and/or serum prostate specific antigen abnormalities [20–22]. First time prostate biopsies reveal cancer in about 38% of patients [23]. Clinical investigators have consistently reported that the false-negative rate of a single systematic sextant biopsy is approximately 25% for clinically significant prostate cancers (i.e., tumors greater than 0.5cc in volume) [24–26]. Keetch et al. [27] concluded that men with a persistently elevated serum PSA level after an initial prostate biopsy should undergo at least one additional biopsy to exclude the presence of prostate cancer. Obtaining biopsies directed at the prostatic peripheral zone, they noted that the positive rate for one, two, three, and four sets of repeated quadrant or sextant biopsies was 34%, 19%, 8%, and 7%, respectively. Additional studies based on smaller patient samples have also demonstrated the positive rate for a repeated biopsy to be 28%, 29%, and 12%, respectively [28–30].

Because of the poor specificity of PSA and DRE testing to detect prostate cancer, both the initial and repeated prostate biopsies in most patients will be negative (62–74%). Serum tests with improved specificity for the detection of prostate cancer inherently enhance the selection of patients for prostate biopsy. Numerous clinical and scientific studies have proved that the free to total (f/t) PSA ratio can improve the discrimination between populations of patients with benign prostatic hyperplasia and prostate cancer [31–34]. One recent study of 51 patients who underwent repeated biopsies for prostate cancer found an improved prediction for the diagnosis of cancer using the f/t PSA ratio [35].

McNeal et al. reported that the distribution of prostatic cancers was 68% in the peripheral, 8% in the central, and 24% in the transition zones [36]. In men with previous negative prostatic biopsies and persistently elevated serum PSA concentrations, an important question is whether the persistent serum PSA elevation is caused by undetected cancer in the transition zone.

O'Dowd et al. [37] recently used a population of patients who underwent prostate biopsies processed by a single pathology laboratory to identify a subset of patients with a repeated biopsy performed within 12 months of an initial non-cancer biopsy. The study assessed the cancer diagnosis rate in repeated biopsies of either no evidence of malignancy (NEM), high-grade prostatic intraepithelial neoplasia (HGPIN) [38,39], atypical glands suspicious for cancer (suspicious) [40], or suspicious with HGPIN (Susp-HGPIN). In addition, they selected a subset of patients with fPSA and tPSA result obtained before the repeated biopsy and constructed a multivariate logistic regression model to predict the likelihood of cancer being diagnosed on repeated biopsy.

The study concluded that men who have an initial noncancerous biopsy diagnosis remain at risk of prostate cancer, especially if the initial diagnosis was suspicious or HGPIN. In addition, combining factors such as the initial biopsy diagnosis, family history, digital rectal examination results, prostate gland volume, age, total PSA, and free to total PSA ratio could provide valuable information for predicting the likelihood of cancer [37].

I. PSA, PROSTATE VOLUME, AND REPEAT BIOPSY

Issues related to prostate volume are still prominent when deciding whether to perform a repeat biopsy or not. Given that sextant prostatic systematic biopsies sample only about 90 mm prostate tissue (6 × 15 mm cores), increased prostatic volume may significantly reduce the chance of detecting cancer of significant volume at biopsy [3,5,6].

The wide variation in gland sizes and shapes seems to lead proportionally to more extensive sampling of smaller glands in systematic core biopsies and less extensive or suboptimal sampling of larger prostates, with accompanying significant differences in biopsy yields [7,8]. Several groups have proposed new biopsy strategies, often increasing the number of biopsies and the sectors to be sampled or performing biopsies more laterally. However, controversial data have been reported about the real advantage of these new techniques [9–12]. Concerned by the fact that the original sextant method may not include adequate sampling of the prostate, Norberg et al. found in a prospective study including 512 patients that the standard method left 15% of cancers undetected with the results of a more extensive procedure using 8–10 biopsies [13].

Recently, Djavan et al. prospectively analyzed the influence of the total and transition prostate volumes on prostate cancer detection using two successive sets of sextant biopsies plus two transition zone (TZ) biopsies at each time [41]. A total of 1018 patients were prospectively included. Of the 1018 patients, 344 had CaP diagnosed, 285 after the first set of biopsies and 59 on repeat biopsy. Compared to patients diagnosed with CaP after the first set of biopsies, patients diagnosed after the second set had larger total prostate and transition zone volumes (43.1 ± 13.0 cc vs. 32.5 ± 10.6 cc, p < 0.0001 and 20.5 ± 8.3 cc vs. 12.8 ± 6.0 cc, p < 0.0001). Receiver operating characteristic (ROC) curves showed that total and TZ volumes of 45 cc and 22.5 cc, respectively, provided the best combination of sensitivity and specificity for differentiating between patients diagnosed with CaP after the first from those diagnosed after a second set.

In patients with total prostate volume above 45 cc and TZ above 22.5 cc, a single set of sextant biopsies was not sufficient to rule out CaP. A repeat biopsy was to be considered in case of a negative first biopsy.

Evaluating the variation of cancer detection in relation to prostate size through random systematic sextant biopsies, Ulzzo et al. (1995) found that 23%

of the patients had cancer and a large prostate ($\geq$50 cc) compared to a 38% rate in patients with smaller prostates (p < 0.01) [42]. This group concluded that significant sampling error may occur in men with globally large glands, suggesting the need for repeat biopsies if prostate cancer is suspected.

Following analysis of a stochastic computer simulation model developed by Chen et al. to optimize prostate biopsy, a 10-case biopsy scheme incorporating midline peripheral zone and inferior portion of the anterior horn of the peripheral zone improved significant cancer detection to 96% and thus recommended the sampling of these zones in the rebiopsy strategy after prior negative biopsies [43]. Eskew et al. have recommended the use of a 5-region sampling technique to improve the cancer detection rate since 11 cores technique increased the percentage of prostate cancer detected from 26 to 40% over the usual sextant biopsies [10]. The detailed maps of consecutive radical prostatectomies have shown that prostate cancers expand mostly in the transverse direction across the posterior surface of the capsule, followed by the cephalocaudal direction [3]. Directing the biopsies more lateral to the midparasagittal plane might enable practitioners to sample the large group of cancers located more laterally in the peripheral zone (PZ) [3].

The posterior and posterolateral border of compressed fibromuscular tissues caused by the expansion transition zone hyperplasic nodules, observed on transrectal ultrasound (TRUS), serves as an excellent marker for placement of PZ biopsies where more than 70% of cancers originate [3].

Bauer et al. have used a three-dimensional computer-assisted prostate biopsy simulator based on whole-mounted step-sectional radical prostatectomy specimens to compare the diagnostic accuracy of various prostate needle biopsy protocols. These authors found that all the biopsy protocols that use laterally placed biopsies based on the five-region anatomical model are superior to the routinely used sextant prostate biopsy technique [11].

The importance of the total volume on prostate cancer yield by sextant biopsies is generally accepted, but the importance of the transition zone has been less extensively investigated [44].

Djavan and others have already stressed the importance of the transition zone and especially of the transition zone density for predicting prostate cancer in men with serum PSA levels below 10 ng/ml [15,16,45]. The concept is based on the observation that a part of the serum PSA is related to the volume of the benign hypertrophied transition zone.

Lui et al. (1995) reported a 38% cancer detection rate in men undergoing repeat systematic biopsies, of which more than 70% were found in the peripheral zone [46].

Another group has also recently used two consecutive sets of transrectal ultrasound guided sextant biopsies for improving prostate cancer detection [47]. These two sets were performed during the same session. Prostate cancer was detected in 43, 27, and 24% of men with prostate volumes less than 30, 30–50, and greater than 50cc, respectively. In analyzing the second set of biopsies, performed at the same place as the first one, the probability of detecting a prostate cancer was approximately twofold more in men with large prostates than in men with smaller and intermediate-sized prostates.

Letran et al. have analyzed the influence of the peripheral zone volume on prostate cancer yield by sextant biopsies [17]. They measured this zone as the difference between the total and transition zone volume, which in fact is an indirect measurement of the influence of the transition zone. These authors suggested that the total and peripheral zone volumes significantly affected the biopsy yield only when both were above the 75th percentile. This corresponds to the mirror image of the role of the transition zone as observed in the study of Djavan et al., since the peripheral zone was estimated as the difference between the total volume of the prostate and the transition zone.

The explanation Djavan et al. provide for this observation about the role of the transition zone on prostate cancer biopsy yield is the possible displacement of the peripheral zone anatomy by the hyperplastic nodules of the TZ. This would move the area where the prostate cancers occur slightly more laterally. The intrinsic tumor biology does not seem to explain this difference, since these tumors show no obvious clinical or pathological differences.

The debate over the need for more lateral biopsies continues [9,48]. In a study aiming to optimize prostate biopsy strategy using computer-based analysis, Chen et al. (1997) observed that simulation of sextant biopsies demonstrated reliably detected cancer in only 107 of 147 patients (73%) in whom total tumor volume as greater than 0.5 cc [43]. There was little correlation between total length of cancer in biopsy cores and tumor volume. Change of biopsy angle from 30 to 45 degrees did not result in significantly increased detection rates. Placing all biopsies more laterally likewise did not increase overall detection rates. When tumor foci from the 40 cases in which sextant biopsies did not reliably detect tumor were mapped, the authors found that the foci were distributed in areas not biopsied by the sextant method: the transitional zone, midline peripheral zone, and inferior portion of the anterior horn of the peripheral zone. A 10-core biopsy scheme incorporating these areas as well as the posterolateral prostate reliably detected cancer in 141 of 147 patients (96%) with total tumor volumes greater than 0.5 cc.

Regarding lower cancer detection rates in large glands, the same group also found that large prostates were more likely to be biopsied because of an elevated prostate antigen value resulting from benign elements of the gland and not from a significant cancer, since there is a higher proportion of low-volume cancers in these large glands [48]. The influence on PSA levels of the hypertrophied transition zone is in full accordance with findings on the value of the PSA density of the transition zone.

II. PSA, f/t PSA, PSAD, PSA-TZ, PSAV, AND REPEAT BIOPSY

Serum PSA determinations are widely used in the early detction of prostate cancer. PSA-based screening trials have shown that approximately 9% of asymptomatic men have elevated serum PSA values but only about 33% have cancer detected on initial evaluation [49,50]. The question is whether the 66% of men with an initially negative evaluation for cancer have an elevated serum PSA value because of benign prostatic hyperplasia, prostatitis, or undetected cancer in their peripheral or transition zone of the prostate. Keetch et al. [48] have previously shown that cancer detection rates at second or third biopsies were 19 and 8%, respectively [51]. However, their patients underwent serial biopsies of the peripheral zone only. We sought to evaluate this in a multicenter trial.

The recommendation that all patients with normal digital rectal examination and an elevated serum PSA value undergo sextant peripheral zone as well as transition zone biopsies seems logical, given the anatomical distribution of prostate cancer. However, there are few data to support this recommendation for routine prostatic transition zone biopsy.

In this prospective study, 1051 subjects aged 48–77 years were enrolled from January, 1997, through March, 1999, at the Departments of Urology of the University of Vienna, Austria, and of the Erasme Hospital, University Clinics of Brussels, Belgium. The study population consisted of consecutive patients referred for early detection of either CaP or lower urinary tract symptoms. All subjects with a total serum PSA level between 4 and 10 ng/ml were enrolled in the study. Patients were excluded if they had a history of CaP (n = 193), prior prostatic biopsy (n = 144), acute or chronic prostatitis and histological evidence of a prostatic intraepithelial neoplasm of any grade, urinary retention, an indwelling urinary catheter, or a confirmed urinary tract infection. Only 39 patients were excluded because they refused to undergo a repeat biopsy.

Djavan et al. evaluated prospectively the ability of % free PSA, PSAD, and PSA-TZ to increase the sensitivity and specificity of PSA screening. Whereas most previous studies focused on the ability of these PSA parameters to predict the outcome of a first biopsy, they focused on the outcome of a repeat biopsy in men with a total PSA level between 4 and 10 ng/ml and an initial prostatic biopsy that was negative for CaP. Of the 1051 men with a total PSA level of 4–10 ng/ml, the initial biopsy was positive for CaP in 22% (231/1051) of the subjects. The initial diagnosis was BPH in the remaining 820 subjects (Fig. 1). The DRE result was normal in 64.9% (682/1051) and abnormal in 35.1% (369/1051) of subjects, and it was not a significant predictor of CaP (chi-square = 4.5; Pearson correlation p = 0.2121).

Of the 369 patients with abnormal DRE result, additional cores were taken in 254 patients, who had suspicious areas found during TRUS and DRE. The

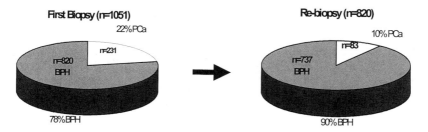

Figure 1 Initial biopsy and repeat biopsy pie charts.

majority of cancers (84%) were detected in peripheral zone, compared to 16% detected in the transition zone.

In general, the complication rate of the repeat biopsy procedure was very low: hematuria was present in 8% of patients (no treatment was necessary), fever was present in 1.7%, and urinary tract infection (UTI) occurred in 3.8% of patients.

Total prostate volume, transition zone volume, and % free PSA were significantly higher in subjects with BPH compared to those diagnosed with CaP ($p < 0.001$, Wilcoxon test). At repeat biopsy the total prostate volume was not significantly different between patients with BPH and CaP. Total PSA, PSAD, and PSA-TZ were all significantly higher in subjects diagnosed with CaP in initial and repeat biopsy ($p < 0.01$, Wilcoxon test).

All 820 subjects diagnosed with BPH after the initial biopsy underwent a repeat prostatic biopsy 6 weeks later. CaP was detected in 10% (83/820) of these subjects (Fig. 1). Compared to the 231 subjects in whom CaP was detected from the initial biopsy, both total prostate volume and transition zone volume were significantly higher ($p < 0.001$, Wilcoxon test) in the 83 subjects with CaP detected in the repeat biopsy sample.

The sensitivity, specificity, and positive and negative predictive values for predicting the repeat biopsy results are shown in Table 1 for each PSA parameter.

Table 1 PSA Results at Specific Cut-Offs for 820 Subjects After Repeat Biopsy

	Cut-off	Sensitivity (%)	Specificity (%)	PPV	NPV
Total PSA	5.5 ng/ml	80	38	0.12	0.95
% Free PSA	30%	90	50	0.16	0.98
PSAD	0.13 ng/ml/cc	74	44	0.12	0.93
PSA-TZ	0.26 ng/ml/cc	78	52	0.15	0.96

Based on the results of a previous study [15], cut-off values were selected that produced good specificity with a sufficiently high level of cancer detection (sensitivity). At a cut-off of 30% and 0.26 ng/ml/cc, respectively, % free PSA and PSA-TZ were the most accurate predictors of a positive repeat biopsy result. Although a similar number of unnecessary repeat biopsies would have been eliminated by either % free PSA or PSA-TZ (approximately 50%), CaP detection was much lower for PSA-TZ (78%) than % free PSA (90%). Table 2 illustrates the decreased specificity that would result by selecting cut-off values that would produce 95% sensitivity for each parameter. At 95% sensitivity, % free PSA would have eliminated the highest percentage of unnecessary repeat biopsies (33.5%).

The ability of each of the PSA parameters to predict the outcome of biopsy results was analyzed further with ROC curves. In both the overall group (initial biopsy results plus repeat biopsy results; Fig. 2) and the repeat biopsy group (Fig. 3), % free PSA and PSA-TZ were the best predictors of CaP. The respective areas under the curve (AUCs) for % free PSA and PSA-TZ were 74.2% and 82.7% in the overall group, and 74.5% and 69.1% in the repeat biopsy group ($p < 0.001$) (Table 3). A combination of initial and repeat biopsy showed 82.7% for PSA-TZ and 74.2% for % free PSA. In fact, % free PSA is a significantly better predictor of repeat biopsy results than PSA-TZ, PSAD, and total PSA.

In multivariate logistic regression analysis for overall biopsy, PSA-TZ, % free PSA, and total PSA were significant predictors for cancer detection ($r = 0.4332$, $p < 0.001$). For the repeat biopsy, only % free PSA and PSA-TZ were significant predictors ($r = 0.2150$, $p < 0.001$) (Table 4).

It is unclear why PSA-TZ was superior to % free PSA when both initial and repeat biopsy results were combined, but not when only the repeat biopsy results were considered. Although Djavan et al. previously reported that measurement of the transition zone volume is accurate and reproducible [19], all TRUS measurements are operator-dependent and, therefore, subject to possible variability. Furthermore, the measurement of the transition zone in small or large prostates sometimes might be difficult. It was reported previously that PSA-TZ was

Table 2 PSA Results at 95% Sensitivity for 820 Subjects After Repeat Biopsy

	Cut-off	Sensitivity (%)	Specificity (%)	PPV	NPV
Total PSA	4.0	95	8.30	0.10	0.93
% Free PSA	38%	95	33.5	0.14	0.98
PSAD	0.09 ng/ml/cc	95	14.7	0.10	0.96
PSA-TZ	0.19 ng/ml/cc	95	21.4	0.12	0.98

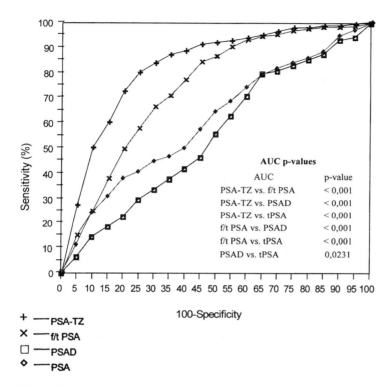

Figure 2 Overall ROC curve for prostate cancer detection. (From Ref. 6.)

not a significant predictor of biopsy results when the total prostate volume was
<30 cc [15].

When comparing % free PSA and PSA-TZ, the use of % free PSA can
eliminate procedures that are more costly and invasive. Of these two parameters,
PSA-TZ is much more expensive and more subjective because it requires the use
of TRUS. For the repeat biopsy group, as well as for the overall group (initial
plus repeat biopsies), the use of % free PSA resulted in a high rate of cancer
detection without a large number of unnecessary biopsies.

With % free PSA results in predicting second biopsy were similar to those
of other groups reporting first biopsy results. In a multicenter study of 773 men
with a total PSA level between 4 and 10 ng/ml (379 with CaP and 394 with
BPH), a % free PSA cut-off of 25% had a sensitivity of 95% and a specificity
of 20% [52]. Another multicenter study of 317 men with a total PSA level between 4.0 and 10.0 ng/ml found that a % free PSA cut-off of 26% detected 95%
of subjects with CaP and eliminated 29% of negative biopsies [44]. In another

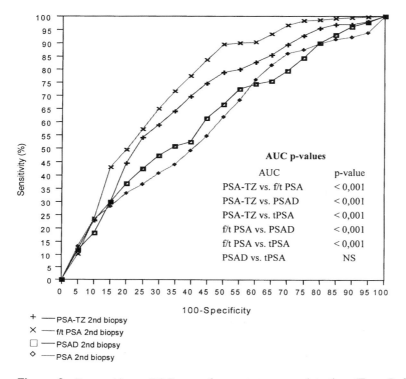

Figure 3 Repeat biopsy ROC curve for prostate cancer detection. (From Ref. 6.)

study of 308 volunteers with an elevated total PSA level (2.5–10.0 ng/ml), a % free PSA cut-off of <20% would have eliminated 45.5% of negative biopsies. When % free PSA was combined with a PSA-TZ density cut-off of >0.22 ng/ml/cc, 54.2% of negative biopsies could have been avoided [53].

Although some previous studies focused on repeat-biopsy results, most have been retrospective trials conducted in relatively small patient populations

Table 3 AUC of the ROC Curves: Overall (Initial + Repeat Biopsy) and Repeat Biopsy

	No. of patients	Total PSA (%)	% Free PSA	PSAD (%)	PSA-TZ (%)
Overall	1051	61.2	74.2	55.1	82.7
Repeat biopsy	820	60.3	74.5	61.8	69.1

Table 4 Multivariate Logistic Regression: Overall (Initial + Repeat Biopsy) and Repeat Biopsy

Overall	Parameter	Estimate	Chi square	Probability
	Intercept	−0.80	3.72	0.05
	t PSA	−0.121	3.71	0.05
	PSA-TZ	6.380	128.5	<0.001
	f/t PSA	−0.085	103.2	<0.001
Whole model test			463.0	<0.001
r = 0.4332				
Repeat Biopsy				
	Intercept	−1.093	10.3	0.0013
	PSA-TZ	2.277	15.6	0.001
	f/t PSA	−0.083	41.8	<0.001
Whole model test			90.5	<0.001
r = 0.2150				

[42–48,54–57]. In one study of 193 men with a negative initial biopsy, 51 (26%) were found to have CaP on repeat biopsy. Of all the PSA parameters tested (total PSA, PSAD, age-referenced PSA, volume-referenced PSA, and PSAV), total PSA and volume-referenced PSA had the highest sensitivity [42]. Another retrospective study in 51 men with a total serum PSA level of 2–15 ng/ml demonstrated a lower median % free PSA value in patients with a positive repeat biopsy compared with those with a negative biopsy (15% vs. 19%, respectively; p = 0.05) [43]. A % free PSA cut-off of 22% yielded a sensitivity of 95% and a specificity of 44% for predicting repeat biopsy results. In a prospective study of 67 men with persistent total PSA elevations and normal DRE, a low % free PSA (<10%) was a powerful predictor of CaP, even after two negative biopsies. In those patients, 11 cases of CaP were identified. The AUC of the ROC curve was 0.93 for % free PSA, compared with 0.69, 0.66, and 0.51 for free PSAD, PSAD, and total PSA, respectively [45].

In another study that used % free PSA to predict repeat biopsy results, CaP was detected in 20 (20%) of 99 men with a total PSA level between 4.1 and 10.0 ng/ml and an initial biopsy that was negative for CaP [47]. Percentage free PSA cut-offs of 28% and 30% had a sensitivity of 90% and 95%, respectively, and a specificity of 13% and 12%, respectively. For PSAD cut-offs of 0.10 and 0.08 ng/ml/cc, the respective sensitivities were 90% and 95%, and the respective specificities were 31% and 12%.

The rate of CaP detected upon repeat biopsy in the present study (10%) was lower than that observed in previous studies, which have ranged from 12 to 30% [23–33]. This difference may be related to the biopsy technique used or to the fact that the repeat biopsy was performed in the present study only 6 weeks after the initial biopsy. The most accurate biopsy technique to be used for repeat biopsies is still a matter of debate. Two issues are still unclear:

When (at which prostate volume) to start increasing the number of cores
By how many cores the total number of cores should be increased per unit of additional prostate volume (e.g., steps of 10 cc or more)

In the current study, the authors intended to analyze the value of PSA-based parameters for prostate cancer prediction on initial and repeat biopsy. Changing the repeat biopsy technique would not allow an accurate comparison, since an increased or decreased detection rate may be due to an altered biopsy technique and not to the predictive value of the parameters analyzed.

In three of the previous studies, the positive repeat biopsy rate was 17% after an interval of 14.7 months between the first and second biopsies [42], 29% after an interval of 19.1 months [43], and 30% after 12.8 months [46]. Other factors that must be considered when comparing studies of the incidence of CaP in repeat biopsies among patients with a negative first biopsy result are:

The range of total PSA levels in the study population, since populations with highly elevated total PSA levels (i.e., >10 ng/ml) may be more likely to have a positive repeat biopsy result
Whether the results were derived from only one repeat biopsy or whether some patients underwent additional biopsies after the first repeat biopsy
Whether all of the patients with an initially negative biopsy result underwent repeat biopsy or whether patients were selected for rebiopsy based on factors such as a persistently elevated total PSA level, a suspicious DRE result, or symptoms suggestive of a prostatic abnormality

Djavan et al. proposed the algorithm shown in Figure 4 for the management of patients whose initial prostatic biopsy results are negative for CaP. All patients with a total PSA level greater than 10 ng/ml should undergo repeat biopsy due to the high likelihood of CaP in patients with persistently elevated total PSA levels. Percentage free PSA and/or PSA-TZ should be determined for patients with a total serum PSA level between 4 and 10 ng/ml. A repeat biopsy should be performed in patients with a % free PSA <30% or a PSA-TZ ≥0.26 ng/ml/cc. The optimal interval between the initial and repeat biopsy is not clear, but an interval between 6 and 12 months is recommended.

At least 10% of patients with a total PSA level between 4 and 10 ng/ml and a negative prostatic biopsy results will be diagnosed with CaP after a repeat biopsy. When using PSA test results to determine which patients should undergo a repeat biopsy, both % free PSA and PSA-TZ enhance the specificity of PSA testing compared to either total PSA or PSAD. A repeat biopsy should be performed in patients with a % free PSA <30% or a PSA-TZ ≥0.26 ng/ml/cc.

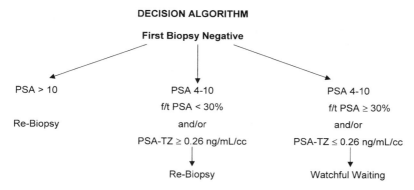

Figure 4 Vienna decision algorithm.

However, PSA-TZ is subject to operator-dependent variability, should only be used in patients with a total prostate volume >30 cc, and is associated with relatively high costs. Although PSA-TZ can be a valuable tool for experienced urologists, most urologists and other physicians will find % free PSA to be the most clinically useful tool for determining which patients initially diagnosed with BPH should undergo a repeat biopsy.

REFERENCES

1. AW Partin, JE Oesterling. The clinical usefulness of prostate specific antigen: update. J Urol 152:1358–1368, 1994.
2. MK Brawer. Prostate-specific antigen: Critical issues. Urology 44:9, 1994.
3. B Djavan, M Susani, B Bursa, A Basharkhah, R Simak, M Marberger. Predictability and significance of multifocal prostate cancer in the radical prostatectomy specimen. Tech Urol 5(3):139–142, 1999.
4. TA Stamey, N Yang, AR Hay, JE McNea, FS Freiha, E Redwine. Prostate-specific antigen as a serum marker for adenocarcinoma of the prostate. N Engl J Med 317: 909–916, 1987.
5. MC Beduchi, JE Oesterling. Percent free prostate-specific antigen: the next frontier in prostate-specific antigen testing. Urology 51(5A Suppl):98–109, 1998.
6. B Djavan, A Zlotta, M Remzi, K Ghawidel, A Basharkhah, CC Schulmann, M Marberger. Optimal predictors of prostate cancer on repeat prostate biopsy: A prospective study of 1,051 men. J Urol 163(4):1144–1148, 2000.
7. WJ Catalona, DS Smith, RL Wolfert, et al. Evaluation of percentage of free serum prostate-specific antigen to improve specificity of prostate cancer screening. JAMA, 274(15):1214–1220, 1995.
8. J Morote, CX Raventos, JA Lorente, et al. Comparison of percent free prostate spe-

cific antigen and prostate specific antigen density as methods to enhance prostate specific antigen specificity in early prostate cancer detection in men with normal rectal examination and prostate specific antigen between 4.1 and 10 ng/mL. J Urol 158(4):502–504, 1997.

9. AR Vashi, KJ Wojno, W Henricks, et al. Determination of the "reflex range" and appropriate cutpoints for percent free prostate-specific antigen in 413 men referred for prostatic evaluation using the AxSYM system. Urology 49(1):19–27, 1997.

10. CH Bangma, JBW Rietbergen, R Kranse, et al. The free-to-total prostate specific antigen ratio improves the specificity of prostate specific antigen screening for prostate cancer in the general population. J Urol 157(6):2191–2196, 1997.

11. MC Bedushi, JE Oesterling. Prostate-specific antigen density. Urol Clin N Am 24(2): 323–332, 1997.

12. M Bazinet, AW Meshref, C Trudel, et al. Prospective evaluation of prostate-specific antigen density and systematic biopsies for early detection of prostatic carcinoma. Urology 43(1):44–51, 1994.

13. HB Carter, JD Pearson. Prostate-specific antigen velocity and repeated measures of prostate-specific antigen. Urol Clin North Am 24(2):333–338, 1997.

14. TD Richardson, JE Oesterling. Age-specific reference ranges for serum prostate-specific antigen. Urol Clin North Am 24(2):339–351, 1997.

15. B Djavan, AR Zlotta, G Byttebier, S Shariat, M Omar, CC Schulman, M Marberger. Prostate specific antigen density of the transition zone for early detection of prostate cancer. J Urol 160(2):411–418, 1998.

16. B Djavan, AR Zlotta, C Kratzik, et al. PSA, PSA density, PSA density of transition zone, free to total PSA ratio and PSA velocity for prostate detection in men with total PSA of 2.5 to 4 ng/mL. Urology 54(3):517–522, 1999.

17. MK Brawer, MC Benson, DG Bostwik, B Djavan, H Lilja, A Semjonow, S Su, Z Zhou. Prostate specific antigen and other serum markers: Current concepts from the World Health Org Consulation authors on Prostate Cancer. Semin Urol Oncol 17(4): 206–221, 1999.

18. B Djavan, C Seitz, M Remzi, et al. Combinations of PSA based diagnostic tests for prostate cancer detection. Techniques Urol 5(2):71–76, 1999.

19. AR Zlotta, B Djavan, T Roumeguere, M Marberger, CC Schulman. The importance of measuring the prostatic transition zone: An anatomial and radiological study. Br J Urol Int 84(6):661, 1999.

20. WJ Catalona, JP Richie, FR Ahamann, et al. Comparison of digital rectal examination and serum prostate specific antigen in the early detection of prostate cancer: Results of a multicenter clinical trial of 6,630 men. J Urol 151:1283–1290, 1994.

21. MK Brawer, MP Chetner, J Beatie, et al. Screening for prostatic carcinoma with prostate specific antigen. J Urol 147:841–845, 1992.

22. SJ Jacobson, DK Datusic, EJ Bergstrahl, et al. Incidence of prostate cancer diagnosis in years before and after serum prostate-specific antigen testing. JAMA 274:1445–1449, 1995.

23. R Orozco, GJ O'Dowd, B Kunnel, et al. Observations on pathology trends in 62,537 prostate biopsies obtained from urology private practices in the United States. Urology 51:186–195, 1998.

24. KK Hodge, JE McNeal, MK Terris, et al. Random systematic versus directed ultrasound guided transrectal core biopsies of the prostate. J Urol 142:71–74, 1989.

25. ME Chen, P Troncoso, DA Johnston, et al. Optimization of prostate biopsy strategy using computer based analysis. J Urol 158:2168–2175, 1997.
26. M Norberg, L Egevad, L Holmberg, et al. The sextant protocol for ultrasound guided core biopsies of the prostate underestimates the presence of cancer. Urology 50: 562–566, 1997.
27. DW Keetch, WJ Catalona, DS Smith. Serial prostatic biopsies in men with persistently elevated serum prostate-specific antigen values. J Urol 151:1571–1574, 1994.
28. WJ Ellis, MK Brawer. Repeat prostate needle biopsy: Who needs it? J Urol 153: 1496–1498, 1995.
29. NE Fleshner, M O' Sullivan, WR Fair. Prevalence and predictors of a positive repeat transrectal ultrasound guide needle biopsy of the prostate. J Urol 158:505–509, 1997.
30. C Roehrborn, GJ Pickens. J Sanders. Diagnostic yield of repeated transrectal ultrasound-guided biopsies stratified by histopathologic diagnoses and prostate specific antigen level. Urology 47:347–352, 1996.
31. AF Prestigiacomo, H Lilja, K Petterson, et al. A comparison of the free fraction of serum specific in men with benign and cancerous prostates: The best case scenario. J Urol 156:350–354, 1996.
32. HB Carter, AW Partin, AA Luderer, et al. Percentage of free prostate specific antigen in sera predicts aggressiveness of prostate cancer a decade before diagnosis. Urology 49:379–384, 1997.
33. AW Partin, WJ Catalona, PC Southwick, et al. Analysis of percent free prostate-specific antigen (PSA) for prostate cancer detection: Influence of total PSA, prostate volume and age. Urology 48 (suppl 6A):55–61, 1996.
34. RW Veltri, MC Miller. Free/total PSA ratios improve differentiation of benign and malignant disease of the prostate: Critical analysis of two different test populations. Urology 53:736–745, 1999.
35. JL Letran, AB Blase, FR Loberiza, et al. Repeat ultrasound guided prostate needle biopsy: Use of free to total PSA ratio in predicting prostatic carcinoma. J Urol 160: 426–429, 1998.
36. JE McNeal, EA Redwine, FS Freiha, TA Stamey. Zonal distribution of prostatic adenocarcinoma: Correlation with histologic pattern and direction of spread. Am J Surg Pathol 12:897, 1988.
37. GJ O'Dowd, M Craig Miller, R Orozco, RW Veltri. Analysis of repeated biopsy results within 1 year after a noncancer diagnosis. Urology 55(4):553–559, 2000.
38. MK Brawer, SA Bigler, OE Sohlberg, et al. Significance of prostatic intraepithelial neoplasia on prostate needle biopsy. Urology 38:103–107, 1991.
39. ML Wills, UM Hamper, AW Partin, et al. Incidence of high-grade prostatic intraepithelial neoplasia in sextant needle biopsy specimens. Urology 49:367–373, 1997.
40. KA Iczkowski, TJ Bassler, VS Schwob, et al. Diagnosis of "suspicious for malignancy" in prostate biopsies: Predictive value for cancer. Urology 51:749–758, 1998.
41. B Djavan, AR Zlotta, M Remzi, K Ghawidel, B Bursa, S Hruby, R Wolfram, CC Schulman, M Marberger. Total and transition zone prostate volume and age: How do they affect the utility of PSA-base diagnostic parameters for early prostate cancer detection? Urology 54(5):846–852, 1999.
42. O Ukimura, O Durrani, RJ Babaian. Role of PSA and its indices in determining the need for repeat prostate biopsies. Urology 50:66–72, 1997.

43. JL Letran, AB Blasé, FR Loberiza, GE Meyer, SD Ransom, MK Brawer. Repeat ultrasound guided prostate needle biopsy: Use of free-to-total prostate specific antigen ratio in predicting prostatic carcinoma. J Urol 160:426–429, 1998.
44. DW Chan, LJ Sokoll, AW Partin, et al. The use of % free PSA to predict prostate cancer probabilities: An eleven center prospective study using an automated immunoassay system in a population with nonsuspicious DER. J Urol 161 (Suppl. A): 353, 1999.
45. TO Morgan, DG McLeod, ES Leifer, GP Murphy, JW Moul. Prospective use of free prostate-specific antigen to avoid repeat prostate biopsies in men with elevated total prostate-specific antigen. Urology 48:76–80, 1996.
46. NE Fleshner, M O'Sullivan, WR Fair. Prevalence and predictors of a positive repeat transrectal ultrasound guided needle biopsy of the prostate. J Urol 158:505–508, 1997.
47. WJ Catalona, JA Beiser, DS Smith. Serum free prostate specific antigen and prostate specific antigen density measurements for predicting cancer in men with prior negative prostatic biopsies. J Urol 158:2162–2167, 1997.
48. DW Keetch, JM McMurtry, DS Smith, GL Andriole, WJ Catalona. Prostate specific antigen density versus prostate specific antigen slope as predictors of prostate cancer in men with initially negative prostatic biopsies. J Urol 156:428–431, 1996.
49. WJ Catalona, DS Smith, TD Ratliff, KM Dodds, DE Coplen, JJJ Yuan, JA Petros, GL Andriole. Measurement of prostate-specific antigen in serum as a screening test for prostate cancer. N Engl J Med 324:1156–1161, 1991.
50. MK Brawer, MP Chetner, J Beatie, DM Buchner, RL Vessella, PH Lange. Screening for prostatic carcinoma with prostate specific antigen. J Urol part 2, 147:841–845, 1992.
51. DW Keetch, WJ Catalona, DS Smith. Serial prostatic biopsies in men with persistently elevated serum prostate specific antigen values. J Urol 151:1571–1574, 1994.
52. WJ Catalona, AW Partin, KM Slawin, et al. Use of the percentage of free prostate-specific antigen to enhance differentiation of prostate cancer from benign prostatic disease. JAMA 279:1542–1547, 1998.
53. W Horninger, A Reissigl, H Klocker, H Rogatsch, K Fink, H Strasser, G Bartsch. Improvement of specificity in PSA-based screening by using PSA-transition zone density and percent free PSA in addition to total PSA levels. Prostate 37:133–137, 1998.
54. JBW Rietbergen, AE Boeken Kruger, RF Hoedemaeker, CH Bangma, WJ Kirkels, FH Schröder. Repeat screening for prostate cancer after 1-year followup in 984 biopsied men: Clinical and pathological features of detected cancer. J Urol 160:2121–2125, 1998.
55. GC Durkan, DR Greene. Elevated serum prostate specific antigen levels in conjunction with an initial prostatic biopsy negative for carcinoma: Who should undergo a repeat biopsy? Br J Urol Int 83:34–38, 1999.
56. M Noguchi, J Yahara, H Koga, O Nakashima, S Noda. Necessity of repeat biopsies in men for suspected prostate cancer. Int J Urol 6:7–12, 1999.
57. DW Keetch, WJ Catalona. Prostatic transition zone biopsies in men with previous negative biopsies and persistently elevated serum prostate specific antigen values. J Urol 154:1795–1797, 1995.

11
PSA and Staging

Jonathan D. Eaton, Grenville M. Oades, and Roger S. Kirby
St. George's Hospital, London, United Kingdom

The accurate staging of disease in men with prostate cancer is important not only for the correct selection of therapy, but also to allow more reliable predictions of prognosis. It also allows comparisons of various forms of therapy in well designed clinical trials. The tumor/node/metastasis TNM classification of staging is the most widely used (Table 1) [1]. Unfortunately, in spite of many recent advances, the precision with which an individual with prostate cancer can be staged remains suboptimal.

For decades digital rectal examination (DRE) was the cornerstone in the diagnosis and assessment of prostatic carcinoma stage. It is, however, generally agreed that a significant level of clinical understaging limits the use of DRE alone. The incidence of unsuspected periprostatic soft tissue invasion after radical prostatectomy in DRE-based staging series is high, ranging from 22 to 63% [2,3]. Extraprostatic extension of prostate cancer in the pathological specimens has been clearly shown to be an unfavorable prognostic finding in patients undergoing radical prostatectomy [4,5]. It is therefore of importance that preoperative staging be as accurate as possible. Despite this, DRE still remains an important part of the diagnosis and clinical staging of prostate cancer.

Serum prostate specific antigen (PSA) has probably become the most useful tumor marker available in clinical practice today, and is now routinely used in the diagnosis, staging, and monitoring of prostate cancer. PSA is more sensitive and more specific than DRE for both the diagnosis and staging of prostate cancer and is increasingly used to detect early, organ-confined disease. The ideal tumor marker is specific to the cancer it originates from, with elevations closely correlated with growth and biological significance. PSA is clearly the most tumor-specific antigen known but it is far from the perfect tumor marker. Since its

Table 1   1992 UICC Tumor-Node-Metastasis Staging System

Primary Tumor
TX   Primary tumor cannot be assessed
T0   No evidence of primary tumor
T1   Clinically inapparent tumor neither palpable nor visible by imaging
T1a   Tumor incidental histological finding in 5% or less of tissue resected
T1b   Tumor incidental histological finding in more than 5% of tissue resected
T1c   Tumor identified by needle biopsy (e.g., because of elevated PSA level)
Note: Tumor found in one or both lobes by needle biopsy, but not palpable or visible by imaging, is classified as T1c.
T2   Tumor confined within prostate
T2a   Tumor involves one-half of a lobe or less
T2b   Tumor involves more than one-half of lobe, but not both lobes
T2c   Tumor involves both lobes
T3   Tumor extends through the prostate capsule
T3a   Unilateral extracapsular extension
T3b   Bilateral extracapsular extension
T3c   Tumor invades seminal vesicle(s)
Note: Invasion into the prostatic apex or into (but not beyond) the prostatic capsule is not classified as T3, but as T2.
T4   Tumor is fixed or invades adjacent structures other than seminal vesicles
T4a   Tumor invades any of the following: bladder neck, external sphincter, rectum
T4b   Tumor invades levator muscles or is fixed to pelvic wall
Regional Lymph Nodes
NX   Regional lymph nodes cannot be assessed
N0   No regional node metastasis
N1   Metastasis in a single lymph node, 2 cm or less in greatest dimension
N2   Metastasis in a single lymph node, more than 2 cm but not more than 5 cm in greatest dimension; or multiple lymph nodes, none more than 5 cm in greatest dimension
N3   Metastasis in a lymph node more than 5 cm in greatest dimension
Metastasis
MX   Presence of metastasis cannot be assessed
M0   No distant metastasis
M1   Distant metastasis
M1a   Nonregional lymph node(s)
M1b   Metastasis in bone(s)
M1c   Metastasis in other site(s)

introduction into clinical diagnosis, numerous investigators have shown that the PSA is organ specific but not disease specific. PSA is produced by both malignant as well as nonmalignant prostate epithelial cells. Both benign prostatic hyperplasia (BPH) and prostate cancer occur in patients of the same age and unfortunately PSA does not appear to have the specificity to differentiate accurately between these two pathological processes. This makes the use of PSA alone in the staging of prostate cancer suboptimal. A combination of abnormal DRE and elevated PSA defines a group of patients at high risk of extraprostatic extension of disease and improves both the sensitivity and specificity of either test alone. As we shall discuss, the accuracy of disease staging can be further improved by combining PSA, Gleason score, and clinical stage (from DRE findings).

In spite of many recent advances, the precision with which an individual patient who has prostate cancer can be staged before therapy still remains suboptimal largely because early extraprostatic extension tends to be microscopic. It is therefore not surprising that imaging techniques such as computed tomography (CT) and magnetic resonance imaging (MRI) have limited accuracy in this context. Progress is being made, however, and future technological advances seem likely to enable us to identify more precisely those patients who have truly localized disease, who are most likely to derive benefit from curative radical therapy.

In this chapter we will try to identify the role of PSA in the staging of prostate cancer and also highlight the new developments that may enhance its future role in the staging of patients with prostate cancer.

I. TOTAL PSA IN THE STAGING OF PROSTATE CANCER

BPH has been crudely estimated to contribute approximately 0.3 ng/ml of PSA per gram of tissue [6], but the exact contribution of BPH tissue to total serum PSA is unknown. Partin et al. [7] have also shown that men with more advanced stage disease have higher-grade, higher-volume tumors that produce less PSA per gram of tumor. These factors make measurement of PSA alone a questionable staging method. However, most investigators agree that total PSA levels correlate reasonably well with pathological stage at both very low (<4.0 ng/ml) and very high (>20 ng/ml) levels. At intermediate PSA values (4.1–19.9 ng/ml), however, which are those levels most likely in patients undergoing definitive therapy, there is a lack of predictive value. Organ-confined rates range from 53 to 67% in men with PSA values between 4.0 and 10 ng/ml, and from 31 to 55.9% for those with PSA values between 10 and 20 ng/ml [8,9]. Thus preoperative PSA, when used by itself on an individual basis, appears to have limited ability to predict accurately the final pathological stage. PSA cannot be relied upon to differentiate patients with organ-confined cancer from those who have extracapsular tumor extension.

In an attempt to determine if the radionuclide bone scan could be eliminated from the routine staging evaluation of patients with newly diagnosed, untreated prostate cancer, Chybowski et al. examined the correlation of tumor grade, local clinical stage, acid phosphatase, prostatic acid phosphatase (PAP), and PSA with bone scan findings [10]. In their review of 521 patients, PSA was the best overall predictor of bone scan findings ($p < 0.00001$). In particular, patients with a low serum PSA concentration (<20 ng/ml) rarely had skeletal metastases. Based on these results, the negative predictive value of a serum PSA concentration less than or equal to 20 ng/ml is 99.7%. Thus, these results suggest that the staging radionuclide bone scan may not always be necessary in newly diagnosed, untreated patients with prostate cancer who have low serum PSA concentrations. Despite this fact many clinicians will still carry out bone scans on patients whose PSA level is between 10 and 20 ng/ml. Indeed, some will perform bone scans on every patient prior to considering radical prostatectomy. This merely highlights the fact that a low PSA level cannot guarantee a patient to be free of extraprostatic disease. In an individual patient total PSA alone is not sensitive enough to stage the disease accurately but may aid in the choice of further staging investigations.

II. PSA DENSITY IN THE STAGING OF PROSTATE CANCER

PSA density (PSAD) is defined as the quotient of serum PSA and prostatic volume (PSAng/ml/prostate volume cc) (see Chapter 4). The concept of PSAD as an adjunct to staging is based on the premise that, under normal circumstances, each epithelial cell (reflected by serum PSA) will require a given amount of stromal support (reflected by prostatic volume) to maintain normal structure and function. Normal prostate tissue and BPH adhere to this rule, whereas malignant tissues, including prostate cancer, do not because the tumor has lost normal architecture and is, as a result, more dense. Stamey et al. [11] demonstrated that prostate cancer contributes 3.5 ng/ml/ml^3 of tissue and BPH contributes only 0.3 ng/ml/ml^3 of tissue, a 10-fold difference. The concept of PSAD as an adjunct to staging is further supported by the observation that benign tumors grow by expansion, whereas malignant tumors grow by expansion and infiltration. Theoretically, cellular proliferation and infiltration affect cell number (PSA) but only minimally affect gland volume, thereby increasing PSAD.

At intermediate PSA levels, the PSA density (PSAD) has been evaluated as a potential approach to improve clinical stage assignment. Benson et al. [12] looked at a series of 328 patients who underwent radical prostatectomy. PSAD was used to predict operative success, defined as favorable pathological findings (no seminal vesicle or lymph node involvement), excision of all tumor with negative margins at the bladder neck and urethra, and an undetectable postoperative PSA level. Eighty percent of patients with a PSAD less than 0.3 ng/ml/ml fulfilled the criteria of operative success, and hence, a PSAD of less than 0.3 ng/ml/ml appeared to be a favourable prognostic factor. However, a high PSAD had a less predictive value, with nearly equal distribution of success and failure among patients with PSAD levels of 0.3 ng/ml/ml or above.

Subsequent investigators evaluated PSAD as a predictor of final pathological stage in 220 patients [13] using postoperative submersion displacement volume to avoid the potential variability of preoperative transrectal ultrasound (TRUS) measurement and incorporated the prostate Gleason score. No patient with both a PSAD greater than 0.3 ng/ml/ml and a Gleason score of 6 or above was found to have a pathologically organ-confined disease.

Although these studies have shown that total PSA and PSAD parallel each other, neither appears to be statistically correlated with Gleason sum or pathological stage. Some authors recommend PSAD determinations in the group of patients with a PSA of 4.1–10.0 ng/ml to increase the sensitivity of cancer detection and identification of those patients with a higher probability of extracapsular disease at the time of surgery. In realistic terms, this measurement will be of little use alone but may have value as part of a predictive nomogram.

III. TRANSITION ZONE PSA IN THE STAGING OF PROSTATE CANCER

Transition zone PSA density (PSAT), an evolution of the PSAD concept, has recently been introduced in an attempt to improve further the accuracy of staging by the measurement of PSAD (see also Chap. 9). PSAT is the ratio between serum total PSA and the volume of the transition zone. PSAT has been hypothesized to have the potential to improve on the accuracy of PSAD.

Zlotta et al. have demonstrated that PSAT is a useful parameter for differentiating between benign disease and prostate cancer in men with a PSA less than 10 ng/ml [14]. In a recent study of 61 consecutive patients with intermediate PSA levels undergoing radical prostatectomy [15], PSAT was superior to total PSA alone and PSAD in predicting pathological stage. In patients with capsular penetration, the areas under the ROC curve were 0.686 for PSA, 0.665 for PSAD, and 0.860 for PSAT. For seminal vesicle invasion, the respective values were 0.712, 0.703, and 0.882.

Improved accuracy of PSAT compared with PSAD was subsequently investigated in a prospective trial of 198 patients who underwent PSAT measurement before radical prostatectomy [16]. In this study, the usefulness of PSAT for differentiating organ-confined prostate cancer from non-organ-confined disease was assessed in men with pretreatment PSA levels less than 10 ng/ml. The ability of PSAT to improve prediction of the final pathological stage with the use of preoperative serum PSA, PSAD, percentage free PSA, DRE, and Gleason score was also assessed. They observed a nearly twofold increase in mean PSAT values in non-organ-confined cancers. The largest difference, as expected, was between patients with and without positive lymph nodes.

Probability plots were created using PSAT, PSAD, percentage free PSA and serum PSA. For predicting extraprostatic extension, PSAT clearly outperformed all other PSA parameters. These encouraging preliminary results warrant evaluation in a larger cohort but suggest that preoperative assessment of the PSAT levels may provide useful information for predicting extraprostatic disease in men with PSA levels less than 10 ng/ml.

IV. PERCENTAGE FREE PSA IN THE STAGING OF PROSTATE CANCER

Total PSA can be reliably measured and differentiated in the serum into free and protein-bound forms. The major portion of circulating PSA is bound to endogenous protease inhibitors, alpha1-antichymotrypsin or alpha2-macroglobulin, whereas a smaller proportion remains free or uncomplexed [17] (see Chaps. 2, 7, 8). Various reports have demonstrated the clinical role of free or uncomplexed PSA in the early detection of prostate cancer [18,19]. Indeed the use of percentage free PSA has been shown to reduce by 20% the rate of negative biopsies in men with a total PSA level between 4.0 and 10.0 ng/ml and still maintain a sensitivity of greater than 90% [18,20].

The use of percentage free PSA for the staging of prostate cancer remains controversial, with many groups publishing conflicting findings. Pannek et al. reported that the use of percentage free PSA might be of interest for prostatic carcinoma staging [21]. In this study, 263 men with clinically localized prostate cancer underwent radical prostatectomy and total and free PSA were measured preoperatively. They found that the percentage free PSA was significantly different between men with organ-confined and those with non-organ-confined tumors (p < 0.0001). This difference was also carried over between those with favorable and unfavorable pathology (p < 0.0001). A cut-off of 15% free PSA provided a 76% and 53% positive and negative predictive value, respectively, for organ-confined disease. Likewise a cut-off of 12% free PSA provided a 72% positive predictive value and 52% negative predictive value for favorable pathology. Arcangeli [22] and Elgamal et al. [23] also reported statistically significance correlation between percentage free PSA and pathological stage. However, other groups contradicted these findings. Henricks [24], Grafen [25], Bangma [26], and Zlotta et al. [16] were all unable to demonstrate a statistical significant correlation between percentage free PSA and pathological stage.

Comparison of the results of the published studies is currently difficult, mainly due to the differences in study populations, study design, definition of pathological outcome, and assays used. Therefore, a final evaluation of the clinical value of percentage free PSA for staging is difficult and the differences observed highlight the difficulty in applying the percentage free PSA for staging prostate cancer on an individual basis [21]. A large multicenter trial, controlling for age, stage, and grade distribution, as well as for a uniform pathological evaluation and comparable total and free PSA assays, is required to elucidate this issue further. Again, it is likely that its measurement will only be of use in combination with other factors as part of a predictive nomogram.

V. PSA VELOCITY IN THE STAGING OF PROSTATE CANCER

PSA velocity, or rate of change in PSA level, has been shown to be a specific marker for the presence of prostate cancer, because most men without prostate cancer have a low rate of change in PSA (less than 0.75 ng/ml/year) [27]. (see also Chap. 5). A persistently rising PSA level suggests disease progression in men with a diagnosis of prostate cancer. Theil et al. [28] retrospectively evaluated the ability of PSA velocity to predict disease stage among a group of patients undergoing radical prostatectomy. Of the 82 patients they were able to evaluate, the mean PSA velocity among men with non-organ-confined prostate cancer (1.88 ng/ml/year) was higher than for men with organ-confined cancer (1.12 ng/ml/yr). The investigators were unable to demonstrate any statistically significant relationship between the PSA velocity and final pathological stage. However, this study was limited in its power by the relatively small number of patients included. This finding was consistent with a previous study by Cadeddu et al. [29], who demonstrated that changes in PSA prior to the diagnosis of prostate cancer were not predictive of later outcome: metastatic disease and death from prostate cancer. These studies all show that although a persistently rising PSA level among men with prostate cancer may reflect disease progression in some cases, PSA velocity prior to a diagnosis of prostate cancer does not appear to reflect disease extent in terms of pathological stage.

VI. REVERSE TRANSCRIPTASE POLYMERASE CHAIN REACTION FOR PSA IN THE STAGING OF PROSTATE CANCER

Reverse transcriptase polymerase chain reaction (RT-PCR) involves the initial conversion of specific mRNA into cDNA followed by the amplification of the

DNA product for analysis by PCR. PSA is secreted primarily by the epithelial cells that line the prostatic acini and ducts and is almost entirely prostate tissue-specific, although PSA gene expression has been identified in a number of other sites such as male and female breast tumors [30] and endometrial tissue [31]. There are significant in vivo data demonstrating that normal prostate cells (and most tumor cells) do not survive in the peripheral circulation [32]. However bloodborne metastasis must by definition be able to survive in order to seed tumor at sites distant to the primary. Taken together, these observations and evidence suggest that the detection of PSA in serum by RT-PCR implies the presence of circulating prostate cancer cells and micrometastatic disease, and could be useful in the staging of prostate cancer. It is, however, important to realize that the presence of tumor cells in the circulation is just one step in the metastatic cascade and these cells may ultimately be cleared from the body without establishing a metastatic site. Animal experiments have suggested that only 0.01% of circulating tumor cells eventually form metastatic deposits [33].

Moreno et al. in 1992 demonstrated that RT-PCR could detect circulating PSA-expressing cells in peripheral blood of patients with prostate cancer [34]. In a study of 12 patients with advanced prostate cancer (stage D) the RT-PCR assay was positive in 4 individuals (2 with stage D1, 1 with stage D2, and 1 with stage D3 disease). All four patients staged as D0 were negative for PSA. In all control patients the RT-PCR assay was negative. Since then a number of studies have been published with highly discrepant results varying from 25 to 80% positive RT-PCR assay in patients with metastatic prostate cancer [35]. Generally, in patients with frank metastasis, the RT-PCR assay was shown to be capable of detecting prostatic cells in the circulation with a high degree of specificity but varying degrees of sensitivity.

A number of studies have shown a significant correlation between positive RT-PCR assay and histological stage. Katz et al. studied a group of 65 patients with clinically localized disease undergoing radical prostatectomy who had a preoperative RT-PCR assay performed [36]. There was a significant correlation between positive findings in the assay and the presence of capsular tumor penetration and positive surgical margins. The authors concluded that the RT-PCR assay was superior to DRE, CT, endorectal MRI, PSA, PSAD, or Gleason score in predicting the true pathological stage of prostate cancer. This and a similar series from the same unit showed sensitivities of around 70% for the assay for predicting extraprostatic disease at the time of surgery, with a specificity of more than 80% [37]. This correlation has not, however, been found in all studies [38].

Other investigators have used this technique to identify prostate cancer cells at other sites. Deguchi et al. detected malignant cells in regional lymph node biopsies of patients with known prostate cancer [39]. RT-PCR was shown to be more sensitive than traditional histological and immunohistochemical methods:

a subset of nodes that were negative for PSA and metastasis by these techniques were positive by RT-PCR. The relevance of this in terms of staging is not theoretically apparent: a positive signal in a lymph node is less likely to indicate a pathological lesion because the node will act as a filtering site for tumorigenic tissue; this may be all that is being demonstrated. Evidence that these findings may be relevant to prostate cancer staging comes from a study by Okegawa et al. [40]. In a series of 38 patients with localized prostate cancer treated with radical prostatectomy they showed that of seven who had a positive RT-PCR assay of their lymph nodes, all went on to experience biochemical recurrence.

Analysis of bone marrow aspirates by RT-PCR has indicated the presence of PSA-expressing cells in the bone marrow of patients with prostate cancer and bone metastasis. RT-PCR of bone marrow aspirates exhibits a good correlation with pathological stage and extracapsular involvment [41].

RT-PCR is an interesting molecular staging method, which enhances the detection of PSA-expressing cells outside the prostate. Current data suggest that it is a very specific but poorly sensitive way to stage patients with prostate cancer. This poor sensitivity may be improved by the concurrent use of markers other than PSA. RT-PCR enhances the detection of PSA-expressing cells in lymph nodes and may allow for more accurate operative staging. Further studies looking at long-term follow-up of patients undergoing curative therapy with positive assays for PSA are awaited with interest. Current evidence suggests that RT-PCR will not replace current staging methods, but it may have a role as a valuable complementary test.

VII. COMBINED MODALITY STAGING OF PROSTATE CANCER

The concept of so-called combined modality staging is not new. It means that all of the clinical factors shown to have independent prognostic significance for the outcome of pathological organ-confined disease are used in determining an individual patient's probability of having pathological organ-confined disease. Partin et al. [42] employed this methodology when generating the probability nomograms for the endpoints of pathological organ-confined disease, extracapsular extension, seminal vesicle involvement, and lymph node involvement. They found that the PSA, biopsy Gleason score, and the clinical stage all contributed independent information in predicting the pathological stage. Further work by Partin et al. [43] on this subject has strengthened the nomograms of the probability of having organ-confined disease with 95% confidence intervals (Table 2). These data were compiled from 4133 surgical cases from 3 separate institutions; PSA, Gleason score, and clinical stage were taken into account. The nomograms

Table 2 Partin's Table: Predicted Probability of Each Pathological Stage Based on Preoperative PSA Level, Clinical Stage, and Gleason Grade in the Biopsy Specimen

Gleason Score	PSA level (ng/ml)								
	0.0–4.0			4.1–10.0			10.1–20.0		
	T1c	T2a	T2b	T1c	T2a	T2b	T1c	T2a	T2b
Organ-confined disease									
5	81	68	57	71	55	43	60	43	32
6	78	64	52	67	51	38	55	38	26
7	63	47	34	49	33	22	35	22	13
8–10	52	36	24	37	23	14	23	14	7
Established capsular penetration									
5	18	30	40	27	41	50	35	50	57
6	21	34	43	30	44	52	38	52	57
7	31	45	51	40	52	54	45	55	51
8–10	34	47	48	40	49	46	40	46	38
Seminal vesicle involvement									
5	1	2	3	2	3	5	3	5	8
6	1	2	3	2	3	5	4	5	7
7	4	6	10	8	10	15	12	14	18
8–10	9	12	17	15	19	24	20	22	25
Lymph node involvement									
5	0	0	1	0	1	2	1	2	4
6	0	1	2	1	2	4	3	4	10
7	1	2	5	3	4	9	8	9	17
8–10	4	5	10	8	9	16	16	17	29

Numbers represent percentage predictive probability.

are able to predict correctly the probability of organ-confined disease in 72.4% of cases.

An addition to the combined modality staging principle is the use of artificial neural networks (ANNs). Artificial neural networks are highly effective and versatile computational models, originally constructed to be analogous with the function of neurons. Using certain methods of parameter optimization, ANNs "learn" to predict output data (e.g., pathological stage) from input data (e.g., PSA, Gleason score) from a given set of preclassified data [44]. Recent applications of neural networks to predict the stage [45] and disease progression [46] indicate that these may be accurate, but further prospective evaluation is required [47]. Such use of artificial intelligence may prove critical for the further use of PSA, and its derivatives, in the staging of prostate cancer.

VIII. CONCLUSIONS

The ability to stage accurately patients with newly diagnosed prostate cancer remains difficult, with even the most sophisticated imaging techniques unable to detect extraprostatic spread in some patients. Partin's nomograms have greatly enhanced the independent prognostic value of serum PSA, DRE, and Gleason score by combining their assessment in individual patients. Improvement in the accuracy of these nomograms will require the addition of more variables. PSA alone is currently limited in its role in the accurate staging of prostate cancer, but it remains one of the most important tumor markers available. Further refinement of its use may still prove critical and highly beneficial

REFERENCES

1. B Spiess, OH Beahrs, P Hermanek, RVP Hutter, O Scheibe, LH Sobin, et al. TNM Atlas: Illustrated Guide to the TNM/pTNM Classification of Malignant Tumours. International Union Against Cancer. Third edition, 2nd revision. Berlin: Springer-Verlag, 1992.
2. GP Haas, et al. Epidemiology of prostate cancer. Cancer J Clin 47:273–287, 1997.
3. JE McNeal, et al. Capsular penetration in prostate cancer: Significance for natural history and treatment. Am J Surg Pathol 14:240–247, 1990.
4. J Epstein, et al. Correlation of pathological findings with progression following radical prostatectomy. Cancer 71:3582, 1993.
5. CR Pound, et al. PSA after anatomic radical retropubic prostatectomy. Patterns of recurrence and cancer control. Urol Clin North Am 24:395, 1997.
6. TA Stamey, et al. PSA as a serum marker for adenocarcinoma of the prostate. N Engl J Med 317:909, 1987.
7. AW Partin, et al. PSA in the staging of localised prostate cancer. Influence of of tumour differentiation, tumour volume and BPH. J Urol 143:747, 1990.
8. P Narayan, et al. The role of TRUS guided biopsy-based staging, preoperative serum PSA, and biopsy Gleason score in prediction of final pathological diagnosis in prostate cancer. Urology 46:205–212, 1995.
9. AW Partin, et al. The use of prostate specific antigen, clinical stage and Gleason score to predict pathological stage in men with localised prostate cancer. J Urol 150:110–114, 1993.
10. FM Chybowski, et al. Predicting radionuclide bone scan findings in patients with newly diagnosed, untreated prostate cancer: prostate specific antigen is superior to all clinical parameters. J Urol 145:313, 1991.
11. Stamey et al. PSA in the diagnosis and treatment of adenocarcinoma of the prostate, 11 radical prostatectomy treated patients. J Urol 141:1076–1083, 1989.
12. MC Benson, et al. PSA and PSAD: Roles in patient evaluation and management. Cancer 74:1667–1673, 1994.

13. M Nishiya, et al. PSAD in patients with histologically proven prostate cancer. Cancer 74:1667–1673, 1994.
14. AR Zlotta, et al. PSAT: A new effective parameter for prostate cancer prediction. J Urol 157:1315, 1997.
15. Y Kurita, et al. Transition zone volume-adjusted PSA value predicts extracapsular carcinoma of the prostate in patients with intermediate PSA levels. Eur Urol 33:32–38, 1998.
16. AR Zlotta, et al. Prostate specific antigen density of the transition zone for predicting pathological stage of localised prostate cancer in patients with serum prostate specific antigen less than 10 ng/ml. J Urol 160:92–98, 1987.
17. H Lilja, et al. PSA in serum occurs predominately in complex with alpha 1-chymotrypsin. Clin Chem 37:1618, 1991.
18. AA Luderer, et al. Measurement of the proportion of free to total PSA improves diagnostic performance of PSA in the diagnostic gray zone of total-PSA. Urology 46:187, 1995.
19. WJ Catalona, et al. Evaluation of percentage of free serum PSA to improve specificity of prostate cancer screening. JAMA 274:1214, 1995.
20. DL Woodrum, et al. Analytical performance of the Tandem-R free PSA immunoassay measuring free PSA. Clin Chem 43:1203, 1997.
21. J Pannek, et al. The use of free PSA for staging clinically localised prostate cancer. J Urol 159:1238, 1998.
22. CG Arcangeli, et al. Correlation of percent free PSA with pathological features of prostate carcinoma. J Urol 155:415A, 1996.
23. AA Elgamali, et al. Free to total PSA ratio as a single test for detection of significant stage T1c prostate cancer. J Urol 156:1042, 1996.
24. WH Henricks, et al. Free to total PSA ratio does not predict extraprostatic spread of prostatic adenocarcinoma. J Urol 155:369A, 1996.
25. M Graefen, et al. Percentage of free PSA does not correlate with pathological outcome. J Urol 155:370A, 1996.
26. CH Bangma, et al. The free to total serum PSA ratio for staging prostate carcinoma. J Urol 157:544, 1997.
27. HB Carter, et al. PSA variability in men without prostate cancer: Effect of sampling intervals on PSA velocity. Urology 45:591, 1995.
28. R Theil, et al. Role of PSA velocity in prediction of final pathological stage in men with localized prostate cancer. Urology 49:716–720, 1997.
29. JA Cadeddu, et al. Relationship between changes in PSA and prognosis of prostate cancer. Urology 42:383, 1993.
30. CM Croce, H Yu, EP Diamandis. Molecular characterisation of prostate-specific antigen mRNA expressed in breast tumours. Cancer Res 54:6344, 1994.
31. J Clements, A Mukhtar. Glandular kallikreins and prostate-specific antigen are expressed in the human endometrium. J Clin Endocrinol Metab 78:1536, 1994.
32. IJ Fidler. Critical factors in the biology of human cancer metastasis: Twenty-eighth GHA Clowes memorial award lerture. Cancer Res. 50:6130, 1990.
33. LA Liotta, J Kleinerman, GM Saidel. Quantitative relationships of intravascular tumour cells, tumour vessels and pulmonary metastasis following tumour implantation. Cancer Res 34: 997, 1974.

34. JG Moreno, CM Croce, R Fischer, M Monne, P Vihko, G Mulholland, LG Gomella. Detection of haematogenous micrometastasis in patients with prostate cancer. Cancer Res 53:6110, 1992.
35. TJ Pelkey, HF Frierson, DE Bruns. Molecular and immunological detection of circulating tumour cells and micrometastasis from solid tumours. Clin Chem 42:1369, 1996.
36. AE Katz, CA Olsson, AJ Raffo, C Cama, H Perlman, E Seaman, KM O'Toole, MC Benson, R Buttyan. Molecular staging of prostate cancer with the use of an enhanced reverse transcriptase-PCR assay. Urology 43(6):765–775, 1994.
37. AE Katz, GM de Vries, MD Begg, AJ Raffo, C Cama, KM O'Toole, R Buttyan, MC Benso, CA Olsson. Enhanced reverse transcriptase-polymerase chain reaction for prostate specific antigen as an indicator of true pathological stage in patients with prostate cancer. Cancer 75(7):1642–8, 1995.
38. P de Cremoux, V Ravery, MP Podgorniak, S Chevillard, M Toublane, N Thiounn, R Tatoud, V Delmas, T Calvo, L Boccon-Gibod. Value of the preoperative detection of prostrate-specific-antigen-positive circulating cells by nested RT-PCR in patients submitted to radical protatectomy. Eur Urol 32:69–74, 1997.
39. C Rinker-Schaeffer, A Partin, W Isaacs, D Coffey, J Isaacs. Molecular and cellular changes associated with the acquisition of metastatic ability by prostate cancer cells. Prostate 25:249, 1994.
40. T Okegawa, K Nutahara, E Higashihara. Detection of micrometastatic prostate cancer cells in the lymph nodes by reverse transcriptase polymerase chain reaction is predictive of biochemical recurrence in pathological stage T2 prostate cancer. J Urol 163:1183–1188, 2000.
41. DP Woods, ER Banks, S Humphreys JW McRoberts, VM Rangnekar. Identification of bone marrow micrometastases in patients with prostate cancer. Cancer 74(9): 2533–40, 1994.
42. AW Partin, et al. The use of PSA, clinical stage and Gleason score to predict pathological stage in men with localised prostate cancer. J Urol 150:110–114, 1993.
43. AW Partin, et al. Combination of PSA, clinical stage and Gleason score to predict pathological stage of localised prostate cancer. A multi-institutional update. JAMA 270:1445, 1997.
44. A Tewari, et al. Artificial intelligence and neural networks: concept, applications and future in urology. Br J Urol 80:53–8, 1997.
45. GP Murphy, et al. Evaluation of prostate cancer patients receiving multiple staging tests, including ProstaScint(R) scintiscans. Prostate 42:145–149, 2000.
46. SR Potter, et al. Genetically engineered neural networks for predicting prostate cancer progression after radical prostatectomy. Urology 54:791–795, 1999.
47. T Mattfeldt, et al. Prediction of prostatic cancer progression after radical prostatectomy using artificial neural networks: A feasibility study. Br J Urol Int 84:316–323, 1999.

12
PSA and Radical Prostatectomy

Mark R. Feneley and Alan W. Partin
The Johns Hopkins Hospital, Baltimore, Maryland

Prostate specific antigen (PSA) identifies men with clinically significant prostate cancer at a stage when definitive treatment is curative [1]. Its use in screening and early detection has had a dramatic influence on the number of men diagnosed with early-stage prostate cancer and undergoing radical prostatectomy [2]. The likelihood of cure with definitive treatment depends predominantly on pathological stage, and serum PSA levels contribute to the preoperative prediction of pathological stage independently of clinical stage and biopsy grade [3]. PSA also provides the earliest indicator of recurrence in almost all patients who are not cured by definitive measures [4].

I. EPIDEMIOLOGY OF PROSTATE CANCER AND PSA TESTING

Our clinical experience with the use of PSA has been acquired principally within the past 15 years. In 1992, the American Cancer Society recommended the combination of PSA testing and digital rectal examination (DRE) as part of a prostate cancer screening strategy [5], and in 1994 PSA testing was approved by the Food and Drug Administration (FDA). Prostate cancer has become the most frequently diagnosed noncutaneous malignancy in American men owing to the increase in diagnosis of early-stage disease [6], and, as a result, a growing number of men are being treated [7,8]. The standard of definitive treatment offered by radical prostatectomy has become widely recommended by urologists for management of early-stage disease [2,9], particularly following description by Walsh of the anatomic surgical approach that has allowed operative morbidity to be reduced without compromising cancer cure [2,9,10].

In the United States, the incidence of prostate cancer increased dramatically, during the early part of the PSA era, from 84:100,000 in 1984 to a peak of 190:100,000 in 1992, predominantly reflecting an increasing diagnosis of early-stage disease in younger men. Eighty percent of this increase is accounted for by moderately differentiated disease (Gleason score 5–7), although well- (Gleason score 2–4) and poorly differentiated (Gleason score 8–10) disease have followed similar trends [11]. This increase has since yielded to a gradual decline that may be predicted from population exposure to screening.

II. RADICAL PROSTATECTOMY AND THE IMPORTANCE OF PREOPERATIVE PSA

PSA has been shown to be a reliable means of identifying men with prostate cancer in whom definitive treatment achieves excellent disease control [12]. Screening with DRE and PSA represents the most certain means for detecting disease at a curable stage and thereby reducing mortality [1]. Outcome studies indicate the prognostic importance of clinical stage [13,14], as well as pathological stage and ultimately organ-confined pathology, for identifying those patients least likely to develop metastatic disease [15,16]. Unfortunately, at least half of palpable (stage T2) clinically organ-confined cancers are understaged, and organ-confined disease based on pathological staging can only be established definitively in men treated by radical prostatectomy at the time of surgery [3,17].

PSA offers a reliable means of detecting cancer before it becomes palpable by DRE (stage T1c), facilitating treatment at an earlier pathological stage [16]. PSA detection has been suggested to provide a lead time in diagnosis of around 4–6 years [18,19]. Nevertheless, more than one-third of PSA-detected tumors are still associated with established capsular penetration or more extensive extraprostatic disease at pathological examination [20].

Preoperative serum PSA levels correlate with tumor stage [21], and risk of subsequent recurrence in men having radical prostatectomy [12,22]. In immunohistochemical terms, there is a decrease in PSA production in higher-grade carcinomas [23]. However, since these tend to be larger neoplasms, serum PSA level generally correlates directly with grade. Serum PSA is also affected by coexisting benign pathological findings and prostatic manipulation. Because of these factors, the value of PSA alone for predicting stage in the individual patient is limited.

The Gleason grade of tumor on needle biopsy specimens relates to risk of non-organ-confined disease, pathological stage, and probability of cure [3,15, 24,26]. Whereas high-grade tumor (Gleason score $\geq$ 7) is associated with substantial risk of extraprostatic disease, seminal vesicle invasion, or lymphatic metastases [27,28], biopsies containing small foci (Gleason score ≤ 7) often indicate a greater likelihood of organ-confined disease [29].

The risk of underestimating pathological stage has therefore been defined by nomograms incorporating clinical stage, PSA level, and biopsy Gleason score. These were initially defined on the basis of the single-institution experience at Johns Hopkins Hospital [30], and subsequently have been validated in a multi-institutional setting [3]. Pathological stage prediction relates also to other biopsy-derived parameters including the distribution of cancer and its core extent [26,28].

The benefit of early diagnosis depends entirely on the therapeutic advantage that is gained, and is most clearly defined by cure. Cure is most reliably obtained in men with organ-confined cancer, and therefore this represents the optimal stage for treatment. Unfortunately, even in men with pathologically organ-confined cancer, a minority may not be cured owing to the presence of microscopic disease beyond the prostate at the time of surgery. Accordingly, an alternative nomogram based on clinical stage, PSA, and biopsy Gleason score has been created to predict PSA relapse within 5 years of radical prostatectomy, using a model in which non-organ-confined cancer may be considered curable [31]. Although PSA relapse may indicate that cure has not been achieved, biochemical recurrence has a notoriously variable relationship to the course of subsequent clinical disease, and does not preclude the possibility of prolonged disease-free survival.

III. DETECTION OF CANCER RECURRENCE AFTER RADICAL PROSTATECTOMY

The first indication of disease recurrence after radical prostatectomy is invariably the return of detectable serum PSA levels, which justifies regular testing in follow-up [4]. In the absence of measurable clinical symptoms or radiographic evidence of disease, this is referred to as biochemical relapse. Using conventional PSA assays with a lower limit of detection at 0.1 ng/ml, serum levels greater than 0.2 ng/ml measured on more than one occasion may be taken as an indication of recurrent or residual disease, particularly when there is an incremental increase [32]. Although ultrasensitive assays with thresholds as low as 0.001 ng/ml may provide an additional lead time of almost 2 years for the detection of recurrence [33–36], low levels of serum PSA from other sources such as the periurethral glands may be misleading [37].

PSA relapse after radical prostatectomy occurs in 20–30% of men by 5 years and in 25–50% by 10 years, and varies significantly between reported series [12,38,42]. The risk of developing biochemical relapse relates independently to preoperative PSA, final pathological stage, and whole-tumor Gleason score [12,15,43,44]. These postoperative parameters have therefore been used to define prognostically distinct risk groups [42,43,45,46]. Biomarker expression in radical prostatectomy specimens may also relate to biological behavior and provide additional prognostic information, but is not generally incorporated into clinical algorithms [45,47,48]. For individual patients, the course of disease following treatment is notoriously variable and difficult to predict.

Since an excellent prognostic assessment can be made on the basis of preoperative clinical evaluation and definitive pathological examination, PSA testing is not generally warranted until 1–3 months following radical prostatectomy [49]. Furthermore, PSA detected within less than 1 month after surgery is difficult to interpret owing to the possibility that preoperative levels are incompletely cleared [50]. In patients who achieve and maintain undetectable PSA postoperatively, long-term follow-up should be recommended since subsequent biochemical relapse may take more than 10 years to become manifest [4].

IV. EVALUATION OF PREOPERATIVE PSA, BIOPSY GLEASON SCORE, AND RISK OF PSA RELAPSE IN MEN WITH STAGE T1c CANCER

The risk of PSA relapse after radical prostatectomy for clinical stage T1c cancer has previously been shown to relate to pathological stage. It is greatest in those patients with positive surgical margins, lymph node and/or seminal vesicle involvement, and, among the remainder, recurrence correlates with tumor grade and extent of extraprostatic disease [15]. High preoperative serum PSA levels also increase the risk of PSA relapse, consistent with the relationship of PSA to more advanced stage and larger tumors [12]. Since over 90% of men with stage T1c cancer have Gleason score 7 or less, and noncurable cancer is not reliably predicted by grade alone in this range [3], we examined how the combination of preoperative PSA and biopsy Gleason score may contribute to the risk of PSA relapse in men with stage T1c disease. We have thereby defined a group of substage categories for further prognostic stratification of this stage.

PSA relapse was actuarially examined in 757 men, median age 59 years (range, 33–73; mean 57), with clinical stage T1c prostate cancer having radical prostatectomy performed by a single surgeon at The Johns Hopkins Hospital between 1989 and 1998. Patients who had received neoadjuvant or immediate adjuvant therapy were not included in this analysis. On pathological staging, 21 (2.8%) had lymph node metastases, 30 (4.0%) had seminal vesicle involvement, and 251 (33%) had organ-confined disease. Median follow-up was for 3 years (range, 1–9; mean 3 years). Kaplan-Meier actuarial survival analysis shown in Figure 1 indicated that the risk of PSA relapse was significantly lower in men with organ-confined cancer than in men with more advanced disease. The influence of tumor grade on risk of PSA relapse is shown in Figure 2. Among preoperative

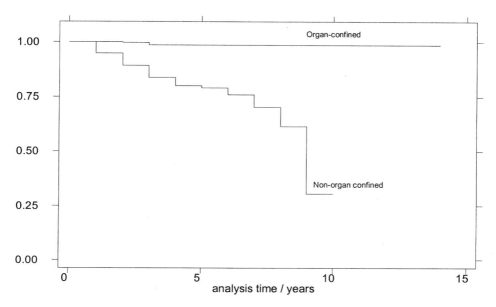

Figure 1   Kaplan-Meier actuarial survival estimates for patients with stage T1c prostate cancer by organ-confined status.

variables, the risk of PSA relapse increased with higher biopsy Gleason score (Table 1).

The combination of biopsy Gleason score and preoperative PSA was examined as a means of identifying patients who subsequently developed PSA relapse, using the receiver operating characteristics (ROC) of these parameters to determine optimum cut-offs. In men with biopsy Gleason score ≤ 7, the proportion of relapse-free patients identified by preoperative PSA below the evaluated cut-off increased with higher PSA cut-offs (sensitivity). The proportion of men with PSA relapse predicted by the reverse criteria (i.e., biopsy Gleason score ≥ 8 or PSA above a given cut-off) decreased with higher PSA cut-offs (specificity): this is shown by the ROC data in Table 2. Using biopsy Gleason score ≤ 6 rather than biopsy Gleason score ≤ 7 with preoperative PSA, greater specificity was obtained for the same sensitivity levels (Table 2). Since biopsy Gleason < 6 has poor sensitivity for predicting PSA-free survival, it did not represent a useful cut-off (not shown). Based on the ROC data predicting PSA-free survival by the combination of preoperative PSA and biopsy Gleason score cut-offs at 6 and 7, the optimal PSA cut-off was shown to be 12.0 ng/ml. The optimal Gleason score cut-off at this PSA level was provided by maximum biopsy Gleason score of 6 (Table 2).

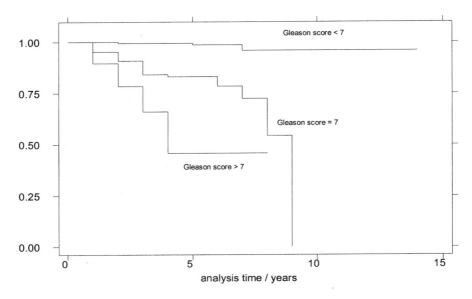

Figure 2   Kaplan-Meier actuarial survival estimates for patients with stage T1c prostate cancer by final Gleason score.

The combination of Gleason score < 7 and preoperative PSA < 12.0 predicted PSA-free survival with a sensitivity of 521/706 (74%) and specificity of 43/51 (84%). This cut-off combination (Gleason score < 7 and preoperative PSA < 12.0) also provided the best positive predictive value for PSA-free survival, with a positive predictive value (PPV) of 521/529 (98%). Kaplan Meier survival analysis demonstrated the increased risk of PSA relapse in men with either biopsy Gleason > 6 or PSA ≥ 12.0, logrank test p < 0.0001 (Fig. 3).

Table 1   Pattern of Relapse by Biopsy Gleason Score After Radical Prostatectomy for Stage T1c Disease

Biopsy Gleason score	Number	Number with PSA relapse (%)	Actuarial 5 year PSA-free survival (%)
<6	80	2 (2.5)	97
6	545	22 (4)	92
7	118	22 (19)	80
>7	14	5 (36)	32

Table 2 Receiver Operating Characteristics of PSA Cut-Offs in Combination with Biopsy Gleason Score for Predicting PSA-Free Survival

Sensitivity for 5 year PSA-free survival		PSA cut-off (less than; ng/ml)	Specificity for 5 year PSA-free survival	
Gleason ≤7	Gleason ≤6		Gleason ≤6	Gleason ≤7
0.12	0.11	4.0	0.96	0.96
0.26	0.24	5.0	0.94	0.94
0.42	0.38	6.0	0.90	0.88
0.55	0.49	7.0	0.86	0.82
0.66	0.58	8.0	0.86	0.78
0.73	0.65	9.0	0.84	0.67
0.78	0.69	10.0	0.84	0.59
0.82	0.72	11.0	0.84	0.59
0.84	0.74	12.0	0.84	0.59
0.87	0.76	13.0	0.78	0.49
0.88	0.77	14.0	0.75	0.45
0.89	0.78	15.0	0.67	0.37

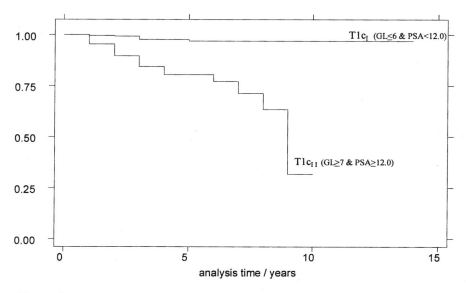

Figure 3 Kaplan-Meier actuarial survival estimates for patients with stage T1c prostate cancer substaged by biopsy Gleason score (GL) and preoperative PSA.

These data closely approximate the excellent stratification provided by pathological stage seen in Figure 1.

The risk of relapse associated with biopsy Gleason score less than 7 and preoperative PSA *at least* 12.0 ng/ml related to non-organ-confined disease and underestimation of whole tumor grade. In the 96 men fulfilling this criteria combination, PSA relapse was predicted by non-organ-confined stage with sensitivity of 16/16 (100%) and specificity of 47/80 (59%). In the same group of 96 men, biopsy undergrading (biopsy Gleason score < 7 for whole tumor Gleason score ≥ 7) had a sensitivity of 13/16 (81%) and specificity of 53/80 (66%) for predicting PSA relapse.

These results indicate that in men with stage T1c cancer, biopsy Gleason score less than 7, and preoperative PSA less than 12.0 ng/ml, the risk of PSA relapse is extremely low (<2%). In men with higher PSA levels, the increased risk of relapse relates to underestimation of whole tumor grade as well as understaging. These findings are consistent with previous observations that have correlated the risk of undergrading with preoperative serum PSA levels [51] and more advanced stage [52].

Previous studies have also shown that cancer of Gleason score 7 or higher is an adverse prognostic factor in men undergoing radical prostatectomy for clinically localized disease, particularly in those with lymph node metastases, seminal vesicle involvement, or positive surgical margins [15]. These Gleason scores in biopsy cores are likewise frequently associated with non-organ-confined disease [53–55]. Focal Gleason 7 cancer in a single biopsy, however, may not necessarily preclude curable disease [29], and some tumors are overgraded in biopsy material. In patients with biopsy Gleason 7 undergoing radical prostatectomy, 13–26% may have whole tumor Gleason score 6 disease [29,56].

Our data suggest stage T1c prostate cancer treated by radical prostatectomy may be subclassified to identify a category of patients at low risk for PSA relapse. This risk was defined in our analysis by the combination of biopsy Gleason score < 7 and PSA < 12.0 ng/ml. Relapse in men with Gleason score 6 and

Table 3 Substratification of Stage T1c Prostate Cancer as $T1c_I$ and $T1c_{II}$ by Preoperative Criteria to Identify Patients with Low or High Risk of PSA Relapse

	$T1c_I$	$T1c_{II}$
Biopsy Gleason score	≤6	≥7
Serum PSA (ng/ml)	<12.0	≥12.0
5 year actuarial PSA-free survival (%)	98	77
10 year actuarial PSA-free survival (%)	96	27

PSA 12.0 ng/ml or greater was associated with underestimation of tumor grade and non-organ-confined disease. Owing to potential selection bias of the studied population, prospective studies in a multi-institutional setting will be required to validate the predictive value of substaging criteria. Table 3 shows the preoperative criteria for substratification of men with clinical stage T1c cancer.

V. EVALUATION OF DISEASE RECURRENCE ASSOCIATED WITH PSA RELAPSE

PSA relapse following radical prostatectomy can be associated with prolonged survival [32,57] and in the majority of patients, it precedes recurrence of clinical disease. Bone scan and pelvic computed tomography are indicated to exclude metastatic or local recurrence that may warrant treatment, even in the absence of symptoms or physical signs of recurrence. Clinically detectable disease in the absence of detectable PSA is rare [58], and usually associated with high-grade disease [59,60]. Symptoms or suspicion of clinical disease should be specifically and irrespectively investigated.

When PSA relapse is first detected and investigated, most individuals have otherwise no clinically detectable disease. They can therefore be managed expectantly with careful follow-up and annual staging investigations. Many will remain free of clinical disease for substantial lengths of time (even without therapeutic intervention) and the benefit of further therapeutic intervention during this period is unproven.

After PSA relapse, recurrence of clinical disease may eventually be detected as distant metastases, local recurrence, or both. At Johns Hopkins Hospital, actuarial rates for isolated PSA relapse, metastatic recurrence, and local recurrence reported at 10 years are 18%, 9%, and 8%, respectively, and for any of these recurrences at 10 years it was 32% [12]. Metastatic disease was indicated by positive findings on bone scan or radiological evidence of lymphadenopathy. Local recurrence was defined as a palpable abnormality of the prostatic fossa (with or without biopsy confirmation) associated with detectable PSA or positive biopsy.

The principal significance of PSA relapse for individual patients relates to cancer-specific and metastasis-free survival. The natural history of postradical prostatectomy PSA and progression from PSA relapse to metastatic disease was recently examined at Johns Hopkins Hospital [4]. Among 1997 men treated by radical prostatectomy, 304 patients with PSA relapse were managed expectantly until metastatic disease occurred. Of these 304 men, 34% developed metastatic disease, at a median interval of 8 years, indicating that PSA relapse may be associated with prolonged survival. The median time from metastatic disease to death was less than 5 years. An interesting finding was that metastatic progression correlated with the rate of development of metastatic disease. In this study, overall 10 and 15 year cancer-specific survival rates were 94% and 91%, respectively, and metastasis-free survival rates were 87% and 82%, respectively.

In men with clinical recurrence after radical prostatectomy, factors associated with this representing metastatic failure included the timing of PSA relapse, Gleason score, and PSA doubling time as well as the presence of lymph node metastases or seminal vesicle invasion at the time of surgery [12]. Relapse within 2 years or Gleason score ≥8 was associated with metastatic pattern of failure in around 90% of cases. The significance of PSA velocity greater than 0.75 cc/year was shown by Partin et al. [61], to predict metastatic failure. The value of this concept has been confirmed independently in a study that showed metastatic progression was associated with doubling times less than 6 months [62]. In patients with lymph node metastases or seminal vesicle involvement, clinical recurrence was associated with distant metastases in 93% and 84% respectively. In those with positive surgical margins, fewer than 50% had local recurrence without metastases.

In practice, the significance of positive surgical margins in men without lymph node metastases or seminal vesicle invasion relates to whole tumor grade [4]. Men with Gleason score ≤ 4 have retained an excellent prognosis irrespective of margin status. Men with Gleason score 8 or 9 have a 35% probability of 10 year PSA-free survival and, for them also, outcome is independent of margin status [15,63]. Surgical margin status, however, is significant in determining outcome for men with Gleason score 7 disease [12,64].

In men with local recurrence, PSA recurrence almost invariably precedes the development of a palpable abnormality in the prostatic fossa [65]. Furthermore, the finding of a palpable abnormality does not necessarily predict cancer on biopsies from the region of the urethrovesical anastomosis, since it may be due to local fibrosis or residual benign prostatic tissue [66]. Residual prostatic tissue (indicating incomplete prostatectomy) may contribute to serum PSA as well as compromising cure. For patients with undetectable PSA, the benefit of follow-up DRE may be limited to a very small minority in whom the palpable abnormality occurs prior to PSA relapse and for which additional treatment would be beneficial.

Imaging with transrectal ultrasound or computed tomography has limited accuracy for determining local recurrence and scan abnormalities are not sufficiently specific or sensitive to detect tumor recurrence [67]. Although positive prostatic fossa biopsy may be associated with positive margin status [67], margin status does not predict that PSA relapse is due to local recurrence [61]. A role for either prostatic radioimmunoscintigraphy using a radiolabeled antibody to prostate membrane-specific antigen (PMSA) or endorectal coil MRI is yet to be established in clinical practice [68,69]. PMSA scan findings suggesting isolated local recurrence may identify patients who are most likely to have disease curable by salvage treatment, but complete response to radiation is not precluded by scan findings suggesting disease beyond the prostatic fossa [70].

VI. IMPLICATIONS FOR TREATMENT OF PSA RELAPSE

Local recurrence may be treated by radiation; the absence of systemic disease raises the possibility of cure [71–79]. The relative merits of adjuvant radiation to the prostatic fossa following surgery in patients who may be at risk of local recurrence or salvage radiation for established local recurrence are debated and unresolved. Prospective randomized trials will eventually be required to determine the optimal timing of postoperative radiation and its influence on subsequent PSA free survival, metastatic control, actuarial disease-specific survival, and morbidity.

Follow-up of adjuvant radiation therapy for patients with suspected or biopsy-proven local recurrence suggest that treatment may be locally effective and well tolerated [80–82]. Following complete PSA response to salvage radiation, PSA-free rates at 5 years range between 10 and 45% [76,77]. Morbidity is usually early, self-limiting, and responsive to treatment. Urinary incontinence is rarely affected by post-operative radiation provided postsurgical urinary incontinence has resolved. Late morbidity relates to concerns about proctitis, cystitis, and urinary incontinence [74,75,78,83–85].

PSA responses following postoperative radiation should be interpreted cautiously at the present time, and long-term follow-up is required before initial expectations can be confirmed to be meaningful. At a pragmatic level, the presence of local disease may be inferred by a complete PSA response to radiation, reported in 50 to more than 90% of patients. PSA response, however, does not exclude the possibility of systemic disease that may become manifest years later. The benefit of adjuvant or salvage radiation must therefore be considered in terms of long-term biochemical relapse-free survival and underlying impact on morbidity and metastatic progression of local recurrence. Several reports indicate that initial PSA response may not be durable [76,77,86].

Prospective randomized trials are currently needed to determine the optimal timing of salvage therapy in relation to surgery, need for biopsy evidence of recurrence, and optimal absolute PSA value [62,84,87]. Present experience suggests that preradiation PSA level may be predictive of response [88]. Where outcome descriptions are available, these may then be related to tumor parameters and prognostic factors [79]. The use of radiation sensitizers, including temporary androgen deprivation, may theoretically improve therapeutic responses in specific situations, but their advantage is unproven [89]. At the present time, the overall efficacy of salvage radiotherapy for disease control and its specific effect on metastatic progression of truly localized recurrence is unknown.

Androgen deprivation offers systemic treatment, but prior to the development of distant metastases it is controversial and of uncertain benefit [90,91]. It also incurs significant immediate and long-term side effects. Although the adverse effects may be reduced, at least to some extent, by intermittent androgen withdrawal, unknown outcome and potentially significant costs remain concerns [92]. Treatment decisions for men with PSA relapse need to be made on the basis of applied oncological principles, descriptions of therapeutic outcome and potential morbidity, as well as recently acquired knowledge of the natural history of biochemical recurrence.

VII. CONCLUSION

The risk of PSA relapse in men with localized prostate cancer treated with radical prostatectomy relates to clinical stage, preoperative PSA, pathological stage, and tumor Gleason score. In men with stage T1c prostate cancer detected by PSA, biopsy Gleason score less than 7 with preoperative PSA less than 12.0 ng/ml indicates a low risk of subsequent relapse, and potentially represents a new substage category (T1c$_I$ and T1c$_{II}$). In patients not fulfilling these criteria, the risk of PSA relapse relates to pathological stage and tumor Gleason score.

The natural history of PSA relapse following radical prostatectomy has begun to be better defined. Many patients with untreated PSA relapse have a substantial metastases-free survival, and, for these individuals, observation need not necessarily yield to early intervention because of anxiety associated with a PSA level reaching an arbitrary clinical threshold. There are currently no clear guidelines for the treatment of PSA relapse without clinically demonstrable disease. The benefit of treatment in men who either have clinical recurrence or at risk of developing clinical recurrence requires evaluation in future randomized trials.

REFERENCES

1. WJ Catalona, DS Smith, TL Ratliff, JW Basler. Detection of organ-confined prostate cancer is increased through prostate-specific antigen-based screening. JAMA 270: 948–954, 1993.
2. WF Gee, HL Holtgrewe, ML Blute, et al. 1997 American Urological Association Gallup survey: Changes in diagnosis and management of prostate cancer and benign prostatic hyperplasia, and other practice trends from 1994 to 1997. J Urol 160:1804–1807, 1998.
3. AW Partin, MW Kattan, EN Subong, et al. Combination of prostate-specific antigen, clinical stage, and Gleason score to predict pathological stage of localized prostate cancer. A multi-institutional update. JAMA 277:1445–1451, 1997.

4. CR Pound, AW Partin, MA Eisenberger, DW Chan, JD Pearson, PC Walsh. Natural history of progression after PSA elevation following radical prostatectomy. JAMA 281:1591–1597, 1999.
5. C Mettlin, G Jones, H Averette, SB Gusberg, GP Murphy. Defining and updating the American Cancer Society guidelines for the cancer-related checkup: prostate and endometrial cancers. Ca Cancer J Clin 43:42–46, 1993.
6. SH Landis, T Murray, S Bolden, PA Wing. Cancer statistics, 1999. CA Cancer J Clin 49:8–31, 1999.
7. MS Litwin, DJ Pasta, ML Stoddard, JM Henning, PR Carroll. Epidemiological trends and financial outcomes in radical prostatectomy among Medicare beneficiaries, 1991 to 1993 [published erratum appears in J Urol 1998 Dec; 160(6 Pt 1):2164] J Urol 160:445–448, 1998.
8. LM Ellison, JA Heaney, JD Birkmeyer. Trends in the use of radical prostatectomy for treatment of prostate cancer. Eff Clin Pract 2:228–233, 1999.
9. GL Lu-Yao, D Mckerran, J Wasson, JE Wennberg. An assessment of radical prostatectomy: Time trends, geographic variation, and outcome. JAMA 269:2633–2636, 1993.
10. PC Walsh. Radical retropubic prostatectomy with reduced morbidity: An anatomic approach. NCI Monogr 7:133–137, 1988.
11. JL Stanford, RA Stephenson, LM Coyle, et al. Prostate Cancer Trends 1973–1995, SEER Program, NCI. NIH Pub. No. 99-4543. National Cancer Institute, Bethesda, MD, 1999.
12. CR Pound, AW Partin, JI Epstein, PC Walsh. Prostate-specific antigen after anatomic radical retropubic prostatectomy. Patterns of recurrence and cancer control. Urol Clin North Am 24:395–406, 1997.
13. GS Gerber, RA Thisted, PT Scardino, et al. Results of radical prostatectomy in men with clinically localized prostate cancer. JAMA 276:615–619, 1996.
14. RV Iyer, AL Hanlon, WH Pinover, GE Hanks. Outcome evaluation of the 1997 American Joint Committee on Cancer staging system for prostate carcinoma treated by radiation therapy. Cancer 85:1816–1821, 1999.
15. JI Epstein, AW Partin, J Sauvageot, PC Walsh. Prediction of progression following radical prostatectomy. A multivariate analysis of 721 men with long-term follow-up. Am J Surg Pathol 20:286–292, 1996.
16. CG Ramos, GF Carvalhal, DS Smith, DE Mager, WJ Catalona. Clinical and pathological characteristics, and recurrence rates of stage T1c versus T2a or T2b prostate cancer. J Urol 161:1525–1529, 1999.
17. GW Chodak, P Keller, HW Schoenberg. Assessment of screening for prostate cancer using the digital rectal examination. J Urol 141:1136–1138, 1989.
18. SJ Jacobsen, SK Katusic, EJ Bergstralh, et al. Incidence of prostate cancer diagnosis in the eras before and after serum prostate-specific antigen testing. JAMA 274:1445–1459, 1995.
19. PH Gann, CH Hennekens, MJ Stampfer. A prospective evaluation of plasma prostate-specific antigen for detection of prostatic cancer. JAMA 273:289–294, 1995.
20. JI Epstein, PC Walsh, M Carmichael, CB Brendler. Pathologic and clinical findings to predict tumor extent of nonpalpable (stage T1c) prostate cancer. JAMA 271:368–374, 1994.

21. TA Stamey, N Yang, AR Hay, et al. Prostate-specific antigen as a serum marker for adenocarcinoma of the prostate. N Engl J Med 317:909–916, 1987.
22. P Kupelian, J Katcher, H Levin, C Zippe, E Klein. Correlation of clinical and pathologic factors with rising prostate-specific antigen profiles after radical prostatectomy alone for clinically localized prostate cancer. Urology 48:249–260, 1996.
23. AW Partin, HB Carter, DW Chan, et al. Prostate specific antigen in the staging of localized prostate cancer: Influence of tumor differentiation, tumor volume and benign hyperplasia. J Urol 143:747–752, 1990.
24. RA Badalament, MC Miller, PA Peller, et al. An algorithm for predicting nonorgan confined prostate cancer using the results obtained from sextant core biopsies with prostate specific antigen level. J Urol 156:1375–1380, 1996.
25. E Kleer, JJ Larson-Keller, H Zincke, JE Oesterling. Ability of preoperative serum prostate-specific antigen value to predict pathologic stage and DNA ploidy. Influence of clinical stage and tumor grade. Urology 41:207–216, 1993.
26. DG Bostwick, J Qian, E Bergstralh, et al. Prediction of capsular perforation and seminal vesicle invasion in prostate cancer. J Urol 155:1361–1367, 1996.
27. JI Epstein, GD Steinberg. The significance of low-grade prostate cancer on needle biopsy. A radical prostatectomy study of tumor grade, volume, and stage of the biopsied and multifocal tumor. Cancer 66: 1927–1932, 1990.
28. ML Wills, J Sauvageot, AW Partin, R Gurganus, JI Epstein. Ability of sextant biopsies to predict radical prostatectomy Urology 51:759–764, 1998.
29. XJ Yang, K Lecksell, SR Potter, JI Epstein. Significance of small foci of Gleason score 7 or greater prostate cancer on needle biopsy. Urology 54:528–532, 1999.
30. AW Partin, J Yoo, HB Carter, et al. The use of prostate specific antigen, clinical stage and Gleason score to predict pathological stage in men with localized prostate cancer. J Urol 150:110–114, 1993.
31. MW Kattan, JA Eastham, AM Stapleton, TM Wheeler, PT Scardino. A preoperative nomogram for disease recurrence following radical prostatectomy for prostate cancer. J Natl Cancer Inst 90:766–771, 1998.
32. PH Lange, CJ Ercole, DJ Lightner, EE Fraley, R Vessella. The value of serum prostate specific antigen determinations before and after radical prostatectomy. J Urol 141:873–879, 1989.
33. WJ Ellis, RL Vessella, JL Noteboom, et al. Early detection of recurrent prostate cancer with an ultrasensitive chemiluminescent prostate-specific antigen assay. Urology 50:573–579, 1997.
34. TA Stamey, HC Graves, N Wehner, et al. Early detection of residual prostate cancer after radical prostatectomy by an ultrasensitive assay for prostate specific antigen. J Urol 149:787–792, 1993.
35. H Yu, EP Diamandis, PY Wong, et al. Detection of prostate cancer relapse with prostate specific antigen monitoring at levels of 0.001 to 0.1 microG./L. J Urol 157: 913–918, 1997.
36. A Haese, E Huland, M Graefen, et al. Ultrasensitive detection of prostate specific antigen in the followup of 422 patients after radical prostatectomy. J Urol 161:1206–1211, 1999.
37. EP Diamandis, H Yu. Nonprostatic sources of prostate-specific antigen. Urol Clin North Am 24:275–282, 1997.

38. H Zincke, JE Oesterling, ML Blute, et al. Long-term (15 years) results after radical prostatectomy for clinically localized (stage T2c or lower) prostate cancer. J Urol 152:1850–1857, 1994.

39. M Ohori, JR Goad, TM Wheeler, et al. Can radical prostatectomy alter the progression of poorly differentiated prostate cancer? J Urol 152:1843–1849, 1994.

40. JG Trapasso, JB DeKernion, RB Smith, F Dorey. The incidence and significance of detectable levels of serum prostate specific antigen after radical prostatectomy. J Urol 152:1821–1825, 1994.

41. WJ Catalona, DS Smith. 5-year tumor recurrence rates after anatomical radical retropubic prostatectomy for prostate cancer. J Urol 152:1837–1842, 1994.

42. MW Kattan, TM Wheeler, PT Scardino. Postoperative nomogram for disease recurrence after radical prostatectomy for prostate cancer. J Clin Oncol 17:1499–1507, 1999.

43. AV D'Amico, R Whittington, SB Malkowicz, et al. The combination of preoperative prostate specific antigen and postoperative pathological findings to predict prostate specific antigen outcome in clinically localized prostate cancer. J Urol 160:2096–2101, 1998.

44. P Kupelian, J Katcher, H Levin, et al. External beam radiotherapy versus radical prostatectomy for clinical stage T1–2 prostate cancer: Therapeutic implications of stratification by pretreatment PSA levels and biopsy Gleason scores. Cancer J Sci Am 3:78–87, 1997.

45. JJ Bauer, RR Connelly, IA Sesterhenn, et al. Biostatistical modeling using traditional variables and genetic biomarkers for predicting the risk of prostate carcinoma recurrence after radical prostatectomy. Cancer 79:952–962, 1997.

46. AW Partin, S Piantadosi, MG Sanda, et al. Selection of men at high risk for disease recurrence for experimental adjuvant therapy following radical prostatectomy. Urology 45:831–838, 1995.

47. JN Netto, ML Lima, MA Guedes, et al. Elevation of prostate specific antigen in cardiac surgery with extracorporeal cardiopulmonary circulation. J Urol 159:875–877, 1998.

48. AM Stapleton, P Zbell, MW Kattan, et al. Assessment of the biologic markers p53, Ki-67, and apoptotic index as predictive indicators of prostate carcinoma recurrence after surgery. Cancer 82:168–175, 1998.

49. J Oh, JW Colberg, DK Ornstein, et al. Current followup strategies after radical prostatectomy: A survey of American Urological Association urologists. J Urol 161:520–523, 1999.

50. AW Partin, JE Oesterling. The clinical usefulness of prostate specific antigen: update 1994. J Urol 152:1358–1368, 1994.

51. M Kojima, P Troncoso, RJ Babaian. Use of prostate-specific antigen and tumor volume in predicting needle biopsy grading error. Urology 45:807–812, 1995.

52. PH Lange, P Narayan. Understaging and undergrading of prostate cancer. Argument for postoperative radiation as adjuvant therapy. Urology 21:113–118, 1983.

53. SA Kramer, J Spahr, CB Brendler, et al. Experience with Gleason's histopathologic grading in prostatic cancer. J Urol 124:223–225, 1980.

54. JI Epstein, MJ Carmichael, AW Partin, et al. Small high grade adenocarcinoma of the prostate in radical prostatectomy specimens performed for nonpalpable disease: Pathogenetic and clinical implications. J Urol 151:1587–1592, 1994.

55. DF Paulson, PV Piserchia, W Gardner. Predictors of lymphocytic spread in prostatic adenocarcinoma. Uro-Oncology Research Group Study. J Urol 123:697–699, 1980.

56. DM Steinberg, J Sauvageot, S Piantadosi, JI Epstein. Correlation of prostate needle biopsy and radical prostatectomy Gleason grade in academic and community settings. Am J Surg Pathol 21:566–576, 1997.

57. FM Jhaveri, CD Zippe, EA Klein, PA Kupelian. Biochemical failure does not predict overall survival after radical prostatectomy for localized prostate cancer: 10-year results. Urology 54:884–890, 1999.

58. AW Partin, CR Pound, JQ Clemens, JI Epstein, PC Walsh. Serum PSA after anatomic radical prostatectomy. The Johns Hopkins experience after 10 years. Urol Clin North Am 20:713–725, 1993.

59. DE Goldrath, EM Messing. Prostate specific antigen: Not detectable despite tumor progression after radical prostatectomy. J Urol 142:1082–1084, 1989.

60. TK Takayama, JN Krieger, LD True, et al. Recurrent prostate cancer despite undetectable prostate specific antigen. J Urol 148:1541–1542, 1992.

61. AW Partin, JD Pearson, PK Landis, et al. Evaluation of serum prostate-specific antigen velocity after radical prostatectomy to distinguish local recurrence from distant metastases. Urology 43:649–659, 1994.

62. A Patel, F Dorey, J Franklin, JB de Kernion. Recurrence patterns after radical retropubic prostatectomy: Clinical usefulness of prostate specific antigen doubling times and log slope prostate specific antigen. J Urol 158:1441–1445, 1997.

63. M Ohori, TM Wheeler, MW Kattan, et al. Prognostic significance of positive surgical margins in radical prostatectomy specimens. J Urol 154:1818–1824, 1995.

64. JI Epstein, CR Pound, AW Partin, PC Walsh. Disease progression following radical prostatectomy in men with Gleason score 7 tumor. J Urol 160:97–100, 1998.

65. CR Pound, OW Christens-Barry, RT Gurganus, et al. Digital rectal examination and imaging studies are unnecessary in men with undetectable prostate specific antigen following radical prostatectomy. J Urol 162:1337–1340, 1999.

66. JEJ Fowler, J Brooks, P Pandey, LE Seaver. Variable histology of anastomotic biopsies with detectable prostate specific antigen after radical prostatectomy. J Urol 153:1011–1014, 1995.

67. JA Connolly, K Shinohara, JCJ Presti, PR Carroll. Local recurrence after radical prostatectomy: Characteristics in size, location, and relationship to prostate-specific antigen and surgical margins. Urology 47:225–231, 1996.

68. D Kahn, RD Williams, MJ Manyak, et al. 111Indium-capromab pendetide in the evaluation of patients with residual or recurrent prostate cancer after radical prostatectomy. The ProstaScint Study Group. J Urol 159:2041–2046, 1998.

69. JM Silverman, TL Krebs. MR imaging evaluation with a transrectal surface coil of local recurrence of prostatic cancer in men who have undergone radical prostatectomy. AJR 168:379–385, 1997.

70. D Kahn, RD Williams, MK Haseman, et al. Radioimmunoscintigraphy with In-111-labeled capromab pendetide predicts prostate cancer response to salvage radiotherapy after failed radical prostatectomy. J Clin Oncol 16:284–289, 1998.

71. JF McCarthy, WJ Catalona, MA Hudson. Effect of radiation therapy on detectable serum prostate specific antigen levels following radical prostatectomy: Early versus delayed treatment. J Urol 151:1575–1578, 1994.

72. F Haab, A Meulemans, L Boccon-Gibod, et al. Effect of radiation therapy after radical prostatectomy on serum prostate-specific antigen measured by an ultrasensitive assay. Urology 45:1022–1027, 1995.

73. LJ Coetzee, V Hars, DF Paulson. Postoperative prostate-specific antigen as a prognostic indicator in patients with margin-positive prostate cancer, undergoing adjuvant radiotherapy after radical prostatectomy. Urology 47:232–235, 1996.

74. E Medini, I Medini, PK Reddy, SH Levitt. Delayed/salvage radiation therapy in patients with elevated prostate specific antigen levels after radical prostatectomy. A long term follow-up. Cancer 78:1254–1259, 1996.

75. SE Schild, SJ Buskirk, WW Wong, et al. The use of radiotherapy for patients with isolated elevation of serum prostate specific antigen following radical prostatectomy. J Urol 156:1725–1729, 1996.

76. JD Forman, K Meetze, E Pontes, et al. Therapeutic irradiation for patients with an elevated post-prostatectomy prostate specific antigen level. J Urol 158:1436–1439, 1997.

77. JA Cadeddu, AW Partin, TL DeWeese, PC Walsh. Long-term results of radiation therapy for prostate cancer recurrence following radical prostatectomy. J Urol 159:173–178, 1998.

78. T Do, RG Parker, C Do, et al. Salvage radiotherapy for biochemical and clinical failures following radical prostatectomy. Cancer J Sci Am 4:324–330, 1998.

79. TM Pisansky, TF Kozelsky, RP Myers, et al. Radiotherapy for isolated serum prostate specific antigen elevation after prostatectomy for prostate cancer [In Process Citation]. J Urol 163:845–850, 2000.

80. MS Anscher, LR Prosnitz. Postoperative radiotherapy for patients with carcinoma of the prostate undergoing radical prostatectomy with positive surgical margins, seminal vesicle involvement and/or penetration through the capsule. J Urol 138:1407–1412, 1987.

81. PH Lange, DJ Lightner, E Medini, PK Reddy, RL Vessella. The effect of radiation therapy after radical prostatectomy in patients with elevated prostate specific antigen levels. J Urol 144:927–932, 1990.

82. JE Montie. Significance and treatment of positive margins or seminal vesicle invasion after radical prostatectomy. Urol Clin North Am 17:803–812, 1990.

83. JD Forman, J Velasco. Therapeutic radiation in patients with a rising post-prostatectomy PSA level. Oncology 12:33–39, 1998.

84. MM Morris, KC Dallow, AL Zietman, et al. Adjuvant and salvage irradiation following radical prostatectomy for prostate cancer. Int J Radiat Oncol Biol Phys 38:731–736, 1997.

85. JJ Wu, SC King, GS Montana, et al. The efficacy of postprostatectomy radiotherapy in patients with an isolated elevation of serum prostate-specific antigen. Int J Radiat Oncol Biol Phys 32:317–323, 1995.

86. P Link, FS Freiha, TA Stamey. Adjuvant radiation therapy in patients with detectable prostate specific antigen following radical prostatectomy. J Urol 145:532–534, 1991.

87. R Rogers, GD Grossfeld, M Roach, et al. Radiation therapy for the management of biopsy proved local recurrence after radical prostatectomy. J Urol 160:1748–1753, 1998.

88. CH Crane, TA Rich, PW Read, et al. Preirradiation PSA predicts biochemical

disease-free survival in patients treated with postprostatectomy external beam irradiation. Int J Radiat Oncol Biol Phys 39:681–686, 1997.

89. SM Eulau, DJ Tate, TA Stamey, MA Bagshaw, SL Haniak. Effect of combined transient androgen deprivation and irradiation following radical prostatectomy for prostatic cancer. Int J Radiat Oncol Biol Phys 41:735–740, 1998.

90. The Medical Research Council Prostate Cancer Working Party Investigators Group. Immediate versus deferred treatment for advanced prostatic cancer: Initial results of the Medical Research Council Trial. Br J Urol 79:235–246, 1997.

91. MA Eisenberger, PC Walsh. Early androgen deprivation for prostate cancer? [editorial; comment]. N Engl J Med 341:1837–1838, 1999.

92. R Kurek, H Renneberg, G Lubben, E Kienle, UW Tunn. Intermittent complete androgen blockade in PSA relapse after radical prostatectomy and incidental prostate cancer. Eur Urol 35 Suppl 1:27–31, 1999.

13
PSA and Radiation Therapy

Juanita Crook
University of Toronto, Toronto, Ontario, Canada

Prostate specific antigen (PSA) is generally accepted as one of the most valuable tumor markers in oncological practice. Although imperfect for screening, once the diagnosis of prostate cancer has been established, serum PSA is the dominant determinant of outcome and has helped to decipher the wide variety of biological aggressiveness seen in tumors of similar T-stage or Gleason score. Knowledge of the pretreatment baseline PSA level is essential to informed decision making and treatment selection. After radiotherapy is completed, serum PSA declines slowly to a nadir that is indicative of treatment efficacy. Postnadir PSA stability is indicative of cure.

I. PSA AS A PRERADIATION PROGNOSTIC FACTOR

Tumor staging in its broadest sense goes beyond a simple tumor/node/metastasis (TNM) classification to include all the known tumor-related prognostic variables that determine outcome, not only to provide an indication of prognosis but also to aid decision making, evaluate the results of treatment, and permit exchange of information. In the prePSA era, palpation of T-stage (PRE) was the primary means of classifying tumors and deciding appropriate treatment. It is still a major criterion in selecting patients for radical prostatectomy, although it clearly fails to differentiate tumors of widely different biological aggressiveness. Pisansky et al. [1] reported that in a data set of 500 patients treated by external radiotherapy, 23% of stage T2b tumors had biochemical recurrence within 5 years. However, when stage T2b was examined in subgroups based on grade and pretreatment PSA, the risk of failure in the subgroups ranged from 0 to 88%. Tumor grade or Gleason score, when added to T-stage, significantly improves the ability to predict ultimate treatment success or failure. Although both these traditional parameters are significant when considered individually, they pale beside the predictive power of the pretreatment PSA.

In univariate analysis the influence of pretreatment PSA on outcome is considerable. Table 1 compares results from five published series and shows remarkable similarity in outcome among the PSA strata. For pretreatment PSA ≤ 4 ng/ml, the 3–5 year biochemical "no evidence of disease" (bNED) rates range from 79 to 90%, dropping to 6–35% for PSA > 20 ng/ml. PSA is commonly treated as a "grouped" variable for these analyses, the groupings naturally compensating for the nonlinear distribution of pretreatment PSA values (PSA < 4 ng/ml, 4–10 ng/ml, 10–20 ng/ml, and >20 ng/ml). If PSA is to be treated as a continuous variable for analysis, it has been suggested that because of the skewed distribution of values, it should be transformed to its natural log [1,2].

Actuarial biochemical disease-free survival according to pretreatment PSA category for Kuban's series [3] of 652 patients is shown in Figure 1: for Crook's series [4] of 498 patients in Figure 2; and for Zietman's series [5] of 161 patients in Figure 3. All three investigators used different definitions of biochemical failure, with Kuban being the most liberal (PSA > 4.0 ng/ml) and Zietman the most strict (PSA > 1.0 ng/ml 2 years or more after radiotherapy, or an increase of >10% in the first 2 years). Crook chose an intermediate definition of PSA > 2.0 ng/ml and >1 ng/ml above the nadir. Patients in the different pretreatment PSA categories have similar relative differences in biochemical disease-free survival in the three series, but the more restrictive standard for determination of failure shifts the curves to the left by 12–18 months, since patients meet these criteria earlier in follow-up.

The dominant role of PSA as a prognostic factor may be due in part to its inherent lack of subjectivity. Although not all prostate cancers have the same capacity for PSA production, serum PSA is the most objective of the pretreatment prognostic factors. Clinical palpation T-stage is prone to interobserver variation, and biopsy Gleason score is subject to institutional differences [6] and sampling error. Although all three factors remain significant predictors of outcome in univariate analyses [1,7–9], when subjected to the rigors of multivariate analysis, the traditional factors of clinical palpation stage and Gleason score may become less strongly predictive and in some series are no longer significant [8,10,11]. Carefully performed multivariate analyses of large groups of patients with adequate follow-up help to determine the interdependence of the various factors and their relative importance [9]. With enough data and experience, these factors can be combined to create homogenous prognostic subgroups of known outcome.

Shipley [6] has combined data from seven institutions for a total of 1765 men with T1b, T1c, or T2 tumors treated with external beam radiotherapy between 1988 and 1995. Recursive partitioning analysis using pretreatment PSA,

Table 1 Biochemical Disease-Free Rates at 3–5 Years According to Pretreatment PSA Category

PreTx PSA (ng/ml)	5 yr bNED (3)	5 yr bNED (4)[a]	4 yr bNED (5)	5 yr bNED (25)	3 yr bNED (8)	5 yr bNED (40)
n = N	652	498	161	502	500	371
0–4	69%	90%	81%	83%	85%	79%
4.1–10	58%	62%	43%		81%	67%
10.1–20	57%	26%	31%	27%	59%	57%
20.1–50	20%	18%	6%	13%	35%	27%
>50			0			0

[a] Pretreatment PSA groupings 0–5 ng/ml, 5.1–10 ng/ml, 10.1–20 ng/ml, and > 20 ng/ml.

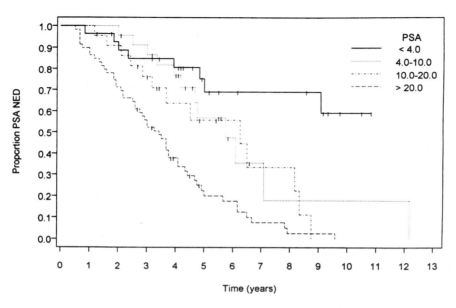

Figure 1   Actuarial biochemical disease-free survival according to pretreatment PSA category for 652 patients. bNED is defined as an elevated PSA > 4.0 ng/ml. (From Ref. 3.)

palpation T stage, and Gleason score yielded four distinct prognostic subgroups. Group 1 included all patients with a PSA level < 9.2 ng/ml. The estimated bNED rate at 5 years was 81%. Group 2 was also defined based on PSA alone and included those patients with pretreatment PSA in the range of 9.2–19.7 ng/ml, for whom the 5 year bNED rate was 69%. The remaining two groups combined Gleason score and PSA to create group 3 with a PSA > 19.7 and Gleason score 2–6 (5 year bNED rate: 47%), and group 4 with PSA > 19.7 and Gleason score 7–10 (5 year bNED rate: 29%). Tumor stage did not play a role in determination of the cut-off points, possibly because the analysis was limited to early-stage T1–2 tumors. Despite the complexity of the analysis, it was only marginally superior to the predictive value of PSA alone when examined in the categories <10 ng/ml (5 year bNED: 81%), 10–<20 ng/ml (5 year bNED: 68%), 20–<30 ng/ml (5 year bNED: 51%), and ≥30 ng/ml (5 year bNED: 31%) (see Fig. 4).

In an analysis of 500 patients, Pisansky et al. [1] found pretreatment PSA, palpation T stage, and Gleason score to be independently predictive of outcome at 5 years. A multiple prognostic index for estimating therapeutic outcome was created using logistic regression analysis. The increasing risk of treatment failure with increasing baseline PSA is plotted in a log-linear fashion and can be read

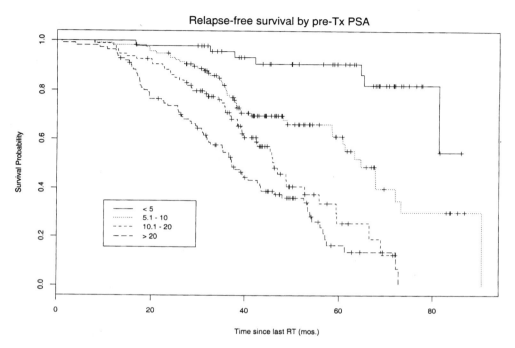

Figure 2   Actuarial relapse-free survival according to pretreatment PSA category for 498 patients. Relapse-free survival is defined according to ASTRO consensus criteria, plus negative results of prostate biopsy. (From Ref. 4.)

off three sets of curves. Figure 5a shows the risk of relapse at 5 years for stage T1a–T2a with each of the Gleason score groupings 2–4, 5–6, and 7–10 graphed separately. Figure 5b shows a similar analysis for stage T2b/c, and Figure 5c for stage T3/4.

Zagars et al. [9] analyzed 938 men treated with radiotherapy, 90% of whom received conventional doses. Mean follow-up was 43 months. In multivariant regression, pretreatment PSA, T-stage and Gleason score were each independently highly significant, correlating with every endpoint. Pretreatment PSA was the most significant variable for rising PSA and local failure, while T stage was the most significant in predicting metastatic failure. All three factors were used to create a six-tier prognostic grouping, shown in Table 2.

The mechanism by which these prognostic variables influence the outcome of radiotherapy is complex, but is related to the interplay of tumor volume, radioresistance, and the risk of subclinical metastatic spread. Partin et al. [12] have published the pathological correlates of the known pretreatment prognostic variables, palpation T-stage, baseline PSA, and biopsy Gleason score for 4133 men

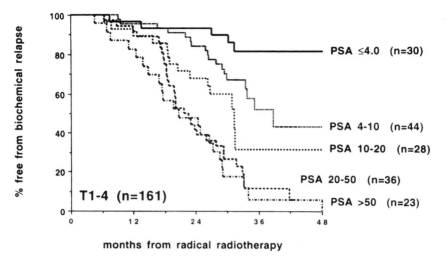

Figure 3 Actuarial freedom from biochemical relapse according to pretreatment PSA group. Failure is defined as an increase of PSA > 10% within 2 years of radiotherapy, or any PSA reading > 1.0 ng/ml after 2 years. (Reprinted from Ref. 5.)

treated with radical prostatectomy at 3 major academic urologic centers in the United States. Pretreatment PSA, palpation T-stage and biopsy Gleason score each contributed significantly to the prediction of pathological, stage in the multi-nominal log-linear regression. The combination of the three variables predicted pathological stage better than any single variable. Using the PSA groupings (0–4.0 ng/ml, 4.1–10 ng/ml, 10.1–20 ng/ml, and >20 ng/ml), and five Gleason score groupings (2–4, 5, 6, 7, and 8–10), nomograms were created for each T-stage to predict the probability of the following pathological endpoints: organ-confined disease, established capsular penetration, seminal vesicle invasion, and lymph node metastases. Although none of these is known to correlate directly with radioresistance, the relationship to tumor volume and distant dissemination is clear.

Figure 4 (a) Estimated rates of freedom from biochemical relapse according to prognostic categories determined by recursive partitioning analysis for 1765 men. Group 1: PSA < 9.2 ng/ml; group 2: PSA 9.2–19.7 ng/ml; group 3: PSA > 19.7 ng/ml and Gleason score 2–6; group 4: PSA > 19.7 ng/ml and Gleason 7–10. (b) Estimated rates of freedom from biochemical relapse according to pretreatment PSA categories. (Reprinted from Ref. 6, with permission.)

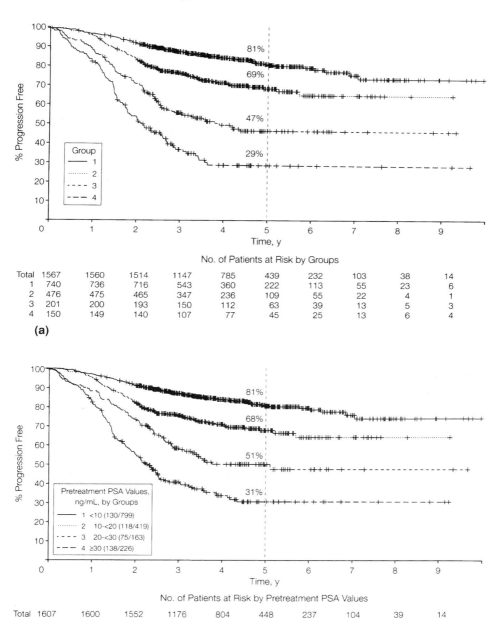

(a)

No. of Patients at Risk by Groups

Total	1567	1560	1514	1147	785	439	232	103	38	14
1	740	736	716	543	360	222	113	55	23	6
2	476	475	465	347	236	109	55	22	4	1
3	201	200	193	150	112	63	39	13	5	3
4	150	149	140	107	77	45	25	13	6	4

No. of Patients at Risk by Pretreatment PSA Values

Total	1607	1600	1552	1176	804	448	237	104	39	14
1	799	795	775	587	387	233	119	57	23	6
2	419	418	407	303	209	98	49	20	4	1
3	163	162	158	126	93	50	25	10	5	3
4	226	225	212	160	115	67	44	17	7	4

(b)

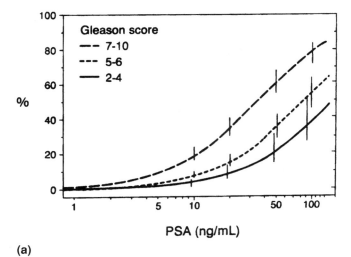

(a)

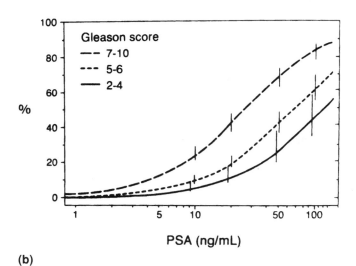

(b)

Figure 5 Risk of any relapse within 5 years according to pretreatment PSA level and Gleason score. Vertical lines represent the 95% confidence intervals for PSA values of 10, 20, 50, and 100 ng/ml. (a) Stage T1a–T2a. (b) Stage T2b–c. (c) Stage T3–4. (From Ref. 1, with permission.)

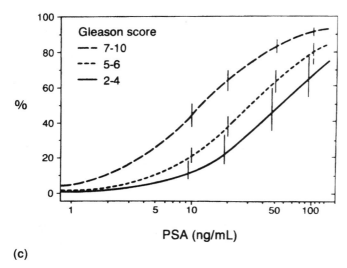

(c)

Figure 5 *Continued.*

Not all patients with seminal vesicle invasion or extracapsular extension will fail primary treatment and show a rising PSA within 5 years. D'Amico et al. [13] reported on 1654 men with stage T1c–T2 prostate cancer treated either by radical prostatectomy (n = 892) or definitive radiotherapy (n = 762), using the same 3 variables to predict biochemical recurrence. Biopsy Gleason score was classified into the same five groupings as in the Partin analysis [2–4,5, 6,7,8–10], and PSA categories were similar. All three variables were independent predictors of PSA failure within 2 years of definitive treatment, for both radiation- and surgically treated patients (Fig. 6). Although the follow-up is short,

Table 2 Prognostic Categories of Zagars et al. [4] Based on Multivariate Regression Analysis of 938 Men

Category	T stage	PSA (ng/ml)	Gleason score	Relapse rate (%)
1	T1/T2	<4.0	2–6	6
2	T1/T2	≤4.0	7–10	30
		4.1–10.0	2–7	
3	T1/T2	4.1–10.0	8–10	40
		10.1–20.0	2–7	
4	T3/T4	<10		46
5	T3/T4	10.1–20	2–7	57
6	any T	>20.0	Any Gleason	88
		10.1–20.0	8–10	

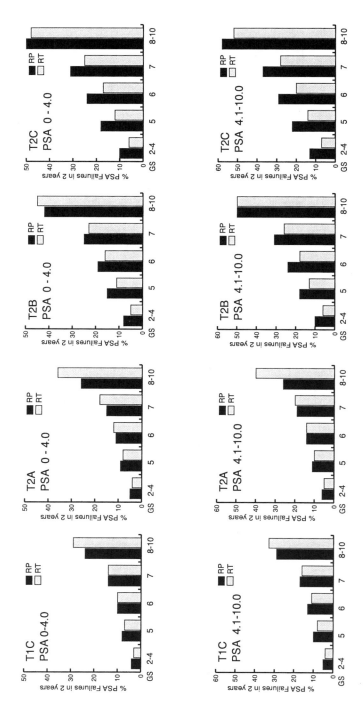

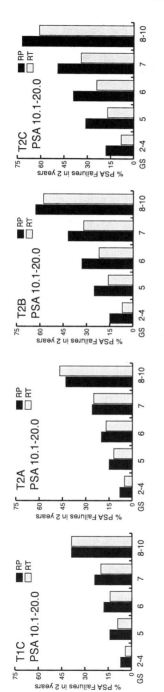

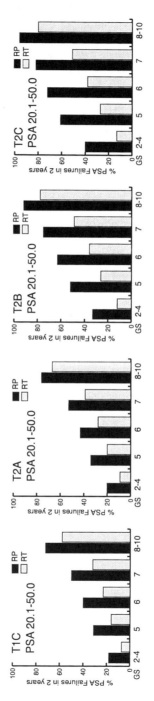

Figure 6 Percentage PSA failure at 2 years for 892 surgically managed patients (RP) compared to 762 radiation-managed patients (RT), according to T stage, Gleason score, and pretreatment PSA. (Adapted from Ref. 13.)

the toll of early failures is impressive. Such knowledge can be used to assess high-risk patients for combined modality treatment that will address the systemic component of their disease. Early PSA failure may eventually with sufficient follow-up, be reflected as reduced cause-specific or overall survival. Zietman et al. [14] reported that second PSA failure is a reliable surrogate end point for death from prostate cancer. In this series, patients were treated with primary radiotherapy and the first PSA failure was managed with hormonal ablation. All patients experiencing a second PSA failure while on hormonal therapy died of prostate cancer at a median time of 27 months.

II. DEFINITION OF BIOCHEMICAL FAILURE

Prior to American Society of Therapeutic Radiation and Oncology (ASTRO)'s consensus guideline in 1997 [15], the definition of biochemical freedom from failure (bNED) was problematic, and over the past decade many definitions have been suggested. Unlike the situation after radical prostatectomy, the patient successfully treated with radiotherapy still has the prostate in situ. Therefore the PSA criteria for cure after radical prostatectomy are inappropriately stringent [16] for the postradiotherapy setting. However, the acceptable range of PSA after radiotherapy is certainly lower than that for an age-matched unirradiated population. Histological examination of the normal irradiated prostate shows marked atrophy of the epithelial glands, with a reduction in the size and number of non-malignant acini [17,18], resulting in a permanent decrease in PSA production.

Ablation of the normal prostatic epithelium appears to be dose-dependent. Willet et al. [19] reported serum PSA readings in a series of 36 men who received incidental radiation to the prostate while being treated for nonprostatic pelvic malignancies. The dose received by the prostate ranged from 45 to 65 Gy. Mean serum PSA level 3 years following radiotherapy was 0.6 ng/ml, but 20% of the men had readings >1.5 ng/ml in the absence of a diagnosis of prostate cancer. This indicates that there is an acceptable range of normal after radiotherapy, but that this range is markedly lower than that for a nonirradiated population. Critz has reported that higher doses of radiotherapy, such as can be delivered with a combination of external beam and brachytherapy will drive the PSA even lower, such that 68% of men achieve a serum PSA of 0.2 ng/ml or lower [20]. Although a lower nadir is associated with an improved chance of maintaining disease-free status, it is probably not necessary to ablate all the normal prostatic epithelium in order to achieve cure.

In 1996, ASTRO convened a consensus conference to examine the emerging data on post radiotherapy PSA [15]. Their aim was to establish a definition for biochemical disease free status that would be clinically relevant to practioners and their patients as well as be applicable to clinical trials and the reporting of data. Serum PSA has become the measure of treatment efficacy. After radiotherapy, serum PSA declines slowly and does not usually reach undetectable levels. The level of the PSA nadir is an important indicator of response to treatment [21], but unfortunately there is no distinct PSA threshold postradiotherapy that differentiates success from failure. Hancock et al. [22] reported on 110 patients followed for an average of 10.7 years, 43 of whom had stable PSA readings. Thirty-three levels were <1.0 ng/ml, but 10 men had stable PSA's > 1.0 ng/ml. Hanks et al. [23] reported 10 year follow-up for the Radiotherapy Oncology Group (RTOG) protocol 7706. This protocol dates from the pre-PSA era and PSA levels were not required in follow-up, but were obtainable for 17 men who were clinically NED. Eleven of the 17 had readings <1.5 ng/ml and six had levels between 1.5 and 3.5 ng/ml. Crook et al. [24] studied PSA profiles after standard dose radiotherapy for 118 men. They reported that benign elevations as high as 2.0 ng/ml may occur and spontaneously decline, but that once the PSA had reached 3.0 ng/ml, an irreversible rising trend was established.

It is clear that PSA stability following the nadir is important and that a steadily rising PSA indicates failure. Some investigators have used definitions based on stability, declaring biochemical failure when there are two or more rising values [11]. Others have used a combination of a threshold level and subsequent stability, such as two rises more than 1 ng/ml above the nadir [25], >1.5 ng/ml and rising on two consecutive readings [23,26], or >2 ng/ml and more than 1 ng/ml above the nadir [7]. Zietman et al. [14] found that after three rises, 87% of men demonstrate a fourth rise.

The ASTRO consensus conference concluded that three consecutive rises in PSA is a reasonable definition of biochemical failure, recommending that the determinations be 3–4 months apart in the first 2 years following radiotherapy, and every 6 months thereafter. The use of three rather than two rises decreases the risk of falsely declaring a failure due to PSA instability due to biological "noise" or fluctuations in PSA of benign cause. Over-call of failure based on two rises may be more of a risk for those tumors with a lower Gleason score (6 or less) [27]. For the purposes of reporting data or clinical trials, failure is backdated to halfway between the nadir and the first rise. It must be emphasized that standardization of the definition of biochemical failure is not justification for early intervention. There may be four or five PSA doublings, before clinical failure is evident [28]. This lead time in declaring failure, over 40 months in the majority of patients [29], may sentence a patient who is otherwise destined to die of intercurrent disease before clinical failure manifests [16] to unnecessary worry or additional treatment. Unless radical local salvage is an option, three consecutive rises in PSA should do no more than signal a potential problem and consign the patient to a closer follow-up schedule.

III. PSA IN THE EVALUATION OF RADIATION RESPONSE

Three potential sources of PSA contribute to a patient's baseline or pretreatment PSA level; normal prostate epithelium, prostate cancer cells within or in the immediate vicinity of the prostate, and disseminated prostate cancer cells. Any of these can contribute to the nadir PSA. For patients who achieve and maintain tumor-free status, the nadir PSA is composed entirely of PSA from the residual benign prostatic epithelium. This nadir is usually in the range of 0.4–0.5 ng/ml and may take 2 years or longer to be achieved. If there are residual viable prostate cancer cells in the prostate following radiotherapy, the PSA will decline until the rate of growth of the surviving cells is greater than the rate of death of those fatally damaged by the radiation. Since the surviving cancer cells are contributing to the nadir, this nadir will be higher and achieved earlier than for those patients in whom all local disease is eradicated (median, 2–3 ng/ml at 17–20 months). If there were disseminated micrometastases at the time of radiotherapy, these will continue to grow exponentially despite successful treatment of the primary tumor. Depending on the relative volumes of local and metastatic disease, continued PSA production by the metastases tends to overwhelm the beneficial effect of the local radiotherapy sooner rather than later, leading to median PSA nadirs in the range of 5–10 ng/ml, occurring at an average of 10–12 months postradiotherapy (Table 3).

The time to nadir has been shown to be inversely proportional to disease-free survival. Lee et al. [26] found that 75% of men whose PSA reached a nadir in <12 months had overt distant metastases by 5 years compared to 25% of those whose PSA nadir was achieved later than 12 months (p < 0.001). Kestin et al. [30] reported that 92% of men whose PSA did not reach a nadir until 36 months remained disease-free compared to 30% of those who reached a nadir in <12 months.

As shown in Table 3, the postnadir doubling time also reflects to some extent the type of failure. Patients with local failures tend to have longer PSA doubling times of 11–14 months [11,31], while distant failures tend to have

Table 3   Failure Pattern According to Level of PSA Nadir, Time to Nadir, and PSA Doubling Time

	PSA nadir (ng/ml)	Time to nadir (months)	PSA doubling time (months)
NED	0.4–0.5	22–33	NA
Local failure	2.0–3.0	17–20	11–13 months
Distant failure	5.0–10.0	10–12	3–6 months

shorter average PSA doubling times of 3–6 months [11,30,31]. Since high-grade tumors have a shorter PSA doubling time [29,31], and increased metastatic potential [32], this may explain the different doubling times for the types of failure. Stamey et al. [33] has suggested that patients failing to respond to radiotherapy demonstrate accelerated tumor growth rates, as indicated by more rapid PSA doubling times. In all probability, the range of PSA doubling times seen in those patients who are not cured by radiotherapy are a reflection of tumor grade, clonogen selection, and pattern of failure.

The slow decline in serum PSA and the long time to PSA nadir can be explained by the fact that radiotherapy does not cause immediate cell death. Unlike the case with ablative treatment modalities such as surgery or cryotherapy, by which cell kill (or extirpation) is completed within the time frame of the treatment, the double-strand DNA breaks produced by radiotherapy permit the cell to survive until it attempts to divide. Postmitotic cell death results from unsuccessful reproduction. Given the long doubling time of many prostate cancers, a fatally damaged cell may survive for 18–24 months before entering mitosis and subsequently dying. In a series of 226 men whose prostates were systematically rebiopsied at intervals following radiotherapy, it was demonstrated that the time to nadir correlates well with the time course of histological resolution of tumor [34].

Although there is no absolute threshold of PSA nadir that differentiates treatment success from failure, the chances of remaining free of recurrence are improved with lower PSA nadirs. Five year freedom from biochemical failure ranges from 75 to 90% for patients achieving a nadir of ≤0.5 ng/ml [10,41,5,20,24], but drops to 50–60% for nadirs of 0.6–1.0 ng/ml (Table 4). The majority of patients with nadirs > 1.0 ng/ml will demonstrate biochemical recurrence within 5 years (Figs. 7, 8). Although it is generally accepted that a PSA nadir ≤ 0.5 ng/ml is desirable, this cannot be taken as an absolute. Up to one-third of patients in some series will remain free of failure, at least in short- and intermediate-term follow-up, despite PSA nadirs > 1.0 ng/ml.

Table 4 Freedom from Biochemical Relapse (bNED) at 3–5 Years after Radiotherapy According to PSA Nadir

PSA nadir	5 yr bNED (4)	4 yr bNED (30)	5 yr bNED (41)	3 yr bNED (26)
N	498	871	314	364
<0.5	75%	78%	90%	93%
0.6–1.0	50%	60%	55%	
1.1–1.9	32%	50%	34%	49%
2.0–3.9	0	20%		16%
>4		9%		

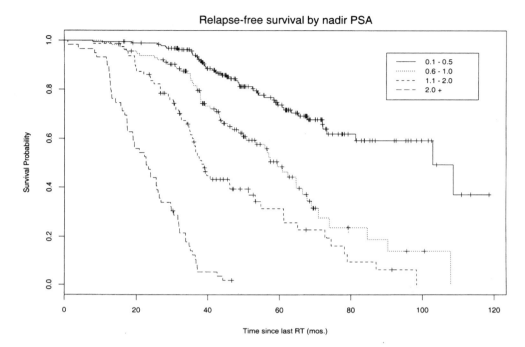

Figure 7 Actuarial relapse-free rate according to nadir PSA group for 498 patients. Relapse defined according to ASTRO consensus guidelines plus negative postradiotherapy biopsy. (From Ref. 4.)

Following radiotherapy, serum PSA provides valuable objective information on the efficacy of treatment. The PSA reading has been examined at many different time points following completion of radiotherapy, but PSA nadir has been found to be the best indicator of response to treatment [35]. The nadir has become an accepted surrogate endpoint that predates clinical failure by four to five PSA doubling times [28], or an average of 40 months [29]. Thus, in the PSA era, most failures are classified as biochemical, and hormonal therapy is instituted before clinical failure manifests. However, one cannot reliably differentiate local from distant failure based on postradiotherapy PSA nadir and time to nadir. For many patients for whom management of recurrence will consist of systemic therapy, the distinction between local and distant failure may be academic. However, if radical local salvage is an option, then postradiotherapy prostate biopsies [36] should demonstrate residual viable tumor.

It is common practice to include postradiotherapy PSA nadir in multivariate analyses with pretreatment prognostic variables such as T-stage, Gleason score,

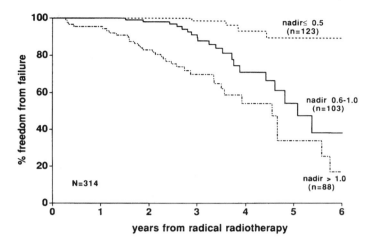

Figure 8 Actuarial freedom from biochemical relapse for T1–2 prostate cancer according to nadir PSA group. Biochemical relapse defined as three consecutive rises > 10%. (From Ref. 41.)

and pretreatment PSA. When these are included in the same model, postradiotherapy PSA nadir is invariably the dominant "predictor" of outcome. This is not surprising considering the close temporal relationship between PSA nadir and the definition of biochemical failure (dated halfway between the nadir and the first rise). However, postradiotherapy PSA nadir should more correctly be considered an indicator of response to treatment than a prognosticator of outcome.

For locally advanced or high-risk disease, neoadjuvant hormonal therapy is often used prior to definitive radiotherapy. An undetectable PSA level prior to radiotherapy makes it impossible to determine a true nadir or time to nadir. If cessation of hormonal therapy at the start of radiotherapy results in a rapid recovery of serum testosterone, the PSA can rise transiently in response to testosterone and subsequently decline once more as the effect of radiotherapy is expressed. This secondary nadir likely has the same prognostic significance as PSA nadir in the absence of neoadjuvant hormonal therapy. Adherence to the ASTRO criteria for biochemical failure, requiring three successive rises at 3–4 month intervals will allow sufficient time for this phenomenon to pass without falsely declaring the patient to have experienced biochemical failure.

Serum PSA provides a reliable endpoint for evaluating the results of radiotherapy. Rising PSA levels postradiotherapy have allowed us to appreciate the frequency with which standard radiotherapy fails to cure patients. It has provided the incentive to initiate improvements in treatment delivery, and the means of assessing their results. PSA as a surrogate endpoint has yielded dose–response data from dose escalation trials within 3–5 years of their completion [37–39], and allows much more rapid progress in the quest to optimize treatment. Nonetheless, it must be remembered that PSA remains a surrogate for response to therapy and cannot replace mature survival data.

IV. CONCLUSION

Pretreatment PSA is an important prognostic factor that combines with the traditional parameters of T stage and Gleason score to create more homogeneous risk groups for prediction of outcome and selection of appropriate therapy. After radiotherapy, serum PSA is a valuable surrogate endpoint and a reliable indicator of treatment efficacy. As the data bases of the past decade mature, the use of serum PSA will be further refined and its durability as an endpoint challenged, and perhaps confirmed.

REFERENCES

1. TM Pisansky, MJ Kahn, GM Rasp, SS Cha, MG Haddock, DG Bostwick. A multiple prognostic index predictive of disease outcome after irradiation for clinically localized prostate carcinoma. Cancer 79:337–244, 1997.
2. TM Pisansky, SS Cha, JD Earle, ED Durr, TF Kozelsky, HS Wieand, JE Oesterling. Prostate-specific antigen as a pretherapy prognostic factor in patients treated with radiation therapy for clinically localized prostate cancer. J Clin Urol 11:2158–2166, 1993.
3. DA Kuban, AM El-Mahdi, PF Schellhammer. Prostate-specific antigen for pretreatment prediction and posttreatment evaluation of outcome after definitive irradiation for prostate cancer. Int J Radiat Oncol Biol Phys 32:307–316, 1995.
4. J Crook, S Malone, Y Bahadur, S Robertson, M Abdollel. Post radiotherapy prostate biopsies: What do they really mean? 5 year results for 498 patients. Int J Radiat Oncol Biol Phys 45:355–367, 2000.
5. AL Zietman, JJ Coeh, WU Shipley, CG Willett, JT Efird. Radical radiation therapy in the management of prostatic adenocarcinoma: The initial prostate specific antigen value as a predictor of treatment outcome. J Urol 151:640–645, 1994.
6. WU Shipley, HD Thames, HM Sandler, GE Hanks, AI Zietman, CA Perez, DA Kuban, SL Hancock, CD Smith. Radiation therapy for clinically localized prostate cancer: A multi-institutional pooled analysis. JAMA 281:1598–1604, 1999.
7. JM Crook, YA Bahadur, RG Bociek, et al. The correlation of pretreatment prostate specific antigen and nadir prostate specific antigen with outcome as assessed by systematic biopsy and serum prostate specific antigen. Cancer 79:328–336, 1997.
8. WR Lee, GE Hanks, TE Schulteiss, BW Vorn, M Hunt. Localized prostate cancer

treated by external-beam radiotherapy alone: serum prostate-specific antigen-driven outcome analysis. J Clin Oncol 13:464–469, 1995.

9. GK Zagars, A Pollack, AC von Eschenbach. Prognostic factors for clinically localized prostate carcinoma: analysis of 938 patients irradiated in the prostate specific antigen era. Cancer 79:1370–1380, 1997.

10. PA Kupelian, J Katcher, H Levin, C Zippe, J Such, R Macklis, E Klein. External beam radiotherapy versus radical prostatectomy for clinical stage T1-2 prostate cancer: Therapeutic implications of stratification by pretreatment PSA levels and biopsy Gleason scores. Cancer J Sci Am 3:78–87, 1997.

11. GK Zagars, A Pollack, VS Kavadi, AC von Eschenbach. Prostate-specific antigen and radiation therapy for clinically localized prostate cancer. Int J Radiat Oncol Biol Phys 32:293–306, 1995.

12. A Partin, ENP Subong, PC Walsh, KJ Wojno, JE Oesterling, MW Kattan, PT Scardino, JD Pearson. Combination of prostate-specific antigen, clinical stage, and Gleason score to predict pathological stage of localized prostate cancer. JAMA 277: 1445–1451.

13. AV D'Amico, R Whittington, SB Malkowicz, J Fondurulia, MH Chen, I Kaplan, CJ Beard, JE Tomaszewski, AA Renshaw, A Wein, CN Coleman. Pretreatment nomogram for prostate-specific antigen recurrence after radical prostatectomy or external-beam radiation therapy for clinically localized prostate cancer. J Clin Oncol 17: 168–172, 1999.

14. AL Zietman, KC Dallow, PA McManus, NM Heney, WU Shipley. Time to second prostate-specific antigen failure is a surrogate endpoint for prostate cancer death in a prospective trial of therapy for localized disease. Urology 47:236–239, 1996.

15. American Society for Therapeutic Radiology and Oncology Consensus Panel. Consensus statement: Guidelines for PSA following radiation therapy. Int J Radiat Oncol Biol Phys 37:1035–1041, 1997.

16. MA Bagshaw, HS Kaplan, H Lebeson. Comments on the treatment of prostate cancer by conventional radiation therapy: An analysis of long-term outcome. Int J Radiat Oncol Biol Phys 32:287–292, 1995.

17. DG Bostwick, BM Egbert, LF Fajardo. Radiation injury of the normal and neoplastic prostate. Am J Surg Pathol 6:541–551, 1982.

18. DJ Grignon, WA Sakr. Histological effects of radiation therapy and total androgen blockade on prostate cancer. Cancer (supplement) 75:1837–1841, 1995.

19. C Willet, H Zietman, W Shipley, JJ Cohen. The effect of pelvic radiation therapy on serum levels of PSA. J Urol 151:1579–1581, 1994.

20. FA Critz, AK Levinson, WH Williams, VD Griffen, DA Holladay. Prostate specific antigen nadir achieved by men apparently cured of prostate cancer by radiotherapy. J Urol 161:1199–1205, 1999.

21. FA Critz, WH Williams, CT Holladay, et al. Post-treatment PSA < 0.2 ng/ml defines disease freedom after radiotherapy for prostate cancer using modern techniques. Urology 54:968–971, 1999.

22. SL Hancock, RS Cox, MA Bagshaw. Prostate specific antigen after radiotherapy for prostate cancer: A reevaluation of long-term biochemical control and the kinetics of recurrence in patients treated at Stanford University. J Urol 154:1412–1417, 1995.

23. GE Hanks, WR Lee, TE Schultiess. Clinical and biochemical evidence of control of prostate cancer at 5 years after external beam radiation. J Urol 154:456–459, 1995.

24. JM Crook, EG Choan, GA Perry, S Robertson, B Esche. Serum prostate-specific antigen profile following radiotherapy for prostate cancer: Implications for patterns of failure and definition of cure. Urology 51:566–572, 1998.

25. GE Hanks, CA Perez, M Kozar, SO Asbell, MV Pilepich, TF Pajak. PSA confirmation of cure at 10 years of T_{1B}, T_2, N_0, M_0 prostate cancer patients treated in RTOG protocol 7706 with external beam irradiation. Int J Radiat Oncol Biol Phys 30:289–292, 1994.

26. WR Lee, AL Hanlon, GE Hanks. Prostate specific antigen nadir following external beam radiation therapy for clinically localized prostate cancer: The relationship between nadir level and disease-free survival. J Urol 156:450–453, 1996.

27. RD Ennis, BK Malyszko, DF Heitjan, MA Rubin, KM O'Toole, AB Schiff. Changes in biochemical disease-free survival rates as a result of adoption of the consensus conference definition in patients with clinically localized prostate cancer treated with external-beam radiotherapy. Int J Radiat Oncol Biol Phys 41:511–517, 1998.

28. AV D'Amico, GE Hanks. Linear regressive analysis using prostate-specific antigen doubling time for predicting tumor biology and clinical outcome in prostate cancer. Cancer 72:2638–2643, 1993.

29. A Pollack, GK Zagars, CS Kavadi. Prostate specific antigen doubling time and disease relapse after radiotherapy for prostate cancer. Cancer 74:670–678, 1994.

30. LL Kestin, FA Vicini, EL Ziaja, et al. Defining biochemical cure for prostate carcinoma patients treated with external beam radiation therapy. Cancer 86:1557–1566, 1999.

31. WR Lee, GE Hanks, A Hanlon. Increasing prostate-specific antigen profile following definitive radiation therapy for localized prostate cancer: Clinical observations. J Clin Oncol 15:230–238, 1997.

32. MJ Zelefsky, SA Leibel, KE Wallner, WF Whitmore, Z Fuks. Significance of normal serum prostate-specific antigen in the follow-up period after definitive radiation therapy for prostatic cancer. J Clin Oncol 13:459–463, 1995.

33. TA Stamey, MK Ferrari, H-P Schmidt. The value of serial prostate specific antigen determinations 5 years after radiotherapy: Steeply increasing values characterize 80% of patients. J Urol 150:1856–1859, 1993.

34. JM Crook, GA Perry, S Robertson, B Esche. Routine prostate biopsies following radiotherapy for prostate cancer: Results for 226 patients. Urology 45:624–632, 1995.

35. E Ben-Josef, F Shamsa, JD Forman. Predicting the outcome of radiotherapy for prostate carcinoma: A model-building strategy. Cancer 82:1334–1342, 1998.

36. JM Crook, YA Bahadur, SJ Robertson, G Perry, B Esche. Evaluation of radiation effect, tumor differentiation, and prostate specific antigen staining in sequential prostate biopsies after external beam radiotherapy for patients with prostate carcinoma. Cancer 27:81–89, 1997.

37. GE Hanks, WR Lee, AL Hanlon, M Hunt, E Kaplan, BE Epstein, B Movsas, TE Schulteiss. Conformal technique dose escalation for prostate cancer: biochemical evidence of improved cancer control with higher does in patients with pretreatment

prostate-specific antigen $\geq$ 10 ng/ml. Int J Radiat Oncol Biol Phys 35:861–868, 1996.

38. PA Kupelian, DS Mohan, J Lyons, EA Klein, CA Reddy. Higher than standard radiation doses ($\geq$ 72 GY) with or without androgen deprivation in the treatment of localized prostate cancer. Int J Radiat Oncol Biol Phys 46:567–574, 2000.

39. A Pollack, GK Zagars. External beam radiotherapy dose response of prostate cancer. Int J Radiat Oncol Biol Phys 39:1011–1018, 1997.

40. DM Preston, JJ Bauer, RR Connelly, et al. Prostate-specific antigen to predict outcome of external beam radiation for prostate cancer: Walter Reed Army Medical Center experience 1988–1995. Urology 53:131–138, 1999.

41. AL Zietman, MK Tibbs, KC Dallow, et al. Use of PSA nadir to predict subsequent biochemical outcome following external beam radiation therapy for T1-2 adenocarcinoma of the prostate. Radiother Oncol 40:159–162, 1996.

14
PSA and Hormonal Therapy

S. Larry Goldenberg, Shane E. La Bianca, and Martin E. Gleave
Vancouver General Hospital/University of British Columbia,
Vancouver, British Columbia, Canada

The hormonal control of prostatic growth, as identified by Huggins and Hodges in 1941 [1], led to dramatic improvements in the management of metastatic prostate cancer. Subsequent advances in the understanding of androgens' effects on prostate growth and development have influenced our knowledge of the basic pathophysiology of benign prostate disease and prostate cancer. This has furthered our ability to diagnose, treat, and monitor malignant disease, particularly through a biological serum marker. By utilizing prostate specific antigen's (PSA's) unique properties as a direct and indirect indicator of prostate activity, rapid progress has been made in prostate disease research, and allowed qualitative and (indirectly) quantitative assessment of prostatic glandular function, further defining the complexity of prostate gland growth and the changes occurring in benign and malignant disease.

Prostatic glandular function is dependent on endocrine, autocrine, and paracrine hormonal stimulation, and, as a result, the serum PSA accurately reflects the basic cellular sequelae of androgen stimulation and deprivation, in both in vitro and in vivo. Its use has revolutionized the management of prostate cancer. For the first time, a serum marker has been available to monitor accurately the biological response to hormonal and other medical and surgical interventions.

This chapter reviews the hormonal regulation and clinical importance of serum PSA. Basic cellular and tissue concepts will be discussed, with examples from both human research and animal models. Because PSA expression is so closely linked to benign disease and prostate cancer, a discussion of the clinical effects of androgens and hormonal therapy on those diseases is required. Nonandrogenic controls will also be discussed, since their effects (both independently and in conjunction with androgens) at both cellular and tissue levels have an

impact on PSA expression in both benign and malignant disease. Although androgen withdrawal therapy is our main focus, we will also discuss the changes in
serum PSA seen with dietary and pharmacological modification, which is an increasingly important concern due to the growing number of men taking dietary
supplements, phytotherapeutics, and 5α-reductase inhibitors. A final brief section
will discuss the effects of androgen replacement on PSA, which, with the increasing use of androgens in men for biochemical hypogonadism, and in young sportsmen for performance enhancement, may have clinical implications for the interpretation of serum PSA levels.

We hope the reader will achieve a better understanding of the relationship
of serum PSA to the hormonal milieu, and thereby appreciate the effects of hormonal therapies in both benign and malignant prostatic disease.

I. REGULATORY MECHANISMS IN PSA SYNTHESIS

A. Gene Regulation of PSA Production

PSA secretion and PSA gene regulation is dependent upon androgens at the cellular level. Androgen is a potent differentiation agent in prostate embryogenesis,
growth, and function, and is required for normal prostate PSA production. Transcriptional activation of the PSA gene by androgen increases PSA mRNA levels,
which, following translation, leads to increased PSA protein synthesis. Initiation
of transcription occurs through binding of transcriptional factors (androgens and
nonandrogenic proteins) to specific DNA-binding domains in the 5 [1] promoter
region of the PSA gene. The androgen receptor (AR) is the major mediating
pathway in this process, and is a member of the superfamily of ligand-responsive
transcription factors [2]. AR contains three major domains: an N-terminal region
involved principally in transcriptional activation; a DNA-binding domain, required for interaction with specific gene sequences as well as transactivation; and
a steroid-binding domain in the C-terminal end of the molecule. Expression of
PSA related genes is androgen-regulated and dependent on androgen binding to
AR (Fig. 1). Transcriptional regulation by AR is mediated by direct binding to
specific enhancer-like DNA sequences in the promoter regions of target genes
termed androgen-responsive elements (ARE). The AR also interacts with general
and specific transcription factors to form stable transcription preinitiation complexes that permit efficient transcription of target genes.

It is likely that transcriptional regulation of PSA gene activity involves
other activators and inhibitors, as well as protein–protein interactions at the same
level. Little is known about the actual mediation of this process, which seems
to be influenced by tissue-specific cofactors [3,4]. PSA synthesis is stimulated
by vitamin D [5], and phorbol esters downregulate the androgen induction of
PSA [6]. Most growth factors have minimal or no effect on PSA mRNA levels

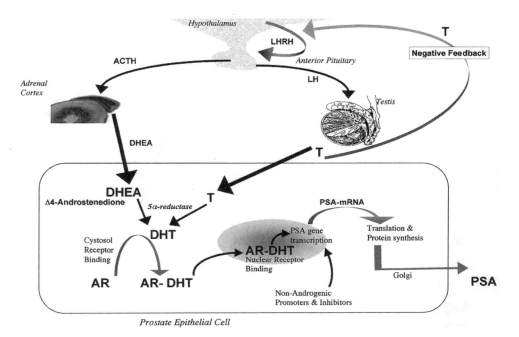

Figure 1   Hormonal regulation of PSA gene expression.

in LNCaP cells over a broad range of concentrations [7]. Epidermal growth factor (EGF) and fibroblast growth factor (FGF) may decrease PSA secretion, while both EGF and transforming growth factor (TGFα) can interfere with the androgen regulation of PSA [8]. Proteins such as insulinlike growth factor (IGF-4) and keratinocyte growth factor (KGF) may also stimulate PSA gene expression via the AR, since their effect can be inhibited by the antiandrogen Casodex [9,10]. Taken together, these observations suggest that PSA gene expression in androgen-dependent tissues is regulated primarily by androgens, but modified by other transcriptional factors through mechanisms that remain poorly understood.

B.   Androgen Regulation of PSA production

The male sex hormones are collectively known as androgens. Testosterone is the principal circulating androgen in men, and the growth of the prostate in man and other species coincides with the rise in serum testosterone (T) at puberty. Castration prior to puberty results in failure of development of the gland [11], as does

5α-reductase II deficiency [12] and mutations of the (AR) [13]. Without androgen stimulation, benign prostate hyperplasia (BPH) likewise does not develop [14], a phenomenon uniquely evidenced in the Russian Caucasus where the Skoptzys practice ritual castration after age 35, and BPH is virtually unknown. Prostate cancer does not develop in eunuchs or other men castrated before puberty.

Testosterone circulates in association with two major plasma proteins: sex hormone-binding globulin and albumin. Only about 2% of the testosterone is unbound and available for target cell uptake. Serum PSA levels are dependent on both circulating and local tissue androgens, the stromal milieu, and, in cases of prostate adenocarcinoma, tumor volume [7,15]. Age-related measurements have determined that PSA levels are testosterone dependent at all ages [16], with serum PSA becoming detectable at puberty with increasing levels of luteinizing hormone (LH) and testosterone [17]. Changes in androgen levels result directly in changes in serum PSA, both at an intracellular level related to gene expression and protein synthesis and at a tissue level related to the number of cells actively producing PSA.

Although testosterone is the major circulating androgen, DHT (the 5α-reduced metabolite) is the major prostatic androgen, with a concentration 20 times higher than T. DHT derives from both testosterone (75%) and adrenal androgens (25%; predominantly DHEA and DHEA-S), taken up by prostatic epithelial cells and stroma. DHT is 1.5–2.5 times more potent than testosterone, although their receptor affinity is similar, and in high enough concentrations testosterone will bind to cytosolic AR and result in stimulation of androgen-dependent pathways. This may account for the persistence of BPH in men treated with 5α-reductase inhibitors, despite the reduction in intracellular DHT levels.

Androgenic regulation of target tissues is characterized by three broadly defined responses: a positive initiation phase, a negative feedback response phase, and, finally, apoptosis [18]. In the presence of androgen, undifferentiated or involuted cells initiate new rounds of DNA synthesis and cell proliferation (i.e., androgen sensitivity), an example of positive gene regulation by androgens [19]. When the tissue becomes normal in size, an inhibitory mechanism comes into play and shuts down DNA synthesis and cell proliferation. This distinctive wearing-off effect is a consequence of negative-gene regulation by androgens, (i.e., transcription is inhibited in the presence of a rising concentration of hormone [20]), and after prolonged androgenic stimulation by negative feedback of androgens on AR production [21].

Changes in prostatic tissue growth and function, as reflected in serum PSA levels, occur in response to changes in androgen stimulation. Withdrawal of androgens induces apoptosis, a form of programmed cell death, in normal, benign hyperplastic, and malignant prostatic epithelial cells, which decreases the size of the prostate by 50–80%, largely through the elimination of epithelial cells. This manifestation of tissue atrophy or androgen dependence [22–24] involves a number of androgen-repressed genes [24,25], which become active when androgens are withdrawn and inactive when replaced. It has been shown in animal models of prostate cancer that immediately after castration, serum PSA levels rapidly decrease by 80% and increase up to 20-fold following androgen supplementation. These immediate changes in serum PSA occur, however, without castration-induced tumor cell death or concomitant changes in tumor volume and reflect instead changes in androgen-regulated PSA gene expression [7], a much more rapid response than cell death.

In the normal prostate, the cycle of androgen-induced cell growth and castration-induced apoptosis and regression can be continued through multiple cycles of androgen replacement and withdrawal. PSA levels closely reflect these changes. Data from animal studies and observations from the long-term follow-up of Chinese eunuchs demonstrate that normal prostatic epithelial cells undergo apoptotic regression and do not develop the ability to regenerate and grow in an androgen-depleted environment [26]. PSA gene expression, as result, remains suppressed. This dependence on androgen stimulation forms the basis for the hormonal therapies used in advanced malignant prostatic disease, and the use of PSA as a marker of tumor activity.

It has been shown in animal models of prostate cancer that both androgens and tumor volume are important codeterminants of circulating PSA levels [7], and that immediately after castration serum PSA levels rapidly decrease by 80% and increase up to 20-fold following androgen supplementation (Fig. 2). Initially PSA synthesis remains androgen sensitive (and therefore suppressed), but progressively PSA production returns to precastration levels in the absence of testic-

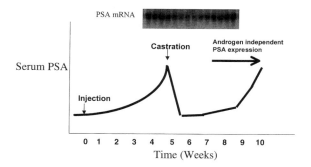

Figure 2   Changes in serum PSA in the LNCaP tumor model mimic the course of human prostate cancer. Serum PSA levels increase in intact male mice after injection are proportional to increases in tumor volume, and decrease rapidly by 80% after castration.

ular androgens, beginning 4 weeks after castration. This heralds the onset of androgen-independent growth.

C. Nonandrogenic Regulation of PSA Production

It is clear that many other coregulators and extracellular factors are involved in the cellular control of PSA production and that stromal–epithelial interactions are very important for both normal and abnormal prostate development. Many of the effects of androgen are mediated by the stroma [27], and androgen only stimulates growth of normal epithelial cells in vitro when cultured with stromal cells [28,29], or other growth factors. An example is in rat prostate cancer models, where tumor growth is accelerated by prostatic stromal and bone fibroblastic factors [8].

With respect to BPH, the major cause of elevated serum PSA levels, evidence suggests that estrogens may have an albeit undefined role in its pathogenesis. Estrogens can exert stimulatory effects on the stroma [30], estradiol potentiates the effects of DHT or Δ4-androstenedione in causing large hyperplastic prostates in dogs, and may enhance hyperplasia by reducing cell death through its effects on DNA synthesis [31]. Activation of the stroma and disregulation of growth factors have likewise been reported, along with observations of increased cytokine expression in stromal tissue, as contributing causes of BPH. The expression of bFGF and TGF-β [32] is heightened, as is the secretion of IGF II-binding proteins and the synthesis of IGF II mRNA by cultured BPH stromal cells [33].

II. ANDROGEN WITHDRAWAL THERAPY AND PSA

A. Historical Review

The ablation of testicular function in the palliative treatment of prostate cancer was first attempted in the 1930s by means of radiation of the testes. This was less effective than surgical removal, which was introduced a decade later [1]. Bilateral orchidectomy has been the gold standard, although more recently medical castration has increased in popularity as a means of avoiding the psychological trauma of surgical castration. Prostatic acid phosphatase was initially used as a marker of disease response, but was primarily restricted to treatment of advanced local and metastatic disease. Since the 1980s, PSA has become the gold standard tumor marker. It now finds its role expanded to include monitoring of patients undergoing neoadjuvant and adjuvant hormonal therapy, treated with radical prostatectomy or radiotherapy, at much earlier stages of disease.

No treatment equals or surpasses androgen ablation in checking the growth of prostate cancer and reducing tumor volume. Biochemical (serum PSA) and objective (radiological, clinical assessment) responses are achieved in 80% of patients as reported in most series [1,34–41]. Withdrawal of androgen induces apoptosis, a form of programmed cell death, in normal and malignant prostatic cells. This fails, however, to eliminate the entire population of malignant cells, and the ultimate course of prolonged androgen withdrawal is androgen-independent disease. This is a complex process involving multiple pathways but at a biochemical level, well before any clinical signs of refractory disease are evident, serum PSA is the first sign of progression to this androgen-independent state.

B. Pharmacologic Agents

Castrate levels of testosterone can be achieved by influencing the pathways of endocrine control of gonadal function as shown below (Fig. 3). Several classes of drugs induce castrate testosterone levels by suppressing the release of luteinizing

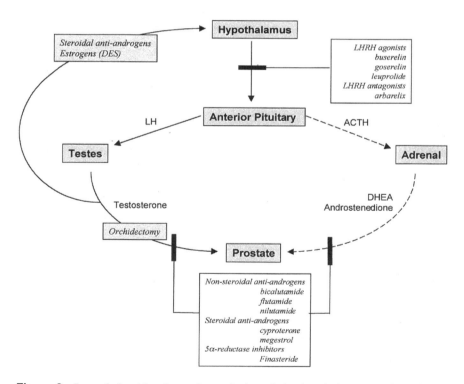

Figure 3   Interrelationships that make up the hypothalamic–pituitary–gonadal axis and regulate prostatic growth via hormonal mechanisms. Inhibiting agents that modify the axis are shown in grey. Dashed lines indicate minor pathways.

hormone from the pituitary. Diethylstilbestrol (DES) suppresses hypothalamic luteinizing hormone-releasing hormone (LHRH) release, and increases levels of sex hormone-binding globulin (SBG); this reduces the serum free testosterone level. DES' low cost and simple dosing (1 mg/day is usually sufficient [34]) must be weighed against the increased risk of thromboembolic disease and cardiovascular complications [34].

LHRH agonists are available as depot subcutaneous or intramuscular injections of varying duration (1–4 months). Normally pulsatile hypothalamic LHRH release stimulates anterior pituitary production of LH. This periodicity is critical and, when altered by continuous administration of luteinizing hormone-releasing hormone LHRH agonist, the control of the pituitary by the hypothalamus is lost. LHRH agonists produce a biphasic response: an initial rise in LH and testosterone levels that may in the presence of metastatic prostate cancer be associated with the ''flare phenomenon'' and symptom exacerbation; this usually lasts around 14 days, and is then followed by a fall in levels [35]. This potential exacerbation of disease can be prevented by the coadministration of an antiandrogen or DES for 1–2 weeks prior to or at the time of LHRH agonist dosing [36].

LHRH antagonists are relatively new agents and current trials [42] are underway to determine their efficacy in comparison to established agents such as LHRH agonists and antiandrogens. They are not associated with the flare phenomenon, making them useful as monotherapy even in advanced metastatic disease in the acute setting.

Antiandrogens compete with androgens for androgen receptor sites in target tissues. The two groups, nonsteroidal and steroidal antiandrogens, have differing mechanisms of action and different effects on serum testosterone levels. Nonsteroidal antiandrogens (flutamide, bicalutamide, nilutamide) have no direct gonadotropic effects, and therefore do not alter serum testosterone levels. Although monotherapy for prostate cancer is not recommended [36], recent data suggest that bicalutamide may be equivalent to orchidectomy when administered at higher doses [37], and its use as a second-line therapy is increasing. Steroidal antiandrogens—cyproterone (CPA) and megestrol—have progestational activity in addition to antiandrogenic action at peripheral receptors: they thus inhibit secretion of LH and decrease testosterone production [36]. A combination of CPA and low-dose DES achieves similar androgen ablation to LHRH agonists, at one-third of the cost [39].

5α-reductase inhibitors, such as finasteride, inhibit the conversion of serum T and dihydroepiandrosterone (DHEA) to DHT in target tissue cells. By lowering intraprostatic DHT, but not affecting serum T levels, these drugs can block both the testicular and adrenal androgen pathways. The resultant intracellular androgen deprivation results in inhibition of prostatic cell proliferation, and activation of prostatic cell death signals or apoptosis [43]. This androgenic blockade is incomplete as intraprostatic testosterone rises up to fivefold, and in these concentrations may have androgenic effects of its own.

C. General Responses to Androgen Deprivation

In the normal and benign prostate, androgen deprivation results in glandular involution and reduction in volume. This comes about by an induction of programmed cell death (PCD) or apoptosis. Figure 4 shows the cell cycle in schematic form and demonstrates the process of recruitment of quiescent G_0 prostatic glandular cells into a pathway of programmed (apoptotic) cell death. PCD does not require cells to be dividing or in the proliferative phase, as shown in numerous animal experiments looking for the typical molecular markers of entry into the proliferative cell cycle [44]. Thus, prostate epithelial cells can exist in one of three phases: metabolically active but not dividing or dying; undergoing division ($G_0 \rightarrow$ mitosis); or undergoing cell death ($G_0 \rightarrow$ apoptosis). Initiation of apoptosis following androgen deprivation is a feature of both BPH and androgen-sensitive or-depen-

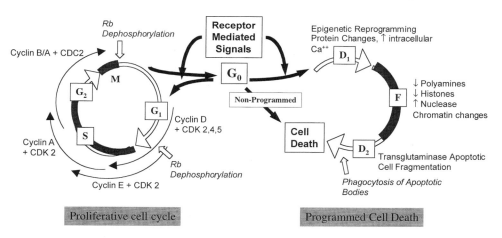

Figure 4 Recruitment of quiescent G_0 epithelial cells into a cell death pathway involves three phases. D_1: epigenetic reprogramming: mRNA expression changes; and altered membrane, intracellular protein synthesis, and increased calcium-magnesium levels; F: decreased intranuclear histone and polyamine content, nuclease activation, and DNA fragmentation. D_2: apoptotic cellular fragmentation and phagocytosis by macrophages or neighbouring epithelial cells. (From Pharmacology, Biology, and Clinical Applications of Androgens: Current Status and Future Prospects. Proceedings of the 2nd International Androgen Workshop. Long Beach, CA, 1995, Wiley-Liss, Inc.)

Table 1 Effects of Androgen Withdrawal on Prostate Size

Androgen inhibitor	Mean % ↓ in prostate volume (method)	Average time for maximal size decrease (months)	Double-blind randomized clinical trials
Surgical castration	30% (TRUS)	3–6	No
Steroidal antiandrogens (CPA)	30% (TRUS)	3–6	No
Flutamide	40% (TRUS)	3–6	No
LHRH agonists	30% (TRUS)	3–6	No
5α-reductase inhibitors (finasteride)	20% (MRI)	3–6	Yes

dent prostate cancer, but not of androgen-independent prostate cancer cells. The quantitative effects of androgen deprivation on prostate size have been studied extensively, and comparison of different methods of androgen deprivation reveals very similar (20–40%) reductions regardless of method used (Table 1).

Finasteride has been shown to be clinically useful in maintaining volume reduction in double-blind clinical trials. Serum PSA in these men falls by up to 50% [45], and current recommendations advise that measured serum PSA in men taking finasteride should be doubled to bring it in line with readings from similar age-matched men not taking the drug, and allow application of age-specific PSA reference ranges. Neoadjuvant hormonal therapy (NHT) has also, likewise been shown to decrease prostatic volume, with longer periods of hormonal withdrawal being more effective. Eight months of NHT resulted in 46% volume reduction on transrectal ultrasound (TRUS), compared to 37% for 3 months treatment in a randomized unblinded phase III trial (CUOG).

D. Hormone-Naïve Prostate Cancer

Use of PSA in the early detection of prostate cancer has produced a stage migration and a 50% decrease in the incidence of stage D_2 disease in recent years [46]. Increasingly, men are diagnosed with rising PSA following curative therapies, and prior to the identification of any soft tissue or bony disease ("biochemical failure"). This has significant implications in terms of long-term outcome of androgen withdrawal therapy using PSA as a marker of disease, since most survival data are derived from patients with predominantly bulky D_2 disease. Survival following treatment is inversely proportional to serum PSA levels prior to treatment, the PSA level being a direct indicator of tumor load, and therefore one would intuitively expect better outcome with early treatment.

Up to 80% of men with metastatic (D_2) prostate cancer exhibit objective clinical and biochemical responses to androgen ablation. Despite this, the overall median progression free survival is only 2–3 years [38,40,41]. Cancers become androgen-independent after a variable period of time (averaging 24 months), and progression inevitably occurs. Serum PSA is the best and most useful indicator of response and prognosis in these patients. Almost all treated patients have an initial rapid response: decreases in serum PSA to the normal range in approximately 70% of men. This may take as long as 32 weeks, and the level of serum PSA reached by this time (the PSA nadir) is a good prognostic indicator of the durability of clinical response. Nadir PSA levels greater than 4 µg/ml after 6 months of therapy are associated with poorer outcome (median survival of 18 months) compared to levels below 4 µg/ml (median survival of 40 months) [47–49]. Beyond 6 months, and in the remaining 30% of men whose disease does not normalize after institution of androgen withdrawal, the serum PSA level will decrease temporarily and then increase. If a plateau is reached it will be short-lived or stabilize outside of the normal range. This is usually an early sign of progression to androgen independence, although in more than 90% of men it may predate any clinical symptoms and recurrence by 6–12 months [47].

Androgen withdrawal therapy cannot cure metastatic prostate cancer because of an inherent inability to eliminate the more lethal, skeletal component of the disease. In a series of 51 patients treated with cyproterone acetate plus low-dose DES, 41 of 49 patients (84%) with evaluable soft tissue disease (local and metastatic) responded with reduction in tumor volume [50]. In contrast, significant improvement occurred in only 13 (27%) of the 48 initially abnormal bone scans. This difference clearly demonstrates the relative resistance of skeletal metastases to potent androgen withdrawal therapy, as has also been noted by other investigators [51]. Soloway et al. documented that patients with fewer than six metastatic deposits on their bone scan had a significantly better 2 year survival than those with more extensive disease [52]. Both the NCI Intergroup study [40] and the EORTC 30853 trial [53] showed that the number and location of bone metastases have a strong effect on treatment outcome. The good-prognosis group, those with five or fewer metastases confined to the axial skeleton, and patients with good performance status, tended to derive the most benefit from treatment.

The response of PSA to androgen withdrawal therapy is somewhat predictable: there is an initial rapid decline (approximately 80%) due to cessation of androgen-regulated PSA gene expression. However, not all men reach their nadir levels at the same time (Fig. 5). Data from neoadjuvant hormonal therapy studies have shown further reductions (up to 50%) after the second month of therapy that reflect continuing prostate epithelial cell apoptosis and decreased cell prolif-

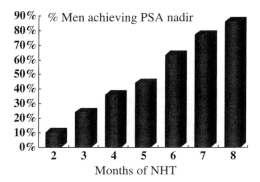

Figure 5   Graph showing percentage of men who reach nadir PSA levels at each month of neoadjuvant hormonal therapy prior to surgery.

eration [7,54] (Fig. 6). The prolonged slow reduction beyond the third month of hormonal therapy, to nadir levels at 8 months, is the basic principle behind long-term neoadjuvant hormonal therapy prior to radical prostatectomy, and will be discussed in detail later.

E.   Androgen-Independent Prostate Cancer

Progression to the androgen-independent state is ubiquitous and is reflected in increasing serum PSA levels after castration. Loss of the androgen dependence of PSA gene regulation during progression to androgen independence (AI) is an example of how an initially androgen-regulated gene becomes activated again in the absence of steroid ligand. Observations in the human prostate LNCaP model suggest that escape from androgen-regulated PSA gene expression may result from LNCaP cells adapting to an androgen-deprived environment through the upregulation of alternative nonandrogenic pathways of signal transduction [55,56], resulting in production of factors capable of transcriptional activation of the androgen receptor. These genetic signals and mechanisms are normally suppressed by the effect of androgens, but in the androgen-deprived environment they become activated. Castration of mice bearing androgen-dependent Shionogi tumors results in a programmatic drift in gene expression initially characterized by upregulation survival or antiapoptotic genes, including Bcl-2, Bcl-xL, and TRPM-2 (Figs. 7, 8).

Cellular and molecular mechanisms that help mediate progression to AI include expansion of preexisting clones of androgen-independent cells (clonal selection) [61,62], upregulation of androgen-repressed adaptive mechanisms capable of aborting the apoptotic process (adaptation) [56,57,59,60], androgen-

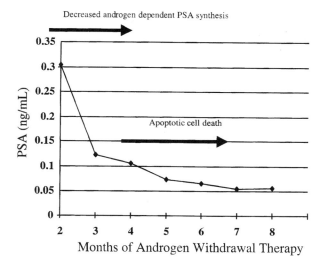

Figure 6 An 80% reduction in serum PSA is seen after 2 months of neoadjuvant hormonal therapy and is the starting point on the y axis. From the third to eighth month of therapy, serum PSA falls a further 50%. (Modified from Ref. 54.)

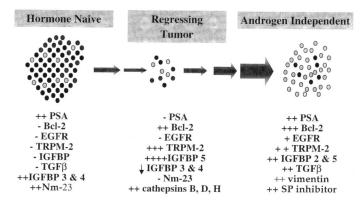

Figure 7 Changes in gene expression in prostate tumors following castration and during AI progression. (From Refs. 57–60.)

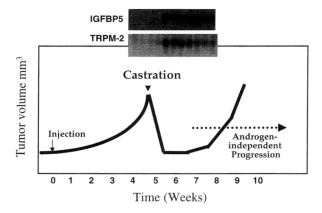

Figure 8   The Shionogi tumor model of androgen independence. Markers of AI progression are apoptosis. TRPM-2 expression, IGFBP 2 & 5, and tumor volume. (From Refs. 59, 60.)

receptor mutations leading to a constitutively active transcriptional factor [63], or production of factors capable of interacting with the androgen receptor (protein–protein interactions) [64]. A complete review of these mechanisms is beyond the scope of this chapter, but all are likely to be variably operative in heterogeneous tumors such as prostate cancer. This tumor heterogeneity reflects a multifocal origin, adaptive (epigenetic) responses to environmental stimuli, and/or genetic instability and provides the basis for AI progression in various subpopulations of cells. Clonal expansion of AI cells after castration cannot be prevented by current therapeutic strategies because of resistance to traditional cytotoxic chemotherapies. However, it may be possible to inhibit or modulate the adaptive changes in gene expression precipitated by androgen ablation through the differentiating influence of androgen.

One interesting phenomenon seen in patients taking long-term antiandrogen therapy is the change in serum PSA following the cessation of antiandrogen therapy. Although first reported as the flutamide withdrawal syndrome [36], it is also seen in approximately 20% of patients after discontinuation of treatment with other steroidal and nonsteroidal antiandrogens, and is characterized by up to a 50% decrease in serum PSA after discontinuation of the drug. This phenomenon highlights the complexity of the androgen–AR interaction, and the changes that occur in tumour receptor biology. Antiandrogens, which have a partial antagonist activity, may become partial agonists during progression to androgen independence, resulting from subtle changes in AR structure and protein–protein interactions.

F. Intermittent Androgen Suppression

Progressively earlier intervention raises the prospect of very long periods of androgen deprivation attended by clinical side effects that reduce quality of life. Early on, androgen withdrawal results in hot flushes, loss of libido, impotence, and general fatigue. Long-term castration leads to bone demineralization, anemia, lipid disorders, and muscle wasting. Most importantly, biological processes, such as the upregulation of previously androgen-repressed survival genes, result in the emergence of androgen-independent growth.

Intermittent androgen suppression (IAS) may be conceived of as a potentially valuable treatment option if immediate hormone therapy is truly superior to delayed treatment [65] and if adaptive (rather than clonal selection alone) mechanisms are involved in the process of androgen-independent progression [66–70]. The idea of inducing repeated regressions of androgen-dependent malignancy arose from the observation that the involution of prostate tissue brought on by castration is an active process involving the rapid elimination of a large number of epithelial cells.

As in human prostate cancer, PSA levels in LNCaP human prostate tumor model are androgen regulated and directly proportional to tumor volume [7,8,71,72]. After castration, serum and tumor-cell PSA levels decrease by 80% and remain suppressed for 3–4 weeks before increasing again. With intermittent testosterone withdrawal and replacement in castrated mice bearing LNCaP tumors, a three-fold delay in the development of androgen-independent regulation of the PSA gene was observed [73]. By 15 weeks after castration, PSA levels in the continuous androgen suppression group had increased 7.0-fold above pre-castration levels, compared to only 1.9-fold in the IAS-treated group.

The intermittent regulation of serum testosterone levels for therapeutic purposes in patients with prostate cancer was first attempted with cyclic administration of estrogenic hormone [74]. Nineteen patients with advanced prostate cancer received diethylstilbestrol until a clinical response was clearly demonstrated; it was then withheld until symptoms recurred. One additional patient was treated with flutamide using a similar schedule. The mean duration of initial therapy was 30 months (range, 2–70 months). Subjective improvement was noted in all patients during the first 3 months of treatment. When therapy was stopped, 12 of 20 patients relapsed after a mean interval of 8 months (range, 1–24 months) and all subsequently responded to readministration of drug. Therapy-induced impotency was reversed in 9 of 10 men within 3 months of the break in treatment. An improved quality of life was achieved owing to the reduced intake of diethylstilbestrol, and no adverse effects on survival were apparent.

The first nonsteroidal antiandrogens became available around the same time as this study, and most clinical research focussed on the combined use of LHRH agonists and antiandrogens. Little attention has been given to the reversibility of action of LHRH agonists, the significance of which is far-reaching. The potential for a full recovery from therapy makes it possible to alternate a patient between periods of treatment and no treatment. Furthermore, serial serum PSA measurements, which were not available at the time of the study by Klotz et al. [74], permit accurate monitoring of disease activity and serve as trigger points for stopping and restarting therapy. In response to this androgenic stimulus, atrophic cells are recruited into a normal pathway of differentiation where the risk of progression to androgen-independence is reduced. With the associated movement through the division cycle, the cells become preapoptotic again, making it possible to repeat therapy.

Trigger points for reinstitution of androgen withdrawal therapy are similar among investigators reporting on their IAS experience [75–80]. Although the optimal time remains undefined and empirical, time off therapy should be long enough to permit normalization of improved quality of life and testosterone-induced tumor cell differentiation. Reexposure of tumor cells to testosterone during the off-treatment cycles of IAS is critical to the underlying hypothesis and rationale behind IAS. Furthermore, recovery of testosterone between treatment cycles is necessary for recovery of sexual function, reduced side effects, and normal sense of well-being. Until more information is obtained, PSA trigger points are regarded as tentative settings only. Trigger points are individualized and factors that are considered include pretreatment PSA levels, stage, PSA velocity, presence of symptoms, and tolerance of androgen ablation therapy. In general, in patients with metastatic disease and high pretreatment PSA levels, therapy is restarted when PSA increases to 20 µg/L; in patients with locally recurrent disease and moderately elevated pretreatment PSA levels, therapy is restarted when PSA reaches 6–15 µg/L, and earlier for recurrences after radical prostatectomy.

Three year results of IAS in 47 patients using reversible medical castration and serum PSA as trigger points were initially reported by Goldenberg et al. [75] in 1995, and updated to include 87 patients in 1999 [81]. Fifty have now been evaluated for at least 3 years, with study range from 40 to 126 months, and a mean of 65 months. Forty-one had clinically localized and 29 had metastatic disease at accrual. Mean initial serum PSA level was 110 µg/L. Treatment was initiated with combined androgen blockade and continued for an average of 9 months. Because prognosis is poor in patients who do not achieve normal PSA levels after androgen ablation, only patients with PSA nadir levels below 4 µg/L are eligible for the IAS protocol. Medication was withheld until serum PSA increased to mean values between 10 and 20 µg/L. This cycle of treatment and no treatment was repeated until the regulation of PSA became androgen independent (Fig. 9). The off-treatment period in all cycles was associated an improvement in sense of well-being, and the recovery of libido and potency in the men who reported normal or near-normal sexual function before the start of therapy. The average time off therapy (percentage time off therapy) for cycles 1, 2, 3,

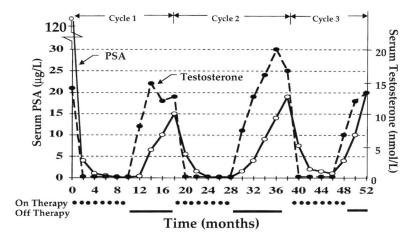

Figure 9 Intermittent androgen suppression cycles: note close correlation between serum T and PSA throughout the trial period. (From Ref. 75.)

and 4 was 15 months (54%), 10 months (48%), 8 months (45%), and 7 months (40%), respectively. The study group included nine patients treated because of a rising PSA level following radiation therapy for locally advanced cancer. These patients have been off therapy for an average of 22 and 13 months in the first 2 treatment cycles, respectively. Six patients with rising PSA levels following radical prostatectomy and with follow-up exceeding 36 months, have been off therapy for an average of 19 and 11 months in the first 2 treatment cycles, respectively. Twenty-three of 87 patients have progressed to androgen independence at a median of 32 months of treatment and 13 have died cancer-specific deaths at a median of 48 months.

Observations from this study suggest that IAS does not have a negative impact on time to progression or survival, both of which are similar to continuous combined therapy. However, phase III randomized studies are required to assess accurately the effects of intermittent treatment on these critical parameters. IAS improves quality of life by permitting recovery of libido and potency, increasing energy levels, and enhancing sense of well-being during off-treatment periods. The animal and preliminary clinical studies have helped to identify groups of patients who are most likely to benefit from IAS, to determine optimal duration of treatment, and to suggest trigger points on when to restart therapy again. The therapeutic strategy and trigger points in each situation is guided by serum PSA. IAS may offer a ''way out'' of the immediate vs. delayed treatment controversy, balancing the benefits of immediate androgen ablation with reduced treatment-related side effects and expense. More information will become available from prospective randomized clinical trials of IAS that have been initiated in Canada, the United States, and Europe.

G. Sequential Androgen Blockade

Another approach to reducing the side effects of therapy is the concept of sequential androgen blockade proposed by Fleshner and Trachtenberg [82,83]. By inhibiting conversion of testosterone to DHT, the relative potencey of flutamide as an androgen receptor antagonist is increased, and the usual side effects of androgen ablation are avoided because testosterone levels are not reduced. Twenty-two sexually active men with stages C and D1 prostate cancer were treated with finasteride 5 mg daily and flutamide 125–250 mg three times daily. Mean serum PSA decreased from 42.9 to 3.6 µg/L and 2.9 µg/L at 3 and 6 months, respectively, and the response was durable to 24 months. Potency was preserved in 86% of patients; however, gynecomastia is a significant problem in many men. Further follow-up and comparative studies are necessary to determine whether time to progression or survival is adversely affected.

H. Neoadjuvant Hormonal Therapy

The rationale for neoadjuvant hormonal withdrawal therapy (NHT) evolved from the observation of high positive margin rates following radical prostatectomy and the desire to reduce the risk of biochemical (and ultimately clinical) recurrence. The availability of potent, reversible, and well-tolerated forms of medical castration and use of serum PSA as a marker of response to therapy make its application prior to localized therapy appealing. The role of NHT prior to radical prostatectomy remains controversial; some clinicians argue that downsizing occurs without downstaging and any apparent downstaging results from difficulty in pathological evaluation of the neoadjuvantly treated prostatectomy specimen [84–86].

Most clinical studies report decreases in positive margin rates of up to 50% following 3 months of neoadjuvant therapy [87–91]. Soloway et al. [90] reported that 3 months of leuprolide acetate and flutamide prior to radical prostatectomy significantly decreased positive margin rates from 42% in the control group to 18% in the neoadjuvant-treated group. Results from the Canadian Uro-Oncology Group using 3 months of cyproterone acetate also demonstrated a 50% reduction in positive margin rates [91]. The ability of neoadjuvant therapy to reduce biochemical and local recurrence is the ultimate goal; this has not been determined from these studies because of lack of statistical power and long-term follow-up. The U.S. Intergroup [92] and Canadian Uro-Oncology Group [93,94] studies have not demonstrated any difference in PSA recurrence rates at 36 months follow-up.

The failure of 3 months of neoadjuvant therapy to reduce PSA recurrence rates in these phase III studies may result from insufficient duration of neoadjuvant therapy. Although downsizing occurs after 3 months of neoadjuvant therapy, serum PSA levels do not reach nadir or undetectable levels in most patients after this period of time (Figs. 5, 6). Serum PSA levels decrease rapidly and dramatically after institution of androgen withdrawal therapy due to cessation of androgen-regulated PSA gene expression and apoptosis [95,96]. Further decreases in serum PSA after the second month likely reflect continued apoptotic prostate epithelial cell death and decreased tumor cell proliferation, which leads to further reduction in tumor volume [96]. Changes in serum PSA during neoadjuvant therapy provide objective biochemical information to gauge tumor response and identify patients whose condition is not responding favorably. The above data suggest that optimal duration of neoadjuvant therapy may be longer than 3 months.

Androgen ablation therapy is rarely curative in patients with osseous metastases; however, 10% of patients with D2 disease do survive longer than 10 years after castration. Furthermore, clinical observations suggest that soft tissue disease responds more favorably to androgen ablation with more frequent and durable complete responses than osseous metastases [96,97]. Patients with stage D1 lymph node-only disease have a median survival more than twice that of patients with D2 osseous disease [98]. Adjuvant androgen ablation therapy following radical prostatectomy in patients with regional lymph node metastases results in long-term (15 year) survival in 30%, which suggests that a significant proportion of patients with low-volume soft tissue metastases may be cured with surgery and immediate androgen ablation [98,99]. One would anticipate that a similar proportion of patients with clinically localized tumors and unrecognized subclinical metastases whose disease would ultimately recur after radical prostatectomy alone may also be cured by neoadjuvant androgen ablation, as long as the course of therapy is long enough. Furthermore, it is logical to assume that maximal tumor regression is achieved when PSA reaches its nadir level, and that these patients will do best postoperatively, because of decreased tumor volume and reduced rates of margin positive disease [97]. Indeed, recent work has demonstrated improved long-term survival with 8 months of NHT in men with localized prostate cancer undergoing radical prostatectomy [100].

Evidence from the Shionogi rat model suggests that neoadjuvant therapy followed by surgery may be more effective in delaying androgen independent progression than surgery followed by adjuvant therapy [101] (Fig. 10). The group that underwent surgery after castration had significantly longer tumor-free survival. This concurs with the concept of NHT in clinical disease reducing margin positive rates and subsequent risk of local recurrence after radical prostatectomy.

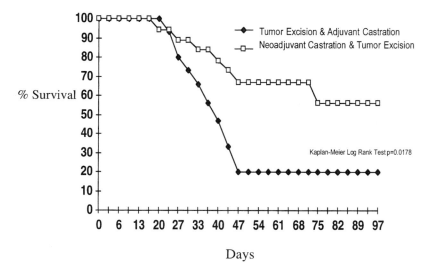

Figure 10 Neoadjuvant castration reduces local recurrence rates in the Shionogi tumor model. Tumors were grown to 1–2 g before rats were randomized to either wide tumor excision followed by castration on local recurrence (group 1), or neoadjuvant castration for 10 days followed by wide tumor excision (group 2). Androgen-independent progression (study end point) occurred in 80% of group 1 at median 36 days, and 44% of group 2 at median 42 days. Tumor-free survival was greater in group 2 (56% vs. 20%; p < 0.05), as shown by Kaplan-Meier curves. (From Ref. 101.)

PSA levels should fall rapidly in response to NHT, according to the well-established patterns seen in clinical practice (see Fig. 6). In certain cases, however, serum PSA levels may not fall rapidly enough, or to adequately low nadir levels in response to NHT, despite achieving castrate levels of testosterone. Specifically, in high-risk localized disease such as clinical T3 tumors, high PSA (>20), or high Gleason score (≥7), reassessment after initial treatment with NHT may identify those patients at higher risk of margin-positive disease or gross lymph node involvement, and who may benefit more from external beam radiation treatment and hormonal withdrawal.

III. PSA CHANGES ASSOCIATED WITH DIETARY MANIPULATION

Increasing interest in recent years in herbal and natural therapies has created a burgeoning industry aimed at the prevention and treatment of prostate cancer using dietary supplements. Of most interest are the phytoestrogens (coumestans, isoflavonoids, flavonoids, and lignans), which have effects in varying degrees but similar in many ways to androgen withdrawal therapy. Commonly prescribed agents include soy derivatives, PC-SPES, Saw palmetto, and, more recently, lycopenes.

A. Dietary Phytoestrogen Consumption

Epidemiological studies over the past 25 years have identified the Western diet as having a primary association with cancer and chronic disease. In contrast to Asian diets, an aspect not found in Western diets that may be causal in this relationship is the relatively low intake of phytoestrogens. Over 90% of Asian children have consumed soy products, many starting before the age of 18 months, a factor that may be critical in the relationship of soy phytoestrogens and disease prevention [102].

The weak natural estrogens genistein and diadzein found in high concentrations in soy are believed to have anticarcinogenic, antiproliferative, hypocholesterolemic, and favorable hormone-altering capacities. Quantitatively, they are the most important environmental estrogens when their hormonal potency is assessed in vitro. They exert their estrogenic activity by interacting with estrogen receptors (ERs) in vitro. They may also act as antiestrogens by competing for the binding sites of estrogen receptors or the active site of the estrogen biosynthesizing and metabolizing enzymes, such as aromatase and oestrogen-specific 17 beta-hydroxysteroid oxidoreductase (type 1). Identification of subtypes of estrogen receptors [103], may help to explain these two opposing mechanisms of action.

Although higher levels of serum testosterone have not been found consistently in men with prostate cancer, lower rates of disease have been seen in eunuchs and castrated men, along with significant changes in the hormonal regulation of prostate cells and apoptosis-related effects [9,12,24]. Although Asian men have similar incidences of latent and small prostate cancers, compared to Western men, the difference in mortality rates is startling [104,105]. One of the reasons may be the high consumption of soy products, since Asian men tend to have higher serum levels and urinary excretion of phytoestrogens. Additionally, prostate size and PSA do not appear to increase with age as dramatically in Asian men [106,107].

Animal model data suggest a significant effect of phytoestrogens on human prostate cancer cells. LNCaP tumors grown in nude mice fed a diet rich in rye and soy are smaller and secrete less PSA than tumors grown in mice on control diets. Addition of fat to the diet of the treatment group reduced the positive effects on prostate cancer growth [108]. Biochanin A, a precursor of genistein, along with other phytoestrogens has also been shown to inhibit growth of both hormone-sensitive and-insensitive prostate cancer cell lines [109].

PC-SPES, a mixture of eight different herbs (including *Serenoa repens*, the saw palmetto), has been advocated as an alternative for the treatment of prostate cancer. It is known to have potent oestrogenic activity, although not because of estrogens such as estrone, estradiol, or DES. Several in vitro and in vivo studies have shown an inhibitory effect upon prostate cancer cell growth, testosterone, and serum PSA level. De la Taille et al. [110] showed that alcohol extracts of PC-SPES had a dose-dependent effect (in vitro) in decreasing growth of hormone-sensitive (LNCaP) and hormone-independent (LNCaP-bcl-2, PC-3, and DU145) prostate cancer cell lines (less effect seen in the latter group). PSA gene and AR expression has also been shown to decrease in LNCaP cultures [111] in response to PC-SPES treatment. Recent work [27] in a nonrandomized clinical human trial has shown up to 65% reduction in serum PSA at 2 months, and 67% reduction at 6 months of treatment with PC-SPES. Testosterone levels likewise fall in conjunction with PSA, but rapidly reverse 2–6 weeks after treatment stops [112].

Phytoestrogens (especially lignans found in flaxseed) have also been shown to inhibit 5α-reductase [113], which may be a partial explanation for the lower levels of this enzyme in Japanese men, and subsequently a lower risk for prostate cancer. PSA levels in these men, as mentioned before, are lower compared to age-matched white men [107] and may reflect the action of phytoestrogens on prostate size because of this action, as well as a partial estrogenic activity.

B. Dietary Lycopene Consumption

Several human studies have observed a direct association between retinol (vitamin A) intake and risk of prostate cancer [114], other studies have found either an inverse association or no association of intake of beta-carotene (the major provitamin A) with risk of prostate cancer [115]. An evaluation of the Health Professionals Follow-Up Study has detected a lower prostate cancer risk associated with the greater consumption of tomatoes and related food products. Tomatoes are the primary dietary source of lycopene, a non-provitamin A carotenoid with potent antioxidant activity. Certain foods containing tomatoes or extracts thereof have higher lycopene concentrations than others.

In the 1995 National Cancer Institute study [114], of 46 vegetables and fruits or related products assessed by questionnaire, four were significantly associated with lower prostate cancer risk. Of the four, tomato sauce (p for trend = 0.001), tomatoes (p for trend = 0.03), and pizza (p for trend = 0.05), but not strawberries, are primary sources of lycopene. Combined intake of tomatoes, tomato sauce, tomato juice, and pizza (which accounted for 82% of lycopene intake) was inversely associated with risk of prostate cancer (multivariate RR = 0.65) when consumed more than 10 times vs. less than twice per week. The association with advanced (stages C and D) prostate cancers was less strong (multivariate RR = 0.47). Other measured carotenoids were unrelated to risk of prostate cancer.

Lycopenes have also been found in the prostate at concentrations that are biologically active in laboratory studies [116]. The implications of these studies are that an increase in vegetable and fruit consumption may reduce cancer incidence, but that tomato-based foods may be especially beneficial regarding prostate cancer risk. The association between serum PSA and lycopenes, has yet to be elucidated. However, on an intuitive basis, if lycopenes have an impact on prostate cancer biology, then PSA production and metabolism should be influenced to some degree.

C. Androgen Supplementation and PSA

There is no current evidence that the endocrine status of men affects the initiation of prostate cancer, or has an impact on the prevalence of precursor lesions. It is likewise not known if exogenous androgen supplementation (as opposed to circulating endogenous androgens) can influence the multistep processes involved in cancer promotion that result in the different phenotypic appearances of prostate cancer.

Androgens do, however, stimulate established prostate cancer in a dose-dependent fashion, as evidenced by animal trials [117,118]. Furthermore, testosterone given to patients with metastatic prostate cancer can result in severe rapid onset of pain at bony metastatic sites [119], presumably due to sudden increases in proteolytic proteins secreted by the prostate cancer. The response of serum PSA in the latter trial was not characterized, since the trial was conducted before the use of PSA became widespread. A more recent study, however, does show an interesting finding: men receiving 200 mg testosterone enanthate intramuscularly ([IM] weekly) as part of an investigation into a male contraceptive regimen maintained high serum testosterone and DHT levels throughout the treatment period. There was no significant rise in serum PSA levels associated with this treatment [120].

One would expect that if androgens are given to a man with a normal PSA level and no evidence of prostate cancer, then provided that serum testosterone does not rise above normal levels, the serum PSA should remain stable and be an ongoing predictor of early disease. If, however, serum testosterone does decrease with age, and older men are hypogonadal and therefore receive androgen supplementation, will increasing their serum testosterone levels to the "normal" range stimulate the silent prostate cancer they have been harboring? Serum PSA in the presupplementation "hypogonadal" state may not be as good a differentiator of benign from malignant prostatic disease. This question has yet to be answered. Current guidelines recommend that any man who would be treated with androgens for hypogonadism undergo DRE and measurement of PSA. If his PSA is above 4, or above age-referenced range limits, he should undergo a biopsy.

The question of monitoring PSA while a patient is receiving androgen supplementation is even more vexed. Provided pretreatment PSA was in the normal
age-specific reference range, the current consensus is DRE and PSA annually,
and a rate of PSA change of <0.75 µg/L/year over 2 years should be considered
normal, irrespective of the use of exogenous androgens [121].

Androgen and other performance-enhancing substance use in elite athletes
has become widespread since the 1970. Although the effects on hepatic metabolism, development of hepatic tumors, and secondary sexual physical characteristics have been well documented based on case studies, no single significant long-
term follow-up of these athletes has been undertaken to ascertain the health risks.
Most athletes use androgens and other agents intermittently, then go through
periods of withdrawal (from levels of supranormal stimulation). In addition, most
usage occurs in the late teens and early adulthood, rather than in the ages of
increasing prostate cancer risk. This cycling of the hormonal mileau may not be
sufficient to result in any significant hypothalamic–pituitary–gonadal suppression or stimulation, which would increase the risk of stimulating latent cancer
or inducing prostate cancer lesions. The corollary is that a significant number of
North American sportsmen who use androgens, are in a high risk group, that is,
Afro-American males, who have a higher incidence of prostate cancer and disease
that tends to develop at a younger age.

REFERENCES

1. C Huggins, and CV Hodges. Studies on prostate cancer: I. Effect of castration,
   estrogen, and androgen injection on serum phosphatases in metastatic carcinoma
   of the prostate. Cancer Res 1:293, 1941.
2. MA Carso-Juria, WT Schrader, BW O'Malley. Steroid receptor family: Structure
   and functions. Endocr Rev 11:201–220, 1990.
3. PS Rennie, N Bruchovsky, KJ Leco, PC Sheppard, SA McQueen, et al. Characterisation of two cis-acting DNA elements involved in the androgen regulation of the
   probasin gene. Mol Endocrin 7:23–36, 1993.
4. AJ Adler, A Scheller, Y Hoffman, DM Robins. Multiple components of a complex
   androgen-dependent enhancer. Molec Endocrin 5:1587–1596, 1991.
5. GJ Miller, GE Stapleton, JA Ferrara, MS Lucia, S Pfister, et al. The human prostatic
   carcinoma cell line LNCaP expresses biologically active, specific receptors for 1-
   24 hydroxy-vitamin D3. Cancer Res 52:515–520, 1992.
6. PE Andrews, CY-F Young, BT Montgomery, DJ Tindall. Tumour promoting pho-
   bol ester down regulates the androgen induction of PSA in a human prostatic adenocarcinoma cell line. Cancer Res 52:1525–1529, 1992.
7. ME Gleave, JT Hsieh, H-C Wu et al. Serum PSA levels in mice bearing human
   prostate LNCaP tumors are determined by tumor volume and endocrine and growth
   factors. Cancer Res 52:1598–1605, 1992.

8. ME Gleave, JT Hsieh, CA Gao, AC von Eschenbach, LWK Chung. Acceleration of human prostate cancer growth in vivo by factors produced by prostate and bone fibroblasts. Cancer Res 51:3753–3761, 1991.

9. P Henttu, P Vihko. Growth factor regulation of gene expression in human prostatic cell line LNCaP. In: P Henttu, ed. Acta Univ. Ouluensis series D medica 252: Prostate Specific Antigen and Prostatic Acid Phosphatase. University of Oulu, Section V, pp 1–21, 1992.

10. Z Culig, A Hobisch, MV Cronauer, C Radmayr, et al. Androgen receptor activation in prostatic tumour cell lines by ILGF-4, KGF and EGF. Cancer Res 54:5474–5478, 1994.

11. R Moore: Benign hypertrophy and carcinoma of the prostate. Surgery 16:152–167, 1944.

12. J Imperato-McGinley, RE Peterson, T Gautier, E Sterla. Male pseudohermaphroditism with 5α-reductase deficiency: A model for the role of androgens in both the development of the male phenotype and the evolution of a male gender identity. J. Steroid Biochem 11:637–645, 1979.

13. MJ McPhaul, M Marcelli, S Zoppi, JE Griffen, JD Wilson. The spectrum of mutations in the androgen receptor gene that cause androgen resistance. J Clin Endocrinol Metab. 76:17–23, 1993.

14. C Huggins, and R Stevens. The effect of castration on BPH in man. J Urol 43:705.

15. TA Starney, JN Kabalin, M Ferrari, N Yang. Prostate specific antigen in the diagnosis and treatment of adenocarcinoma of the prostate. IV. Anti-androgen treated patients. J Urol 141:1088, 1989.

16. DA Goldfarb, BS Stein, M Shamozadeh, RO Petersen. Age related changes in tissue levels of prostatic acid phosphatase and PSA. J Urol 136:1266–1269, 1986.

17. JGH Vieira, SK Nishida, AB Pereira, et al. Serum levels of PSA in normal boys throughout puberty. J Clin Edocrinol Metab 78:1185–1187, 1994.

18. N Bruchovsky, EM Brown, CM Coppin, SL Goldenberg, JC Le Riche, NC Murray, PS Rennie. The endocrinology and treatment of prostate tumor progression. In: DS Coffey, N Bruchovsky, WA Gardner, Jr, MI Resnick, JP Karr, eds. Current Concepts and Approaches to the Study of Prostate Cancer. New York: Alan R Liss, 1987, pp 348–387.

19. M Beato, G Chalepakis, M Schauer, EP Slater. DNA regulatory elements for steroid hormones. J Steroid Biochem, 32:737, 1989.

20. JFR Kerr, CR Winterford, BV Harmon. Apoptosis: Its significance in cancer and cancer therapy. Cancer 73:2013, 1994.

21. DA Wolf, T Herzinger, H Hermekin, et al. Transcriptional and post-transcriptional regulation of human androgen receptor expression by androgen. Mol Endocrinol 7:924–928, 1993.

22. PS Rennie, N Bruchovsky, R Buttyan, M Benson, and H Cheng: Gene expression during the early phases of regression of the androgen-dependent Shionogi mouse mammary carcinoma. Cancer Res, 48:6309, 1988.

23. TJ McDonnell, P Troncoso, SM Brisbay, et al. Expression of the protooncogene bcl-2 in the prostate and its association with emergence of androgen-independent prostate cancer. Cancer Res 52:6940, 1992.

24. F Neumann, M Humpel, T Senge, B Schenck, and U Tunn. Cyproterone acetate:

Biochemical and biological basis for treatment of prostatic cancer. In: by GH Jacobi, R Hohenfellner, eds. Prostate Cancer. Baltimore: Williams & Wilkins, 1982, p 269.

25. HI Scher, WK Kelly. Flutamide withdrawal syndrome: Its impact on clinical trials in hormone-refractory prostate cancer. J Clin Oncol, 11:1566, 1993.

26. CP Wu and FL Gu. The prostate in eunuchs. EORTC Genitourinary Group Monograph 10-Urologic Oncology: Reconstructive Surgery, Organ Preservation, and Restoration of Function. New York: Wiley-Liss, Inc., 1992, pp 249–255.

27. GR Cunha, ET Alarid, T Turner, AA Donjacour, EI Boutin, et al. Normal and abnormal development of the male genitourinary tract. J Androl 13:465–475, 1992.

28. S-M Chang, LWK Chung. Interaction between prostatic fibroblast and epithelial cells in culture: Role of androgen. Endocrinology 125:2719–2727, 1989.

29. Y Kusama, J Enami, Y Kano. Growth and morphogenesis of mouse prostate epithelial cells in collagen gel matrix culture. Cell Biol Int Rep 13:569–575, 1989.

30. MF El Etreby. Atamestane: An aromatase inhibitor for the treatment of BPH. A short review. J Steroid Biochem. Mol Biol. 44(4–6):565–572, 1993.

31. ER Barrack, SJ Berry. DNA synthesis in the canine prostate: Effects of androgen and estrogen treatment. Prostate 10:45–56, 1987.

32. H Mori, M Maki, K Oishi, M Jaye, K Igarashi, et al. Increased expression of genes for basic fibroblast growth factor and transforming growth factor type-2 in human prostatic hyperplasia. Prostate 16:71–80, 1990.

33. P Cohen, DM Peehl, B Baker, F Liu, RL Hintz, et al. Insulin-like growth factor axis abnormalities in prostatic stromal cells from patients with benign prostatic hyperplasia. J Clin Endocrinol Metab 79:1410–1415, 1994.

34. RL Cox, ED Crawford. Estrogens in the treatment of prostate cancer J Urol 154: 1991–1998, 1995.

35. The Leuprolide Study Group. Leuprolide vs diethylstibestrol for metatstatic prostate cancer. N Engl J Med 311:1281–1286, 1984.

36. N Bruchovsky. Androgens and anti-androgens. In: JF Holland, E III Frei, RC Bast, DW Kufe, DL Morton, RR Weichselbaum, eds. Cancer Medicine, 3rd ed. Philadelphia: Lea & Febiger, 1993, pp 884–896.

37. GR Blackledge. High dose bicalutamide monotherapy for the treatment of prostate cancer. Urology 47(1A suppl):44–47, 1996.

38. PF Schellhammer, R Sharifi, N Block, MS Soloway, P Venner, et al. A controlled trial of bicalutamide vs flutamide, each in combination with LHRH analogue therapy, in patients with advanced prostate cancer. Cancer 78:2164–2169, 1996.

39. SL Goldenberg, N Bruchovsky, ME Gleave, LD Sullivan. Low dose cyproterone acetate plus mini-dose diethylstilbestrol—a protocol for reversible medical castration. Urology 47:882–884, 1996.

40. ED Crawford, MA Eisenberger, DG McLeod, JT Spalding, R Benson, et al. A controlled trial of leuprolide with and without flutamide in prostatic carcinoma. N Engl J Med 321:419–424, 1989.

41. Prostate Cancer Trialists' Collaborative Group. Maximum androgen blockade in advanced prostate cancer: an overview of 22 randomised trials with 3283 deaths in 5710 patients. Lancet 346:265–269, 1995.

42. MB Garnick, K Tomera, W Moseley, et al. Abarelix-Depot, a sustained release

formulation of a potent GnRH pure antagonist in patients with prostate cancer: Initial results and endocrine comparison with superagonists lupron and zoladex. J Endocrinol. Abstr 1998.

43. JC Lamb, H English, PL Levandoski, GR Rhodes, RK Johnson, et al. Prostatic involution in rats induced by a novel 5α-reductase inhibitor, SK&F 105657: Role for testosterone in the androgenic response. Endocrinology 130:685–694, 1992.

44. Y Furuya, JC Walsh, X Lin, WG Nelson, JT Isaacs. Androgen ablation induced programmed cell death of prostatic glandular cells does not involve recruitment into a defective cell cycle or p53 induction. Endocrinology 136:1898–1906, 1995.

45. HA Guess, GJ Gormley, E Stoner, JE Oesterling. The effect of finasteride on prostate specific antigen: Review of available data. J Urol 155:3–9, 1996.

46. JL Stanford, BA Blumenstein, MK Brawer. Temporal trends in prostate cancer rates in the Pacific Northwest. J Urol 155:604A, 1996.

47. N Bruchovsky, SL Goldenberg, K Akakura, PS Rennie. LHRH agonists in prostate cancer: elimination of the flare reaction by pretreatment with cyproterone acetate and low dose diethylstilbestrol. Cancer 72:1685–1691, 1993.

48. JI Miller, FR Ahmanmn, GW Drach, SS Emerson, MR Bottaccini. The clinical usefulness of serum PSA after hormonal therapy of metastatic prostate cancer. J Urol 147:956–961, 1992.

49. DWW Newlin, L Denis, K Vermeylen. Orchiectomy versus goserelin and flutamide in the treatment of newly diagnosed metastatic prostate cancer: Analysis of the criteria of evaluation used in the European Organisation for Research on Treatment of Cancer—Genitourinary Group Study 30853. Cancer 72:3793–3798.

50. SL Goldenberg, N Bruchovsky, PS Rennie, CM Coppin. The combination of cyproterone acetate and low dose diethylstilbestrol in the treatment of advanced prostatic carcinoma. J Urol 140:1460, 1988.

51. SD Fossa, A Heilo, M Lindegaard, A Skinningrud, S Ous. Clinical significance of routine follow-up examinations in patients with metastatic cancer of the prostate under hormone treatment. Eur Urol; 9:262, 1983.

52. H Matzkin, PE Perito, MS Soloway. Prognostic factors in metastatic prostate cancer. Cancer; 72:3788, 1993.

53. LJ Denis, P Whelan, JL Carneiro De Moura, et al. Goserelin acetate and flutamide versus bilateral orchiectomy. Urology; 42:119, 1993.

54. ME Gleave, SL Goldenberg, EC Jones, N Bruckovsky, and LD Sullivan. Biochemical and pathological effects of eight months of androgen withdrawal therapy prior to radical prostatectomy in clinically confined prostate cancer. J Urol 155:213–219, 1996.

55. JT Hsieh, H-C Wu, ME Gleave, et al. Autocrine regulation of PSA gene expression in a human prostatic cancer (LNCaP) subline. Cancer Res 52:2852–2857, 1993.

56. H-C Wu, JT Hsieh, ME Gleave, et al. Derivation of androgen independent human LNCaP prostate cancer sublines: Role of bone stromal cells. Int J Cancer 57:406, 1994.

57. T Nickerson, H Miyake, M Gleave, M Pollack. Castration-induced apoptosis of androgen-dependent Shionogi carcinoma is associated with increased expression of genes encoding insulin-like growth factor binding proteins. Cancer Res 59: 3392–3395, 1999.

58. H Miyake, A Tolcher, M Gleave. Anti-sense Bcl-2 oligodeoxynucleotides enhance taxol chemosensitivity and synergistically delays progression to androgen-independence after castration in the the androgen dependent Shionogi tumour model. J Natl Cancer Inst 92:34–41, 2000.

59. H Miyake, P Rennie, C Nelson, M Gleave. Testosterone repressed prostate message-2 (TRPM-2) is an anti-apoptotic gene that confers resistance to androgen ablation in prostate cancer xenograft models. Cancer Res 60:170–176, 2000.

60. H Miyake, C Nelson, P Rennie, M Gleave. Overexpression of insulin like growthfactor binding protein-5 helps accelerate progression to androgen independence in the human LNCaP tumour model through activation of phosphatidylinositol 3″–kinase pathway. Endocrinology 2000 Jun; 141(6):2257–2265.

61. JT Isaacs, N Wake, DS Coffey, AA Sandberg.: Genetic instability coupled to clonal selection as a mechanism for progression in prostatic cancer. Cancer Res 42:2353–2361, 1982.

62. JT Issacs. The timing of androgen ablation therapy and/or chemotherapy in the treatment of prostatic cancer. Prostate 51:1–17, 1984.

63. WM van Weerden. Animal models in the study of progression of prostate and breast cancers to endocrine independency. In: PMJJ Berns, JC Romijin, FH Schröder eds.), Mechanisms of Progression to Hormone-Independent Growth of Breast and Prostate Cancer New Jersey: Parthenon Publishers, 1991, pp 55–70.

64. ME Taplin, GJ Bubley, TD Shuster, ME Frantz AE Spooner, GK Ogata, HN Keer, SP Balk. Mutation of the androgen receptor in metastatic androgen-independent prostate cancer. N Engl J Med 332:1393–1398, 1995.

65. D Kirk. Immediate versus deferred treatment for advanced disease. In: A Belldegrun, RS Kirby, RTD Oliver, eds. New Perspectives in Prostate Cancer. Oxford: Isis Medical Media Ltd., 1998, pp 283–292.

66. N Bruchovsky, PS Rennie, AJ Coldman, SL Goldenberg, M To, D Lawson. Effects of androgen withdrawal on the stem cell composition of the Shionogi carcinoma. Cancer Res 50:2275–2282, 1990.

67. PS Rennie, N Bruchovsky, K Akakura, et al. Effect of tumour progression on the androgenic regulation of the androgen receptor, TRPM-2 and YPT1 genes in the Shionogi Carcinoma. J Steroid Biochem Mol Biol 40(1/2):31–40, 1994.

68. N Sato, ME Gleave, N Bruchovsky, et al. Intermittent androgen suppression delays progression to androgen-independent regulation of prostate-specific antigen gene in the LNCaP prostate tumour model. J Steroid Biochem Mol Biol 58(2):139–146, 1996.

69. K Akakura, N Bruchovsky, PS Rennie, et al. Effects of intermittent androgen suppression on the stem cell composition and the expression of the TRPM-2 (clusterin) gene in the Shionogi carcinoma. J Steroid Biochem Mol Biol 59(5/6):501–511, 1996.

70. JM Kokontis, N Hay, S Liao. Progression of LNCaP prostate tumor cells during androgen deprivation: Hormone-independent growth, repression of proliferation by androgen, and role for p27 [Kip1] in androgen-induced cell cycle arrest. Mol Endocrinol 12:941–953, 1998.

71. ME Gleave, M Bowden, N Bruchovsky, SL Goldenberg, LD Sullivan. Predictors of time to androgen-independent progression in the LNCaP prostate tumor model. J Urol; 151:241 (abstract), 1994.

72. N Sato, M Gleave, N Bruchovsky, P Rennie, E Beraldi, L Sullivan. A metastatic and androgen-sensitive human prostate cancer model using intraprostatic inoculation of LNCaP cells in SCID mice. Cancer Res; 57:1584–1589, 1997.
73. N Sato, ME Gleave, N Bruchovsky, SL Goldenberg, P Rennie, LD Sullivan. Intermittent androgen suppression delays time to non-androgen regulated prostate specific antigen gene expression in the human prostate LNCaP tumour model. J Steroid Biochem Mol Biol; 58:139–146, 1996.
74. LH Klotz, HW Herr, MJ Morse, WF Whitmore, Jr. Intermittent endocrine therapy for advanced prostate cancer. Cancer; 58:2546–2250, 1986.
75. SL Goldenberg, N Bruchovsky, ME Gleave, LD Sullivan, K Akakura. Intermittent androgen suppression in the treatment of prostate cancer: A preliminary report. Urology; 45:839–845, 1995.
76. ME Gleave, N Bruchovsky, SL Goldenberg, P Rennie. Intermittent androgen suppression: Rationale and clinical experience. In: F. Schroeder, ed. Recent Advances in Prostate Cancer and BPH. London: Parthenon Publishing, 1997, pp 109–121.
77. RT Oliver, G Williams, AM Paris, JP Blandy. Intermittent androgen deprivation after PSA-complete response as a strategy to reduce induction of hormone-resistant prostate cancer. Urology; 49:79–82, 1997.
78. CS Higano, W Ellis, K Russell, PH Lange. Intermittent androgen suppression with leuprolide and flutamide for prostate cancer. A pilot study. Urology; 48:800–804, 1996.
79. Grossfeld GD, Small EJ, Carroll PR. Intermittent androgen deprivation for clinically localized prostate cancer: Initial experience. Urology 51(1):137–144, 1998 Jan.
80. G Theyer, S Houb, A Duer, S Ander, I Haberl, U Theyer, G Hamilton. Measurements of tissue polypeptide-specific antigen and prostate-specific antigen in prostate cancer patients under intermittent androgen suppression therapy. Br J Cancer; 75:1515–1518, 1997.
81. SL Goldenberg, M Gleave, D Taylor. Clinical experience with intermittent androgen suppression for prostate cancer: Minimum 3 year follow up. Mol Urol. 3:287–292, 1999.
82. NE Fleshner, J Trachtenberg. Sequential androgen blockade: A biological study in the inhibition of prostatic growth. J Urol; 148:1928–1931, 1992.
83. NE Fleshner, J Trachtenberg. Combination finasteride and flutamide in advanced carcinoma of the prostate: effective therapy with minimal side effects. J Urol; 154:1642–1646, 1995.
84. MT Macfarlane, A Abi-aad, A Stein, J Danella, A Belldegrun, JB deKernion. Neoadjuvant hormonal deprivation in patients with locally advanced prostate cancer. J Urol. 150:132, 1993.
85. JE Oesterling, PE Andrews, VJ Suman, H Zincke, RP Myers. Preoperative androgen deprivation therapy: Artificial lowering of serum prostate specific antigen without downstaging the tumor. J Urol 149:779, 1992.
86. DF Paulson. Neoadjuvant androgen deprivation therapy prior to radical prostatectomy. Contemp Urology 48:539–540, 1996.
87. CC Schulman. Neoadjuvant androgen blockade prior to prostatectomy: A retrospective study and critical review. Prostate 5:9, 1994.

88. WR Fair, A Aprikian, P Sogani, V Reuter, WF Whitmore. The role of neoadjuvant hormonal manipulation in localized prostate cancer. Cancer 71:1031, 1993.
89. F Labrie, L Cusan, JL Gomez, et al. Down-staging of early stage prostate cancer: The first randomized trial of neoadjuvant combination therapy with flutamide and a luteinizing hormone-releasing hormone agonist. Urology 44:29, 1995.
90. MS Soloway, R Sharifi, Z Wajsman, et al. Randomized prospective study comparing radical prostatectomy alone versus radical prostatectomy preceded by androgen blockade in clinical state B2 (T2bN × M0) prostate cancer. J Urol 154:424–428, 1995.
91. SL Goldenberg, LH Klotz, MAS Jewitt. Canadian Urologic Oncolgy Group. Randomized controlled study of neoadjuvant reversible androgen withdrawal therapy with cyproterone acetate in the surgical management of localized prostate cancer. J Urol 156:873–877, 1996.
92. MS Soloway, R Sharifie, Z Wajsman, D McLeod, D Wood, A Puras-Baes, the Lupron Depot Neoadjuvant Study Group. Randomized prospective study: Radical prostatectomy alone vs. radical prostatectomy proceeded by androgen blockade in cT2b prostate cancer. J Urol 157(4):619A, 1997.
93. SL Goldenberg, L Klotz, MJ Bullock, JR Scrigley, S Laplante, Canadian Urologic Oncology Group. Neoadjuvant cyproterone acetate therapy prior to radical prostatectomy reduces tumour burden and margin positivity without altering 6 and 12 month post-treatment PSA: Results of a randomized trial. J Urol 155:399A, 1997.
94. LH Klotz, SL Goldenberg, M Jewett, J Barkin, M Chetner, et al. CUOG randomized trial of neoadjuvant androgen ablation before radical prostatectomy: 36 month post treatment PSA results. Urology. 53(4):757–763, 1999.
95. ME Gleave, JT Hsieh, H-C Wu et al. Serum PSA levels in mice bearing human prostate LNCaP tumors are determined by tumor volume and endocrine and growth factors. Cancer Res 52:1598, 1992.
96. TA Stamey, JN Kabalin, M Ferrari, N Yang. Prostate specific antigen in the diagnosis and treatment of adenocarcinoma of the prostate. IV. Anti-androgen treated patients. J Urol 141:1088, 1989.
97. ME Gleave, SL Goldenberg, EC Jones, N Bruchovsky, LS Sullivan. Long term neoadjuvant hormone therapy prior to radical prostatectomy: Analysis of outcome by preoperative risk factors. Mol Urol 2(3):171–79, 1998.
98. J Sayer, EI Ramirez, AC von Eschenbach. Retrospective review of prostate cancer patients with lymph node metastases. J Urol 147:52A, 1992.
99. CWS Cheng, EJ Bergstralh, H Zincke. Stage D1 prostate cancer. A nonrandomized comparison of conservative treatment options versus radical prostatectomy. Cancer 71:996–1004, 1993.
100. ME Gleave, SE La Bianca, SL Goldenberg, EC Jones, N Bruchovsky, LD Sullivan. Long-term neoadjuvant hormone therapy prior to radical prostatectomy: Evaluation of risk for biochemical recurrence at 5 year follow-up. Urology 56(2):289–294, 2000 Aug. 1.
101. ME Gleave, N Sato, SL Goldenberg, L Stothers, N Bruchovsky, LS Sullivan. Neoadjuvant androgen withdrawal therapy decreases local recurrence rates following tumour excision in the shionogi tumour model. J Urol 157:1727–1730, 1997.

102. S Makela, R Santti, L Salo, JA McLachlan. Phytoestrogens are partial estrogen agonists in the adult male mouse. Environ Health Perspect 103 Suppl 7:123–127, 1995.

103. A Cassidy. Potential tissue selectivity of dietary phytoestrogens anti-estrogens. Curr Opin Lipidol 10(1):47–52, 1999.

104. NE Breslow, CW Chan, G Dhom, et al. Latent carcinoma of prostate at autopsy in seven areas. Int J Cancer 20:680–688, 1977.

105. R Yatani, I Chigusa, K Akazaki, et al. Geographic pathology of latent prostatic cancer. Int J Cancer 29:611–616, 1982.

106. JE Oesterling, SJ Jacobsen, CG Chute, et al. Serum prostate specific antigen in a community based population of healthy men—establishment of age specific reference ranges. JAMA 270:860–864, 1993.

107. JE Oesterling, Y Kumamoto, T Tsukamoto, et al. Serum prostate prostate specific antigen in a community based population of healthy Japanese men: Lower values than for similarly aged white men. Br J Urol 75:347–353, 1995.

108. A Bylund, JX Zhang, A Bergh, JE Damber, A Widmark, et al. Rye bran and soy protein delay growth and increase apoptosis of human LNCaP prostate adenocarcinoma in nude mice. Prostate 42(4):304–314, 2000.

109. J Hempstock, JP Kavanagh, NJ George. Growth inhibition of prostate cell lines in vitro by phyto-oestrogens. Br J Urol 82(4):560–563, 1998.

110. A de la Taille, OR Hayek, R Buttyan, E Bagiella, M Butchardt, et al. Effects of a phytotherapeutic agent, PC-SPES, on prostate cancer: A preliminary investigation on human cells lines and patients. Br J Urol 84:843–844, 1999.

111. T Hsieh, SS Chen, X Wang, JM Wu. Regulation of androgen receptor (AR) and PSA expression by the androgen responsive human prostate LNCaP cells by ethanolic extracts of the chinese herbal preparation, PC-SPES. Biochem Mol Biol Int 42:535–544, 1997.

112. RS DiPaola, H Zhang, GH Lambert, et al. Clinical and biologic activity of an estrogenic herbal combination (PC-SPES) in prostate cancer. N Engl J Med 339:785–791, 1998.

113. A Evans, K Griffiths, MS Morton. Inhibition of 5α-reductase in genital skin fibroblasts and prostatic tissue by dietary lignans and isoflavonoids. J Endocrinol 147:295–302, 1995.

114. E Giovannucci, A Ascherio, EB Rimm, MJ Stampfer, GA Colditz. et al. Intake of carotenoids and retinol in relation to risk of prostate cancer. J Natl Cancer Inst 87(23):1767–1776, 1995.

115. The Alpha-tocopherol, Beta Carotene Cancer Prevention Study Group. The effect of vitamin E and beta carotene on the incidence of lung cancer and other cancers in male smokers. N Engl J Med 330(15):1029–1035, 1994.

116. SK Clinton, C Emenhiser, SJ Schwartz, DG Bostwick, AW Williams, JW Erdman. Cis-trans Lycopene isomers, carotenoids, and retinol in the human prostate. Cancer Epidemiol. Biomarkers Prev 10:823–833, 1996.

117. WM van Weerden, GJ van Steenbrugge, A van Kreuningen, EP Moerings, FH de Jong, FH Schroder. Assessment of the critical level of androgen for growth response of transplantable human prostatic carcinoma (PC-82) in nude mice. J Urol 145(3):631–634, 1991.

118. A Manni, RJ Santeen, AE Boucher, A Lipton, H Harvey, et al. Androgen depletion and repletion as a means of potentiating the effects of cytotoxic chemotherapy in advanced prostate cancer. J Steroid Biochem 27:551–556, 1987.

119. JE Fowler, EF Whitmore. The response of metastatic adenocarcinoma of the prostate to exogenous testosterone. J Urol 126:372–375, 1981.

120. EM Wallace, SD Pye, SR Wild, FCW Wu. Prostate-specific antigen and prostate gland size in men receiving exogenous testosterone for male contraception. Int J Androl 16:35–40, 1993.

121. DS Smith, WJ Catalona. Rate of change in serum PSA levels as a method for prostate cancer detection. J Urol 152:1163–1167, 1994.

15
PSA and Chemotherapy

Andrea Veatch
University of Washington Medical Center and Fred Hutchinson Cancer Research Center, Seattle, Washington

Celestia Higano
University of Washington, Seattle, Washington

I. INTRODUCTION

The use of chemotherapy in prostate cancer is generally limited to those with hormone-refractory disease. Patients with hormone-refractory prostate cancer (HRPC) have a poor prognosis with a median survival of 9–12 months, a figure that has not been ameliorated by chemotherapeutic intervention to date. HRPC is a general term that describes disease in a heterogeneous spectrum of patients including those with asymptomatic biochemical-only disease (rising prostate specific antigen [PSA] levels with no other evidence of disease), asymptomatic metastatic disease, and extensive symptomatic metastatic disease to the bone, soft tissue, or both. In these categories, however, an elevation in PSA is nearly ubiquitous: only 1–3% of patients with HRPC do not have an elevated serum PSA [1].

A. Measurable Disease

The use of PSA as a marker for progression and response to chemotherapy in the setting of HRPC continues to evolve. Traditional phase II clinical trials use standardized response criteria that include complete response (CR), partial response (PR), stable disease (SD) and progressive disease (PD), defined by radiographically measurable lesions. These response criteria are suboptimal for HRPC because only 20% of patients with this diagnosis have bidimensionally measurable disease with visceral or soft tissue metastases [2], which may not be representative of the remaining patients that have primarily bone metastases or a rising PSA.

B. Osseous Disease

The majority of patients with HRPC have metastases to the bone, but blastic skeletal metastases as measured on bone scan are often difficult to quantify and may underestimate tumor response. Serum PSA levels and bone disease do not always correlate. A rising PSA often precedes bone progression by 6–12 months [3]. Dawson documented a significant lag time between normalization of the PSA and resolution of bone scan abnormalities for patients who experienced a complete remission with combined chemohormonal therapy [4]. In three patients, tumor markers became normal after 3 months; however, bone scans became normal only after 13, 24, 38 months.

In a study by Sissons et al., serial bone scans and PSA levels were available in 59 patients with metastatic prostate cancer [5]. In three cases new bone deposits were observed with unchanged serum PSA values, while rising PSA levels preceded new bone scan lesions in 13 patients and paralleled bone scan findings in the remaining 41 cases. The use of bone scans is optimal only for documenting complete response or disease progression; it is often ambiguous in cases of partial response or when PSA decline is discordant with an additional bone scan lesion.

C. Alternative End Points: PSA

For the reasons reviewed above, clinical trials in HRPC warrant alternative criteria for assessment of chemotherapeutic response including the use of the PSA tumor marker as well as other parameters, such as quality of life. Since Ferro first reported a decline in PSA as a marker of response to treatment with high-dosage estrogen therapy in 1989, nearly every citation in the HRPC literature reports serum PSA as a marker of response to therapy [6].

In contrast to androgen ablation therapy for prostate cancer (80%–90% of patients have a significant clinical and biochemical response), patients with HRPC undergoing chemotherapy usually have a less dramatic decline in PSA. Monitoring serum PSA is nevertheless pervasive in clinical practice as a marker of disease response and progression. Treatment decisions are often driven by changes in PSA when no other evidence of progression or response is obtainable. In clinical trials using chemotherapy for HRPC, however, the use of PSA as a primary end point of objective disease response or progression has not been defined consistently and the degree and duration of PSA change considered significant have varied.

In a survey of respected clinicians who treat HRPC, Dawson et al. [7] reported that 94% would alter their clinical management if survival were significantly improved by a specific intervention. Therefore, the validity of a PSA-based model as a surrogate end point in chemotherapy clinical trials necessitates the prospective establishment of a correlation between PSA decline and survival.

Caution and criticism have been raised against the use of PSA as a measure of therapeutic response following chemotherapy for several reasons. First, PSA secretion by the tumor cell may be affected by some therapy independent of cytotoxicity [8–14]. Second, serum PSA may not represent tumor histology and biology in the same manner as it does in earlier stages of disease [15–18]. Third, serum levels of PSA may vary widely in the temporal course of chemotherapy [4]. Fourth, bias may be introduced in favor of PSA responders.

Ideally, however, the use of an accepted and defined decline in PSA as a measure of response in phase II trials, rather than disease progression or survival, would shorten the duration of clinical trials and allow for a more rapid evaluation of potentially effective chemotherapeutic interventions. Validation of PSA as a definitive end point in a phase III study will strengthen the supposition put forth by numerous phase II studies [19–21] and one phase III study [22] that PSA decline correlates with pain improvement [19], reduction in tumor burden in those patients with measurable disease [20], and survival [20–23].

II. EFFECT OF DRUGS ON PSA EXPRESSION IN VITRO

Concerns about the use of serum PSA decline as a measurable end point in chemotherapy trials stem from the concept that agents may modulate PSA expression, production, and secretion by the tumor cell, and do so independent of cytotoxicity. The PSA gene is modified by androgens and/or ligands bound to the androgen receptors [24–26], hence the rationale for continuing androgen deprivation during chemotherapeutic clinical trials. Chemotherapy and other treatments in the hormone-refractory setting may also alter PSA expression so that serum PSA would not accurately reflect tumor response. Awareness of this principle initially developed from the misinterpretation of PSA response following treatment with suramin.

A. Suramin

Suramin is an antitrypanosomal agent that generated enthusiasm as an element in HRPC therapy following early reports of significant biochemical and clinical responses. While the actual antitumor mechanism of suramin is unknown, it is thought to bind to and inhibit several autocrine growth factors and cytokines.

Preclinical studies [8,9] suggested that suramin inhibited in vitro growth of prostate cancer cell lines inconsistently. Specifically, the androgen-independent (AI) prostate cancer cell line PC-3 and the androgen-dependent (AD) cell line LNCaP-FGC were inhibited; whereas DU 145 and C4-2, two AI prostate cancer cell lines, were not inhibited. Furthermore, PSA levels in the media were initially proportional to cell number; however, when suramin was added to the cells, the PSA concentration relative to cell number significantly decreased and PSA mRNA expression per cell decreased. Further evaluation of the effects of suramin on castrated athymic mice revealed that the ratio of PSA to tumor volume in the mice decreased following treatment.

Despite these preclinical data, early clinical studies reported PSA decline as a measure of response. One study [27] reported that while 12% of patients had a >80% PSA decline from baseline PSA (6/50), the measurable disease PR rate was only 4% (1/28) and no response in bone disease was observed. In another study [28], 38 patients with HRPC were treated with suramin and 1 PR among 21 patients with bone scan only disease was reported, a >50% PSA decline was observed in 21 of 38 patients.

B.   Influence of Other Agents on PSA Expression

In vitro dose escalation studies with vinblastine and adriamycin using LNCaP (androgen-dependent) and PC3 (androgen-independent) human prostate cancer cell lines have been reported [29]. Cell number, intracellular PSA concentrations, and secreted PSA levels were determined daily for 4 days. Untreated cells produced a constant secretion of PSA per cell. LNCaP cells treated with adriamycin or vinblastine had an 80% reduction in cell number and a threefold increase in secreted PSA per cell. PC3 cells had a 97% reduction in cell number and the remaining viable cells had suppressed PSA production. The PSA secretion in response to the chemotherapy agents was therefore inconsistent and could potentially obscure the results of clinical trials.

Carboxy amido-triazole (CAI) inhibits non-voltage-gated calcium channels and was evaluated for potential signal transduction-targeted therapy in HRPC [30]. In a dose-dependent manner, CAI reduces PSA production by LNCaP cells in vitro. Other agents have also been shown to influence PSA expression including phenylacetate and phenylbutyrate [31] and retinoic acid, which upregulate PSA expression [13,14]; prednisone; and vitamin [11].

The optimal approach was suggested by the Clinical Pharmacology Branch of the Division of Clinical Sciences at the National Cancer Institute. Chemotherapeutic agents and their influence on tumor cell PSA mRNA expression, protein production, and secretion should be evaluated in vitro prior to the initiation of clinical studies.

III.   APPROACHES TO USING PSA IN HRPC

PSA has been evaluated as a measure of disease response and progression, albeit inconsistently. Although 94% of 35 established investigators in HRPC who were surveyed by Dawson accepted a decrease of PSA as evidence of response [7], the percentage decline of PSA and the defined time points including 4, 8, and 12 weeks following chemotherapy remain controversial. Additional methods of reporting have included pretreatment PSA, free to total PSA and dynamic models of PSA including doubling time and relative velocity average of PSA.

A. Baseline PSA

Reports have been widely inconsistent with regard to the significance of baseline PSA as a univariate predictor of response to chemotherapy. Kelly et al. report that baseline PSA is not related to survival [23]. Smith et al. [20] report a statistically significant improved survival by univariate analysis with a baseline PSA level of 20 ng/ml or less (p = 0.037); however, a multivariate analysis did not confirm this. Another study [21] reports that patients with a baseline PSA greater than 100 had a median survival of 10.6 months, compared with those with a baseline less than 100 whose median survival was 17.1 months. Absolute baseline PSA levels $\geq$ 150 ng/ml correlated significantly with reduced survival in yet a different study [22].

B. Free to Total PSA

Berruti et al. [32] evaluated the free and free to total PSA ratio in 57 patients with HRPC who received chemotherapy. Twenty patients had a PSA response following chemotherapy, of whom 90% had an increased free to total ratio and 10% had a decreased free to total PSA ratio. Patients with an increase in free to total PSA ratio (primarily resulting from a decrease in total PSA) after chemotherapy had greater survival than those with a decrease or no change (19.8 vs. 15.5 months, p < 0.03). The authors concluded that effective cytotoxic chemotherapy reduces the protein-bound PSA fraction.

C. Dynamic Model of PSA

1. PSA Doubling Time

A dynamic model of PSA may be more useful and improve accuracy. Schmid et al. [33] first suggested the use of PSA doubling time (PSA-DT) as a surrogate end point. Initially these investigators followed the PSAdt in 43 untreated prostate cancer patients for 30 months. The PSA increase was exponential (log-linear) and doubling times were faster for those patients with higher stages and grades of disease. This rise allowed for calculation of PSA doubling time according to the following formula:

$$\text{PSA doubling time} = \frac{(\log 2) \times t}{\log (\text{final PSA}) - \log (\text{initial PSA})}$$

where t is the time from the first to the final PSA determination. PSA-DT was then evaluated by the same Swiss investigators [34] as an end point in an unsuccessful study of 30 patients with HRPC treated with oral idarubicin. Patients were given 35 mg idarubicin on days 1 and 8 of each cycle. Assessment was based on response rates, sequential PSA measurements, toxicity, and quality of life. Three patients had stable disease that correlated with stable PSA; however, the remaining patients all had progressive disease. The median PSA-DT was 2.1 months. Quality of life parameters did not improve in any patient. These studies suggest that the influence of therapy on PSA-DT may provide rapid correlation with efficacy.

2. Average Relative Velocity PSA

Using the dynamic PSA approach, investigators in the Cancer and Leukemia Group B (CALGB) have further refined and validated a two-variable model of PSA using the log PSA and average relative velocity (rvaPSA) [35]. This model can be applied at any time point in a patient's course of HRPC. The rvaPSA was calculated with serial measurements of PSA and defined as $(dy/dt)/y$ where y is PSA and t is time. Data was pooled from 148 patients with HRPC enrolled in CALGB 9181, a study in which patients were treated with low-dose (160 mg/d) or high-dose (640 mg/d) megestrol acetate. The dynamics of PSA and survival were analyzed during the follow-up period in a retrospective manner. Although the treatment showed no effect on survival, the log PSA and rvaPSA correlated significantly with survival ($p = 0.0001$ and $p = 0.0008$, respectively). The PSA level and the rvaPSA formed a two-variable model for survival time that is applicable throughout the course of HRPC with or without the use of chemotherapy.

Vollmer et al. further improved upon this model by adding serial measurements of body weight and serum hemoglobin levels, thereby significantly improving the prognostic value of the model [36]. Retrospective analysis of data collected from 348 patients treated with low-dose hydrocortisone with or without mitoxantrone (CALGB 9182) and low-dose or high-dose megestrel (CALGB 9181) were used to validate the model. The four-variable prognostic score at time t is:

$$0.156 \times [\log PSA (t) - \text{mean} \log (PSA)] + 17.2$$
$$\times [rva(t) - \text{mean rva}] - 3.16$$
$$\times [\log (Hb(t)) - \text{mean} \log (Hb)] - 1.69$$
$$\times [\log(wt (t)) - \text{mean} \log(wt)].$$

Cox proportional hazard analysis for this model reveal that serial measurements for these four variables relates to survival time with p values ranging from 1.2×10^{-15} to 2.1×10^{-5}. Although this prognostic score warrants prospective evaluation, it appears to be a promising and potentially useful measure of treatment effects in phase II and phase III trials as well as providing a useful clinical aid for management strategies.

IV. PSA CORRELATION WITH TUMOR BURDEN, GRADE, AND STAGE

Correlations among tumor volume, tumor differentiation, stage, and histological grade have only been reported for patients with hormone-naïve disease (see Table 1). These results may not translate to meaningful conclusions for the patients with hormone-refractory disease, however. The relationship between serum PSA and HRPC is variable and as the tumor dedifferentiates, PSA levels become less reliable. The serum PSA for patients who continue androgen ablation while on chemotherapy treatment may have a significantly different meaning from a similar value for a patient not on androgen ablation [34] because the production of PSA per cell falls dramatically when androgens are withdrawn. This relationship is less clear when the tumor becomes androgen-independent and therefore few assumptions can be made in the hormone-refractory setting.

Table 1 Serum PSA Correlation with Clinical Stage, Tumor Burden, and Histological Grade

Reference	No. of patients	Parameter	P value
Stamey [18]	78	Log of tumor volume	<0.001
		Microscopic capsular penetration	NS
		Seminal vesicle invasion	NS
		Invasion of pelvic lymph nodes	NS
		Gleason 4 and 5	NS
Partin [15]	347	Tumor volume	<0.01
	350	Surgical stage	<0.001
	331	Gleason score (inverse correlation)	<0.05
Kleen [38]	945	Stage	<0.002–0.007
		DNA ploidy	<0.002–0.005
		Grade	<0.0001–0.005
Kabalin [37]	350	Tumor volume	<0.0001
		Lymph node metastases	0.005
		Gleason grade 4/5	0.004
		Seminal vesicle invasion	NS
		Capsular penetration	0.015
Stein [16]	14	Gleason score up to 9	Not reported

V. PSA RESPONSE AND SURVIVAL

The most clinically meaningful end point in a clinical trial is survival. Therefore, the validity of a PSA-based model as a surrogate end point in chemotherapy clinical trials necessitates the prospective establishment of a correlation between PSA decline and survival. Multivariate retrospective [21,23] and prospective [20,22] analyses of prognostic variables in men with HRPC treated on phase II studies showed that >50% decline in PSA was associated with prolonged survival.

A. Retrospective Analyses

Kelly et al. evaluated PSA levels in 110 patients with HRPC from seven sequential phase II trials using cytotoxic agents alone or in combination at Memorial–Sloan Kettering Cancer Center to determine the prognostic survival significance of posttreatment PSA decline [23]. The authors evaluated 29 different pre- and posttherapy parameters including a posttherapy decline in PSA of 50%. The landmark method [40] was used to avoid bias between responders and nonresponders. Prior treatment regimens, sites of metastasis (measurable vs. nonmeasurable), and pretreatment baseline PSA were not associated with survival.

     Following chemotherapy in 108 evaluable patients, 93 patients did not and 15 patients did achieve >50% decline in PSA level at a predetermined landmark of 60 days. Median survival (8.6 months vs. not reached) was significantly different for the two groups (p = 0.001) despite similar baseline parameters, Karnofsky performance status (KPS) scores, age, and extent of disease. The median number of days to reach >50% decline was 27. In patients whose PSA declined by >50%, the median duration of maintaining the PSA reduction was 167 days. A delayed response in eight patients that reached >50% decline after the landmark time of 60 days (mean, 115 days) was associated with a median survival of 20.8 months.

     Six variables were predictive of longer survival in a univariate analysis: ≥50% reduction in PSA at 60 days, baseline lactate dehydrogenase (LDH) ≤230 U/L, baseline acid phosphatase ≤0.6 U/L, baseline alkaline phosphatase ≤115 U/L, Karnofsky performance status ≥80%, and baseline hemoglobin <13 g/dl. Multivariate Cox regression identified two factors: >50% decline in PSA and the natural log of the initial LDH as the two most significant factors. A multivariate model was developed using the formula:

$$\ln [RR] = 2.1 (Decl\ 50) + 1.09 [\ln (LDH) - 5.45].$$

Decl 50 is 0 if the patient obtains >50% decline in PSA posttreatment and 1 if the patient does not. With this model, the relative risk of death can be calculated based on these two parameters alone. Using this formula, the death rate for those who did not achieve >50% decline in PSA was eight times higher than those who did achieve >50% decline in PSA 60 days following treatment. A Cox score calculated from the above model was used to form low (Cox risk score <2) and high-risk (Cox score >2.0) categories that had statistically significant (p = 0.0001) median survival rates of 17.1 and 8.1 months.

Validation of this model with an independent data set was performed by analyzing 85 patients with HRPC treated at the Norwegian Radium Hospital. There was a threefold increase in the death rate for those who did not achieve a posttherapy PSA decline of 50% or greater. The model classified patients into two distinct risk categories. Median survivals were 10.8 months for the low-risk and 8.5 months for the high-risk groups, which was significantly different p = 0.01.

Investigators at Memorial–Sloan Kettering again evaluated the relationship between posttherapy decline in serum PSA and survival in 1999 and reviewed data from 254 patients with HRPC treated on 11 clinical trials [21]. Treatment protocols included suramin, rhenium-186 hydroxyethylidene disphosphonate, high-dosage Casodex, 13-*cis*-retinoic acid and interferon alfa, edatrexate, and all-*trans*-retinoic acid. The median PSA was 96, median age was 67 years, and median follow-up was 39 months.

The median survival for 26 of 254 patients (10%) who had >50% decline in PSA at 8 weeks was significantly longer than for those who did not (23.6 months vs. 12.3 months, p = 0.0002). Increased survival was also seen for 32 (13%) patients who achieved >50% reduction in PSA by 12 weeks (25.3 months vs. 13 months, p = 0.0001).

A multivariate analysis showed that elevated LDH was a negative prognostic predictor of survival, while increased age and normal serum hemoglobin levels were predictive of longer survival. Using these three parameters in addition to a >50% decline in PSA following treatment, a prognostic model was developed and the risk of death was validated using an independent data set. Data gathered from 541 patients enrolled on one of two phase III studies were then analyzed and classified into one of three equal categories: high-risk, intermediate-risk, and low-risk. The median survival times for these groups were 23, 17, and 9 months for the low-, intermediate-, and high-risk groups, respectively.

The pretherapy rate of PSA rise was not a predictor of survival, although the absolute baseline PSA value did predict survival. Patients with a baseline PSA greater than 100 had a median survival of 10.6 months compared with those with a baseline less than 100, whose median survival was 17.1 months.

B. Prospective Analyses

To analyze further the use of PSA as a marker of response and predictor of survival in chemotherapy clinical trials, Smith et al. prospectively collected PSA levels from 62 patients enrolled in two sequential phase II trials of estramustine and etoposide [20].

In the first trial, patients were given estramustine 15 mg/kg/daily in four divided doses and oral etoposide 50 mg/m^2 in two divided daily doses on days 1–21 for 3 of every 4 weeks. In the second trial, patients were given estramustine 10 mg/kg daily in three divided doses with a similar etoposide dose schedule as the previous trial.

The PSA level obtained every 4 weeks was compared to the pretreatment baseline as a continuous scale relative change, 50% reduction and 75% reduction. A landmark time of 8 weeks was selected to reduce bias towards responders. Sixty-two of 114 patients enrolled on these studies had baseline, 4 week, and 8 week PSA levels. The remainder of patients did not have PSA data available for one or more time points and therefore were not included in the analysis.

A univariate association of patient parameters and survival from the landmark time point of 4 and 8 weeks were assessed by the log-rank test and examined by Kaplan Meier survival plots. Statistically significant improved survival was associated with four factors: pretreatment performance status (p < 0.0001), >75% reduction in PSA level by 8 weeks (p = 0.0094), and a baseline PSA level of 20 ng/ml or less (p = 0.037). Factors that were not predictors of survival in this analysis included ≥50% reduction in PSA at 4 weeks, >75% reduction of PSA at 4 weeks, the presence of measurable disease, pretreatment alkaline phosphatase, and hemoglobin.

The median survival for patients with >50% reduction in PSA at 8 weeks was 91 weeks compared with 38 weeks for those patients without a 50% decrease at 8 weeks (p = 0.0005). Additionally, those patients with >75% decrease in PSA level at 8 weeks had a significantly longer median survival time than those who did not achieve >75% reduction in PSA: 129 weeks vs. 46 weeks (p = 0.0094). Performance status predicted survival where patients with a PS 0 had a median survival of 121 weeks, PS 1 had a median survival of 42 weeks, and PS ≥ 2 or greater had a median survival of 20 weeks (p < 0.0001).

In contrast to calculations of >50% or >75% reduction in PSA, the best predictor for survival in this series was the actual relative change in PSA level at 8 weeks (p = 0.0583) as a continuous variable. A 50% reduction at 8 weeks may be a more useful clinical measure. To determine the best PSA predictor of survival, the authors constructed a Cox regression multivariable model. Using this model, the relative change in PSA level at 8 weeks, pretreatment hemoglobin, and performance status were the most significant prognostic variables. Patients compared with the same performance status who did not achieve >50% reduction in PSA level at 8 weeks had a 1.79 relative risk of death compared with patients with >50% decline in PSA decrease. Furthermore, the >50% decrease in PSA is associated with improved survival independent of performance status and hemoglobin level.

In conclusion, >50% reduction in PSA 8 weeks after initiation of treatment was associated with increased survival and is a better predictor of survival than >50% at 4 weeks and >75% at 4 or 8 weeks. This analysis, however, was not confirmed using an independent data set.

VI. USE OF PSA AS THE PRIMARY END POINT IN CHEMOTHERAPY TRIALS

A. Three Studies from Memorial–Sloan Kettering

In 1990, a phase II study using trimetrexate in HRPC studied the utility of PSA rise or decline following therapy as a marker of tumor progression or response [41]. Trimetrexate is a folate analog initially used as an antimalarial agent and works by inhibiting dihydrofolate reductase and thymidylate synthase and by preventing thymidylate biosynthesis. Five patients achieved a partial remission based on measurable disease response. Serial PSA levels were available for 20 patients, of whom 19 had an abnormal baseline. A correlation between the PSA and measurable disease response was seen in 68% (13/19) of patients. A 50% increase from the patient's minimum value of PSA correlated with disease progression in 90% of cases. A PSA increase by 50% or more from a baseline value on three determinations predated measurable disease progression.

Along the same theme, Schultz reported PSA decline as the primary end point in a phase II study of edatrexate (a synthetic antifolate derivative of aminopterin) in 14 patients with chemotherapy-naïve HRPC [42]. The investigators defined response criteria based on PSA changes. Complete response (CR) was defined as normalization of the PSA for three successive determinations 2 or more weeks apart. Partial response (PR) was defined as a decline in PSA (without normalization) for three successive determinations two or more weeks apart. Stable response was defined as occurring in those patients who did not meet the criteria for PR or progression for at least 90 days. Progression was defined as three consecutive increases in PSA to >50% above the nadir.

The initial intention of the study was to enroll 20 patients. If eight or more PRs were documented using PSA criteria of response, then the agent would be tested in a standard phase II trial of patients with measurable disease. This method ensures that if the PSA response rate is really 20% or lower, there is a probability of less than 5% that the agent would warrant further study on a standard phase II evaluation. One patient had stable disease as measured by <50% decline in PSA for 11 months. One patient was unevaluable. The remaining patients experienced disease progression. Ten patients showed biochemical progression, of whom five had new bone scan lesions. Therefore, in this study, the use of PSA as a marker of response was useful to determine efficiently the lack of activity.

In a third phase II study from Memorial–Sloan Kettering, PSA was used as a clinical trial end point in HRPC assessing the efficacy of estramustine and vinblastine [43]. The study used PSA as a clinical trial end point in HRPC using estramustine and vinblastine with 25 patients, 24 of whom had an elevated PSA at the time of enrollment. Patients were treated with intravenous vinblastine 4 mg/m^2 for 6 consecutive weeks followed by a 2 week rest period. Estramustine 10 mg/kg was administered orally in three divided doses daily for 6 weeks with a 2 week rest period between cycles. Of 25 patients, 13 had >50% decline in

PSA for at least three measurements, 4 of whom (16%) had >80% decline in PSA. Seven patients experienced stabilization of disease and four had disease progression. Of the five patients with bidimensionally measurable disease there were two partial remissions. Unfortunately, this study did not permit a meaningful correlation between measurable disease response and PSA decline. The reduction in PSA could not be correlated with survival due to the low subject number.

B. Kantoff, 1999

A Phase III study [22] compared mitoxantrone and hydrocortisone with hydrocortisone alone by the CALGB in 242 HRPC patients with survival as the primary end point. Patients who achieved a maximum PSA decline ≥50% had a significantly improved (p < 0.001) median survival duration of (20.5 months) vs. those who did not (10.3 months).

VII.   CHEMOTHERAPY IN HRPC: A SUMMARY OF PSA RESPONSES

A.   Estramustine-Based Therapy

Estramustine is a stable conjugate of estradiol and nitrogen mustard that, in addition to effecting castrate levels of testosterone, has antimitotic properties. By binding both tubulin- and microtubule-associated proteins, estramustine induces metaphase arrest by inhibiting microtubule assembly and disassembly. The initial intention of the drug was to facilitate uptake via a steroid receptor, followed by intracellular release of the alkylating agent.

Estramustine has been studied in several trials by the National Prostate Cancer Program (NPCP) and European Organization for Research and Treatment of Cancer (EORTC) as a single agent or in combination with other agents. Single-agent objective response rates have not exceeded 22%. Clinical trials using estramustine in combination with vinblastine, docetaxel, etoposide, and paclitaxel have been more promising, with PSA response rates ranging from 52% to 63% (Table 2).

1.   Estramustine and Vinblastine

In a phase II trial of estramustine and vinblastine [19], 22 of 32 patients had >50% decline in PSA and 22% had >75% decline in PSA. The PSA response correlated closely with pain reduction for a positive predictive value of 85.7%, specificity of 93.7%, and sensitivity of 50%. Of seven patients with bidimensionally measurable nonosseous disease, one had a partial response. Progression-free and overall survival rates for patients with >50% decline in PSA were superior to those without a PSA response (p = 0.027 and p = 0.033, respectively).

Table 2 Estramustine-Based Regimens: Summary of PSA Responses

Estramustine	No. of Patients	>50% PSA decline		#PR/ #measurable disease	Reference
Vinblastine	25	54	13/24	2/5	Seidman [43]
Vinblastine	36	61	22/32	1/7	Hudes [19]
Vinblastine	95	25	22/87	6/30	Hudes [44]
vs. V alone	98	3.2	3/94	2/33	
Etoposide	56	59	30/51	15/33	DiMopoulos [45]
Etoposide	42	52	22/42	9/18	Pienta [46]
Paclitaxel	34	53	17/32	4/9	Hudes [51]
Paclitaxel and carboplatin	26	73	19/26	9/14	Kelly [52]
Docetaxel	17	82	14/17	1/6	Kreis [56]
Docetaxel	34	63	20/32	5/18	Petrylak [57]

Vinblastine is derived from the periwinkle plant and acts primarily on microtubules to cause metaphase arrest. The DU145 HRPC cell line has shown additive cytotoxicity with vinblastine and estramustine in vitro. Based on these preclinical data, and the encouraging phase II studies, a randomized phase III trial of 201 patients with HRPC compared vinblastine (V) to estramustine and vinblastine (EM-V). The primary endpoint was survival. The median survival for the EM-V arm was 11.9 months vs. 9.2 months for the vinblastine alone arm, which suggested, but did not attain, statistical significance (p = 0.08). The time to disease progression was significantly longer (3.7 months vs. 2.2 months) in the EM-V arm (p < 0.0004). A total of 63 patients had bidimensionally measurable soft tissue metastases, 33 treated with V and 30 with EM-V. Partial responses observed in the V arm (6%) vs. in the EM-V arm (20%) were not statistically significant. PSA decline was a secondary endpoint. There was a significantly greater decline in PSA in the EM-V arm that was sustained for at least 3 months (3.2% vs. 25%, p < 0.0001) [44].

2. Estramustine and Etoposide

Estramustine and etoposide have been evaluated in several studies; however, few report a correlation between survival and PSA response. Fifty-six patients were enrolled in a study of oral estramustine and oral etoposide [45]. Of 33 patients with soft tissue disease, 45% had an objective response. Responses occurred at all sites. In all but one patient, measurable disease response was associated with at least a 50% decrease in PSA values. Of 52 patients with osseous disease, 17% had bone scan response and 50% had a stable bone scan. A PSA >50% decline was observed in 59% of patients. The median duration of PSA response was 8 months. The overall median survival was 13 months. Pretreatment PSA did not correlate with survival. The median survival duration of patients who had a >50% PSA decline was 15.7 months vs. 6.9 months in those with less than 50% reduction. None of the patients had clinical disease progression: the PSA response was sustained and all but one patient with measurable response had a PSA response.

In another study [46], 42 patients were treated with etoposide and estramustine. A PSA decline >50% was seen in 52% of patients while 15 (21%) had a >75% decline. There were three complete responses and six partial responses out of the 18 patients with bidimensionally measurable disease. In those 18 men, PSA level decreased by 75% in 5 and 50% in 9 men. In general, a decline in PSA >50% correlated with soft tissue and/or bone scan response; however, two patients with CRs demonstrated only 43% decreases in PSA. Two patients had progressive disease and died and had rapid decline in PSA level. The decreases in PSA did not predict survival. Several patients with a PSA decrease <50% had survival times of longer than 48 weeks.

3. Estramustine and Taxanes

The taxanes inhibit cell proliferation by blocking mitosis, binding to tubulin, and possibly by disrupting microtubule disassembly. The taxanes including paclitaxel and docetaxel have been evaluated extensively in HRPC. Docetaxel is a potent inducer of bcl-2 phosphorylation at nanomolar concentrations whereas paclitaxel requires micromolar concentrations. Bcl-2 phosphorylation abolishes its anti-apoptotic properties [47]. Additionally, docetaxel is twice as efficient as paclitaxel in stabilizing microtubules against cold-induced disassembly [48], and has a slower cellular efflux than paclitaxel thus prolonging the intracellular exposure [49].

Preclinical studies have shown significant antimicrotubule synergy between the taxanes and estramustine in vitro [50]. To evaluate further the estramustine–taxane combination, a phase II trial [51] enrolled 34 patients who received continuous infusion paclitaxel 120–140 mg/m^2 every 3 weeks plus daily oral estramustine. Seven patients had bidimensionally measurable disease of whom three obtained a partial remission. These three patients had a 92%, 71%, and 47% decrease in PSA, respectively. Three patients with stable disease had PSA decreases of 90%, 50%, and 33%. Altogether, 15 of 24 evaluable patients (65%) had >50% decline in PSA and 8 patients had >80% response. At the time of publication, the clinical trial had not reached maturity to report on survival data and therefore was unable to correlate PSA response with survival.

In a promising but toxic phase II study [52], estramustine in combination with carboplatin and paclitaxel showed a PSA >50% decline in 19/26 patients

(73%). Measurable disease regression was seen in 64% (9/14) while 23% (6/26) had a complete normalization of their PSA.

Single-agent paclitaxel has poor activity in HRPC. A study of continuous intravenous infusion (130–170 mg/m2) paclitaxel over 24 hr revealed a partial response rate of 4.3% (1 patient out of 23) [53]. In contrast, docetaxel used as a single agent given every 3 weeks reported >50% PSA decline in 45% and 42% of patients and 28% and 24% objective disease response in two separate studies [54,55].

Results of combination therapy in 17 HRPC patients with estramustine 14 mg/kg/day with dose escalation of docetaxel every 21 days in a dose escalation phase I trial were recently reported [56]. Although efficacy was not the endpoint of this study, 14 patients (82%) had a biochemical response with >50% decline in PSA of 1–11 months' duration. PSA responses were dose-dependent. One of six patients with soft tissue measurable disease had a partial response.

Another study that escalated the dosages of docetaxel from 40 to 80 mg/m^2 on day 2 every 21 days with oral estramustine 280 mg three times daily on days 1–5 in 34 patients with HRPC has been reported [57]. Patients were classified into minimally pretreated (MPT) and extensively pretreated (EPT) subgroups. The overall PSA response >50% reduction rate was 63% (70% for MPT and 50% for EPT). Eight (40%) had a PSA reduction >75% and five patients had normalization of their PSA. Of the 18 patients with bidimensionally measurable disease, 5 had a partial response (27%).

Docetaxel has been incorporated into several schedules including every 3 weeks, daily for 5 days, or as a single 1 hr, 6 hr, or 24 hr infusion. Weekly docetaxel may reduce myelosuppression and nonhematological toxicity, as has been shown in breast cancer [58] while allowing for dose intensification. Trials now underway will further characterize the optimal treatment schedule for docetaxel in HRPC.

B.   Mitoxantrone-Based Therapy

As mentioned previously, responses to cytotoxic chemotherapy in HRPC as measured by traditional endpoints have been both difficult and disappointing. Alternative criteria for assessment have thus been validated including palliative measures such as quality of life, pain, and performance status.

Mitoxantrone is an anthracenedione, a synthetic anthracycline, and does not produce the free radicals thought to be responsible for anthracycline-induced cardiotoxicity.

A large Canadian phase III study [59] randomized 161 symptomatic patients with HRPC to mitoxantrone and prednisone vs. prednisone alone with palliative end points. A preliminary phase II study showed a palliative response in 36% of patients treated with mitoxantrone and prednisone [60]. Palliative responses were seen in 29% of the mitoxantrone and prednisone group vs. 12% of those treated with prednisone alone. Overall survival for the two groups were not significantly different. A decline in PSA of >50% was observed in 22% of patients, treated with prednisone vs. 33% in the arm treated with prednisone and mitoxantrone; however, this was not significantly different. PSA response was not an endpoint of the study. The baseline median PSA was higher in the mitoxantrone and prednisone group (209 vs. 158). PSA was not evaluated consistently among patients: only 134 patients had available measurements at the time of study entry while 111 patients had at least one additional PSA measurement. Despite these limitations, PSA response did correlate with palliative response, but the decline in PSA did not provide useful predictive power for palliative response.

A second phase III study [22] comparing mitoxantrone and hydrocortisone vs. hydrocortisone alone by the CALGB in 242 HRPC patients confirmed the palliative benefits of the Canadian study. Between the two arms, there was no difference in overall survival (12.3 months for M + H vs. 12.6 months for hydrocortisone alone), but the time to disease progression was longer (31 weeks vs. 17 weeks, p = 0.065). Between 28 and 56 days in the combined therapy arm, 19% of patients had >50% decline in PSA vs. 13% of those who received hydrocortisone alone (p = 0.412). A post hoc analysis was performed to analyze maximum PSA decline by arm and found 38% of the M + H arm vs. 22% of the hydrocortisone only arm achieved a maximum serum PSA decline >50%. This analysis, therefore, does not evaluate patients at a predetermined time point allowing for a delayed PSA decline. Partial responses observed in patients with measurable disease occurred in 7% of the M + H group and 4% of the hydrocortisone only group. There were no complete responses and no significant differences in the two groups with respect to measurable disease responses. Some quality of life factors, specifically pain symptoms, were significantly better for the combined therapy group. Absolute baseline PSA levels $\geq$ 150 ng/ml correlated significantly with reduced survival. Also, patients who achieved a maximum PSA decline $\geq$50% had a significantly improved (p < 0.001) median survival duration (20.5 months) vs. those who did not (10.3 months). There was no survival benefit in those patients who achieved >50% decline in PSA compared with those who achieved >80% decline.

VIII. PSA AS A SURROGATE END POINT

The use of percentage decline of serum PSA as a surrogate end point for response following chemotherapy has been argued over for more than a decade. The lack of bidimensionally measurable disease in the majority of patients makes tumor response criteria difficult to evaluate in HRPC.

When comparing survival between PSA responders and PSA nonresponders, bias may be introduced due to the false conclusion that if responders survive significantly longer than nonresponders then the effect of response is to prolong survival. To be labeled a responder, a patient must survive for a certain length of time, thereby introducing selection bias in favor of patients with a more indolent course. These biases are addressed by the use of a landmark analysis [40]. The landmark analysis measures survival at a fixed time (landmark) using patient characteristics known before or at the time of the landmark, thereby reducing bias introduced by length of time during which patient characteristics may change. The landmark analysis has not been consistently applied to clinical trials in HRPC that have used PSA as an end point.

Surrogate end points must demonstrate a statistically significant correlation with other meaningful established end points like survival or palliation. Although measurable tumor response often has little relationship to survival in phase III studies of other malignancies, it is used as a measure of activity in phase II chemotherapy studies. Correlative studies, however, cannot be used as a basis for establishing surrogacy unless the PSA levels are from a randomized study in which a statistically significant difference in arms with respect to the definitive outcome is also reflected in a statistically significant difference in PSA. For these reasons, the US Food and Drug Administration (FDA) has not previously acknowledged PSA as a surrogate marker for prostate cancer response to chemotherapy. Although revised FDA guidelines for the evaluation of cancer therapies for patients with cancer do not specifically mention PSA, the possibility of market approval based on surrogate markers does exist and may be indicated in cases in which postapproval studies establish evidence of patient benefit [62]. Until there are established correlations between patient benefit in terms of other response criteria such as survival, palliation, or prolongation in disease response and this correlates significantly with PSA decline in a prospective randomized Phase III trial, validation of PSA as a surrogate marker remains pending.

IX. CONCLUSION

Scher et al. first suggested the use of postchemotherapy PSA decline as a surrogate marker for response in HRPC [41,43]. The proposal was to use decline in serum PSA as a criterion for activity in a phase II screening trial, thereby rapidly and efficiently assessing preliminary treatment activity by allowing patients with both osseous and soft tissue disease to be included. If the ''PSA trial'' produces a biochemical response (PSA decline of a previously defined percentage at a previously defined time point following therapy), a second, phase II evaluation of treatment efficacy for patients with measurable disease would be undertaken based on traditional measurable disease criteria. Phase III studies would be initiated only if this second phase II evaluation established sufficient promise of efficacy.

Eligibility and response guidelines for phase II clinical trials in HRPC were recently published by the Prostate Specific Antigen Working Group [61]. The panel recommends that PSA be used as an outcome measure to guide further trial development and not as a surrogate marker for survival. The recommendations include that investigators report a PSA decline of 50% that is confirmed 4 weeks or more later and is in reference to a baseline PSA measured within 2 weeks before initiating therapy. If disease progression is demonstrated radiographically concurrent with PSA decline, it is recommended that the PSA decline not be reported.

In summary, caution must be exercised when interpreting PSA response in clinical trials using chemotherapy for several reasons. First, bias may occur in favor of responders when comparing nonresponders to responders for survival. Second, chemotherapeutic agents may alter PSA expression independent of cytotoxicity. Third, PSA expression by androgen-independent tumor cells has not been studied adequately enough that conclusions can be drawn regarding its predictive value for tumor burden, clinical stage, and histological grade. Despite these limitations, PSA is exceptionally feasible tool for clinicians, providing a measurement of tumor activity with minimal intervention. PSA as a method to screen drugs for activity, rather than a surrogate marker for response, is currently the most favorable application.

REFERENCES

1. RJ Cohen, Z Haffejee, GS Steele, SJ Nayler. Advanced prostate cancer with normal serum prostate specific antigen values. Arch Pathol Lab Med 118:1123–26, 1994.
2. WD Figg, K Ammerman, N Patronas. Lack of correlation between prostate specific antigen and the presence of measurable soft tissue metastases in hormone refractory prostate cancer. Cancer Invest 14:513–517, 1996.
3. EH Cooper, TG Armitage, MRG Robinson, DWW Newling, BR Richards, PH Smith, L Denis, R Sylvester. Prostatic specific antigen and the prediction of prognosis in metastatic prostatic cancer. Cancer 66:1025–1028, 1990.
4. NA Dawson, G Wilding, RB Weiss, DG McLeod, WM Linehan, JA Frank, JL Jacob, EP Gelmann. A pilot trial of chemohormonal therapy for metastatic prostate carcinoma. Cancer 69:213–218, 1992.
5. GR Sissons, R Clements, WB Peeling, MD Penney. Can serum prostate-specific antigen replace bone scintigraphy in the follow-up of metastatic prostatic cancer? Br J Radiol 65(778):861–864, 1992.
6. MA Ferro, D Gillatt, MO Symes, PJB Smith. High-dose intravenous estrogentherapy in advanced prostatic carcinoma. Use of prostate specific antigen to monitor response. Urology 34(3):134–138, 1989.

7. NA Dawson. Apples and oranges: Building a consensus for standardized eligibility criteria and end points in prostate cancer clinical trials. J Clin Oncol 16(10):3398–3405, 1998.

8. RV La Rocca, R Danesi, MR Cooper, CA Jamis-Dow, MW Ewing, WM Linhan, CE Myers. Effect of suramin on human prostate cancer cells in vitro. J Urol 145: 393–398, 1991.

9. GN Thalmann, RA Sikes, SM Chang, DA Johnston, AC von Eschenbach, LWK Chung. Suramin-induced decrease in prostate-specific antigen expression with no effect on tumor growth in the LNCaP model of human prostate cancer. J Natl Cancer Inst 88:794–801, 1996.

10. B Seckin, CT Anthony, B Murphy, MS Steiner. Can prostate specific antigen be used as a valid end point to determine the efficacy of chemotherapy for advanced prostate cancer? World J Urol; 14 suppl 1:S26–29, 1996.

11. HI Scher, M Mazumdar, WK Kelly. Clinical trials in relapsed prostate cancer: Defining the target. J Natl Cancer Inst 88:1623–1634, 1996.

12. WJ Wasilenko, AJ Palad, KD Somers. Effect of the calcium influx inhibitor carboxyamido-triazole on the proliferation and invasiveness of human prostate tumor cell lines. Int J Cancer 68:259–264, 1996.

13. DM Peehl, ST Wong, TA Stamey. Vitamin A regulates proliferation and differentiation of human prostatic epithelial cells. Prostate 23:69–78, 1993.

14. R Dahiya, HD Park, J Cusick, RL Vessella, P Narayan. Downregulation of PSA and tumorigenic potential by retinoic acid in prostate cancer cells. Proc Am Assoc Cancer Res 34:ab 1751, 1993.

15. AW Partin, HB Carter, DW Chan, JI Epstein, JE Oesterling, RC Rock, JP Weber, PC Walsh. Prostate specific antigen in the staging of localized prostate cancer: Influence of tumor differentiation, tumor volume and benign hyperplasia. J Urol 143: 747–752, 1990.

16. BS Stein, RO Petersen, S Vangore, AR Kendall. Immunoperoxidase localization of prostate-specific antigen. Am J Surg Pathol 6:553–557, 1982.

17. TF Ford, DN Butcher, JRW Masters, MC Parkinson. Immunocytochemical localization of prostate-specific antigen: Specificity and application to clinical practice. B J Urol 57:50–55, 1985.

18. TA Stamey, N Yang, AR Hay, JE McNeal, FS Freiha, E Redwine. Prostate specific antigen as a serum marker for adenocarcinoma of the prostate. N Engl J Med 317: 909–916, 1987.

19. GR Hudes, R Greenberg, RL Krigel, S Fox, R Scher, S Litwin, P Watts, L Speicher, K Tew, R Comis. Phase II study of estramustine and vinblastine, two microtubule inhibitors, in hormone-refractory prostate cancer. J Clin Oncol 10(11):1754–1761, 1992.

20. DC Smith, RL Dunn, MS Strawderman, KJ Pienta. Change in serum prostate specific antigen as a marker of response to cytotoxic therapy for hormone refractory prostate cancer. J Clin Oncol 16:1835–1843, 1998.

21. HI Scher, WKK Kelly, ZF Zhang, P Ouyang, M Sun, M Schwartz, C Ding, W Wang, ID Horak, AB Kremer. Post-therapy serum prostate specific antigen level and survival in patients with androgen-independent prostate cancer. J Natl Cancer Inst 91:244–251, 1999.

22. PW Kantoff, S Halabi, M Conaway, J Picus, J Kirshner, V Hars, D Trump, EP Winer, NJ Vogelzang. Hydrocortisone with or without mitoxantrone in men with hormone-refractory prostate cancer: Results of the cancer and leukemia group B 9182 study. J Clin Oncol 17:2506–2513, 1999.
23. WK Kelly, HI Scher, M Mazumdar, V Vlamis, M Schwartz, SD Fossa. Prostate specific antigen as a measure of disease outcome in metastatic hormone refractory prostate cancer. J Clin Oncol 11:607–615, 1993.
24. CY Young, BT Montgomery, PE Andrews, SD Qui, DL Bilhartz, DJ Tindall. Hormonal regulation of prostate-specific antigen messenger RNA in human prostatic adenocarcinoma cell line LNCaP. Cancer Res 51(14):3748–3752, 1991.
25. BT Montgomery, CY Young, DL Bilhartz, PE Andrews, JL Prescott, NF Thompson, DJ Tindall. Hormonal regulation of prostate-specific antigen (PSA) glycoprotein in the human prostatic adenocarcinoma cell line, LNCaP. Prostate 21(1):63–73.
26. PH Riegman, RJ Vlietstra, JA van der Korput, AO Brinkmann, J Trapman. The promoter of the prostate specific antigen gene contains a functional androgen responsive element. Mol Endocrinol 5(12):1921–1930, 1991.
27. WK Kelly, HI Scher, M Mazumdar, D Pfister, T Curley, C Leibertz, L Cohen, V Vlamis, A Dnistrian, M Schwartz. Suramin and hydrocortisone: Determining drug efficacy in androgen-independent prostate cancer. J Clin Oncol 13:2214–2222.
28. C Myers, M Cooper, C Stein, R LaRocca, M McClellan, M Walkther, G Weiss, P Choyke, N Dawson, S Steinberg, M Uhrich, J Cassidy, DR Kohler, J Trepel, WM Linehan. Suramin: A novel growth factor antagonist with activity in hormone refractory metastatic prostate cancer. J Clin Oncol 10:881–889, 1992.
29. B Seckin, CT Anthony, B Murphy, MS Steiner. Can prostate specific antigen be used as a valid end point to determine the efficacy of chemotherapy for advanced prostate cancer? World J Urol 14 Suppl 1:S26–29, 1996.
30. WJ Wasilenko, AJ Palad, KD Somers, PF Blackmore, EC Kohn, JS Rhim, GL Wright Jr., and PF Schellhammer. Effects of the calcium influx inhibitor carboxy-amidotrazole on the proliferation and invasiveness of human prostate tumor cell lines. Int J Cancer: 68:259–264, 1996.
31. S Melchior, B Stone, R Santucci, L Brown, L True, J Daniel. Differentiation inducers phenylacetate and phenylbutyrate and their effects in vitro and on the advanced prostate cancer (CaP) xenograft model LUCaP 23.1. Proc Am Assoc Cancer Res 1996; 37:abst 498.
32. A Berrutti, L Dogliotti, G Fasolis, A Mosca, R Tarabuzzi, M Torta, M Mari, D Fontana, A Angeli. Changes in free and free-to-total prostate specific antigen after androgen deprivation or chemotherapy in patients with advanced prostate cancer. J Urol 161 (1):176–181, 1999.
33. HP Schmid JE McNeal, TA Stamey. Clinical observations on the doubling time of prostate cancer. Eur Urol 23 suppl 2:60–63, 1993.
34. HP Schmid, R Maibach, J Bernhard, F Hering, S Hanselmann, H Gusset, R Morant, M Pestalozzi, M Castiglione. A phase II study of oral idarubicin as a treatment for metastatic hormone-refractory prostate carcinoma with special focus on prostate specific antigen doubling time. Cancer 79:1703–1709, 1996.
35. RT Vollmer, NA Dawson, NJ Vogelzang. The dynamics of prostate specific antigen in hormone refractory prostate carcinoma. An analysis of cancer and leukemia group B study 9181 of megestrol acetate. Cancer 83:1989–1994, 1998.

36. RT Vollmer, PW Kantoff, NA Dawson, NJ Vogelzang. A prognostic score for hormone-refractory prostate cancer: Analysis of two cancer and leukemia group B studies. Clin Cancer Res 5:831–837, 1999.

37. JN Kabalin, JE McNeal, IM Johnstone, TA Stamey. Serum prostate-specific antigen and the biologic progression of prostate cancer. Urology 46:65–70, 1995.

38. E Kleer, JJ Larson-Keller, H Zincke, JE Oesterling. Ability of preoperative serum prostate specific antigen value to predict pathologic stage and DNA ploidy. Influence of clinical stage and tumor grade. Urology 41:207–216, 1993.

39. ME Leo, DL Bilhartz, EJ Bergstralh, JE Oesterling. Prostate specific antigen in hormonally treated stage D2 prostate cancer: Is it always an accurate indicator of disease status? J Urol 145, 802–806, 1990.

40. JR Anderson, KC Cain, RD Gelber. Analysis of survival by tumor response. J Clin Oncol 1(11):710–719, 1983.

41. HI Scher, T Curley, N Geller, C Engstrom, DD Dershaw, SY Lin, K Fitzpatrick, J Nisselbaum, M Schwartz, L Bezirdjian, M Eisenberger. Trimetrexate in prostatic cancer: Preliminary observations on the use of prostate-specific antigen and acid phosphatase as a marker in measurable hormone refractory disease. J Clin Oncol 8: 1830–1838, 1990.

42. PK Schultz, WK Kelly, C Begg, C Liebertz, L Cohen, HI Scher. Post-therapy change in prostate specific antigen levels as a clinical trial endpoint in hormone-refractory prostatic cancer: A trial with 10-ethyl-deaza-aminopterin. Urology 44(2):1994.

43. AD Seidman, HI Scher, D Petrylak, DD Dershaw, T Curley. Estramustine and vinblastine: Use of prostate specific antigen as a clinical trial end point for hormone refractory prostatic cancer. J Urol 147:931–934, 1992.

44. G Hudes, L Einhorn, E Ross, A Balsham, P Loehrer, H Ramsey, J Sprandio, M Entmacher, W Dugan, R Ansari, F Monaco, M Hanna, B Roth. Vinblastine versus vinblastine plus oral estramustine phosphate for patients with hormone-refractory prosate cancer: A Hoosier Oncology Group and Fox Chase Network Phase III trial. J Clin Oncol 17:3160–3166, 1999.

45. MA Dimopoulos, C Panopoulos, C Bamia, C Deliveliotis, G Alivizatos, D Pantazopoulos, C Constantiinidis, A Kostakopoulos, I Kastriotis, A Zervas, G Aravantinos, C Dimopoulos. Oral estramustine and oral etoposide for hormone-refractory prostate cancer. Urology 50:754–758, 1997.

46. KJ Pienta, B Redman, M Hussain, G Cummings, PS Esper, C Appel, LE Flaherty. Phase II evaluation of oral estramustine and oral etoposide in hormone refractory adenocarcinoma of the prostate. J Clin Oncol 12(10), 2005–2012, 1994.

47. VT DeVita, S Hellman, SA Rosenberg. Principles and Practice of Oncology. 5th ed. Philadelphia and New York: Lippincott-Raven, 1997, pp. 473–474.

48. JF Diaz, JM Andreu. Assembly of purified GP-tubulin into microtubules induced by taxol and taxotere: Reversibility, ligand stoichiometry, and competition. Biochemistry 32:2747–2755, 1993.

49. JF Riou, C Petitgenet, C Combeau. Cellular uptake and efflux of docetaxel (Taxotere) and paclitaxel (Taxol) in P388 cell line. Proc Am Assoc Cancer Res 35:385, 1994 (#2292).

50. W Kreis, DR Budman, A Calabro. Unique synergism or antagonism of combinations of chemotherapeutic and hormonal agents in human prostate cancer cell lines. Br J Urol 79:196–202, 1997.

51. GR Hudes, F Nathan, C Khater, N Haas, M Cornfield, B Giantonio, R Greenberg, L Gomella, S Litwin, E Ross, S Roethke, C McAleer. Phase II trial of 96-hour paclitaxel plus oral estramustine phosphate in metastatic hormone refractory prostate cancer. J Clin Oncol 15(9):3156–3163, 1997.

52. WK Kelly, P Gaudin, S Slovin, T Curley, J McCaffrey, A Ciolino, G Dalbagni, S Donat, P Scardino, H Scher, P Kantoff, M Smith, W Oh, D Smith, E Small. Paclitaxel (T), estramustine (E), and carboplatin (C) in patients (pts) with advanced prostate cancer (PC). J Urol 177:683, 1999.

53. BJ Roth, BY Yeap, G Wilding, B Kasimis, D McLeod, PJ Loehrer. Taxol in advanced, hormone-refractory carcinoma of the prostate. A phase II study of the Eastern Cooperative Oncology Group. Cancer 72:2457–2460, 1993.

54. D Friedland, J Cohen, R Miller. A phase II trial of taxotere in hormone refractory prostate cancer: Correlation of antitumor activity to phosphorylation of bcl2. Proc Am Soc Clin Oncol 18:322a, 1237, 1999.

55. J Picus, M Schultz, J Cochrane. A phase II trial of docetaxel in patients with hormone refractory prostate cancer (HRPC): Long term results. Proc Am Soc Clin Oncol. 18: 314a, 1206, 1999.

56. W Kreis, DR Budman, J Fetten, AL Gonzales, B Barile and V Vinciguerra. Phase I trial of the combination of daily estramustine phosphate and intermittent docetaxel in patients with metastatic hormone refractory prostate carcinoma. Ann Oncol 10: 33–38, 1999.

57. DP Petrylak, RB Macarthur, J O'Connor, G Shelton, T Judge, J Balog, C Pfaff, E Bagiella, D Heitjan, R Fine, N Zuech, I Sawczuk, M Benson, CA Olsson. Phase I trial of docetaxel with estramustine in androgen-independent prostate cancer. J Clin Oncol 17:958–967, 1999.

58. TM Loeffler, W Freund, C Droge. Activity of weekly Taxotere (TXT) in patients with metastatic breast cancer. Proc ASCO 17:113a, 1998.

59. IF Tannock, D Osoba, MR Stockler, D Scott Ernst, AJ Neville, MJ Moore, GR Armitage, JJ Wilson, PM Venner, CML Coppin, KC Murphy. Chemotherapy with mitoxantrone plus prednisone or prednisone alone for symtomatic hormone-resistant prostate cancer: A Canadian randomized trial with palliative end points. J Clin Oncol 14:1756–1764, 1996.

60. MJ Moore, D Osoba, K Murphy, IF Tannock, A Armitage, B Findlay, C Coppin, A Neville, P Venner, J Wilson. Use of palliative end points to evaluate the effects of mitoxantrone and low dose prednisone in patients with hormonally resistant prostate cancer. J Clin Oncol 12:689–694, 1994.

61. GJ Bubley, M Carducci, W Dahut, N Dawson, D Daliani, M Eisenberger, WD Figg, B Freidlin, S Halabi, G Hudes, M Hussain, R Kaplan, C Myers, W Oh, DP Petrylak, E Reed, B Roth, O Sartor, H Scher, J Simons, V Sinibaldi, EJ Small, MR Smith, DL Trump, R Vollmer, G Wilding. Eligibility and response guidelines for Phase II clinical trials in androgen-independent prostate cancer: Recommendations from the prostate-specific antigen working group. J Clin Oncol 17:3461–3467, 1999.

62. B Clinton, A Gore. Reinventing the Regulation of Cancer Drugs. Washington DC: US Food and Drug Administration, 1996.

16
Human Glandular Kallikrein 2 Protein

George G. Klee
Mayo Foundation, Rochester, Minnesota

Charles Young and Donald Tindall
Mayo Clinic and Mayo Foundation, Rochester, Minnesota

Human glandular kallikrein 2 (hK2) is a homologue of prostate-specific antigen (PSA) with about 80% identity in amino acid sequences [1–4]. HK2 is enzymatically active as a serine protease that can cleave the leader sequence from the precursor form of PSA to make enzymatically active PSA [5]. Like PSA, hK2 exists in multiple forms including complexes with protease inhibitors, precursor forms, and degradation products [3]. The highest concentrations of hK2 are found in prostate tissue and seminal fluid, whereas lower but measurable levels of several forms of hK2 are present in blood. The tissue expressions of hK2 increase progressively from benign to prostatic intraepithelial neoplasia (PIN) to carcinoma as opposed to PSA, which has decreased tissue expression in prostate cancer compared to PIN and benign prostatic hypertrophy [6].

The physiological functions of hK2 and the clinical utility of hK2 measurements are still under investigation. Because of its protease structure, it is logical that hK2 is involved in activation and control of selective proteins. The observation that hK2 can activate PSA raises the intriguing hypothesis that hK2 may be a regulator of PSA activity. However, the metabolic roles of PSA are not well understood, so it is difficult to solve this puzzle.

The clinical utility of hK2 measurements is closely linked to the utility of PSA measurements. The three major uses of PSA measurements all relate to the diagnosis and monitoring of prostate cancer: early detection, monitoring effectiveness of therapy, and monitoring for recurrence. Although PSA is considered to be one of the best clinical tumor markers, there is considerable room for improvement. There is a major overlap in the distribution of PSA concentrations in men with prostate cancer compared to men with benign prostatic diseases and men without prostate disease. This overlap of distribution causes decreased specificity, which leads to an increased number of prostate biopsies in men with borderline elevated values of PSA. Therefore, additional markers would be helpful to add specificity for the early detection of cancer. Also not all men with prostate cancer have elevated PSA levels, so there is an opportunity for developing new markers to improve early disease detection.

A key issue in clinical management of prostate cancer is the prediction of tumor growth rate. Many prostate cancers are indolent and do not cause clinical complications for years or even decades, while other tumors grow aggressively and cause metastasis and death within a few years. PSA concentrations do not correlate well with tumor growth rates. If the more rapidly growing forms of prostate cancer could be identified early, more aggressive treatment could be given to these men, while "watchful waiting" may be more appropriate for patients with slowly advancing disease. Additional markers could be helpful for stratification of prostate cancer patients for prognosis and management.

I. MOLECULAR BIOLOGY

Both PSA and hK2 are members of the human kallikrein family [1–4,15]. The kallikrein proteins are a group of arginine bond-cleaving serine proteases involved in post translational processing of polypeptides to biologically active proteins. The human genome may contain at least five kallikrein genes coding for pancreatic/salivary/renal kallikrein (KLK-1), glandular kallikrein (KLK-2), prostate specific antigen (PSA/KLK-3), prostate/KLK-L1/KLK4, and KLK-L2. According to current nomenclature [11], the pancreatic/salivary/renal kallikrein gene is called hKLK1, while its protein is called hK1; the glandular kallikrein-1 gene is called hKLK2, and its protein hK2; the PSA gene is hKLK3 and its protein hK3 (herein, for the sake of clarity, the more familiar term "PSA" will be retained). The names for protein products of the newest genes, prostase/KLK-L1/KLK4 [17,18] and KLK-L2 [19], remain to be defined. All five of the human kallikrein genes are located as a cluster on chromosome 19q 13.2–13.4 spanning approximate 130 kilobase pairs (Kbp) [9,19]. The hKLK2 gene is located 12 Kbp downstream from the PSA gene in a head to tail orientation, while the hKLK1 gene is located 30 Kbp upstream from the PSA gene in a head to head orientation. Prostase/KLK-L1/KLK4 and KLK-L2 are 25 Kbp downstream of the hKLK2 gene. Their DNA (65–87%) and amino acid (37–78%) sequence homology as well as their similarities in organization (i.e., five exons and four introns) suggest that all five moieties evolved from the same ancestral gene [9,12]. Like PSA, hK2 is prostate specific and androgen regulated [7,14,20]. Unlike its two siblings, hK1 can be found in many tissues but is not expressed in the prostate [8,12], whereas prostase/KLK-L1/KLK4 and KLK-L2 are expressed in many tissues including the prostate [17,18,21].

The hKLK2 gene was first discovered in 1987 by low-stringency hybridization screening of a human liver genomic library using mouse kallikrein (MK-1) as a probe [22]. The complete cDNA was isolated in 1992 [23]. More recently, genes encoding prostase/hK4 [21,24] and TMPRSS2 [25] were reported as androgen regulated.

Androgens, via their nuclear receptors, are the primary transcriptional regulators for expression of hK2 and PSA [26]. Other moieties such as vitamin D3 [27], extracelluar matrix, and growth factors [28,29] may regulate the expression of PSA and/or hK2. A number of growth factors can upregulate PSA expression by activating the androgen receptor in the absence of androgens [30]. Such nonandrogenic stimuli may play a role in continued progression of prostate cancer despite androgen ablation therapy. Our study [31] has recently shown that thyroid hormone can upregulate mRNA transcription for PSA but has no effect on hK2 transcription. DNA sequence analysis of the PSA and hK2 promoter regions has revealed few similarities. In fact, transfection experiments with 5′ deletion constructs of the hK2 and PSA promoters have demonstrated differing transcription capabilities between the two promoters when corresponding areas are compared. Thus, it appears that the differential expression of these two genes, although related, has a genetic basis. In addition, the two also display many differences in primary structure, putative function, enzymatic activity, and regulation of expression.

II. BIOCHEMICAL CHARACTERISTICS

PSA and the deduced sequence of hK2 have substantial homology; however, the sequence of hK2 suggests trypsinlike activity, while PSA is a chymotrypsinlike enzyme. Like PSA, the deduced sequence of hK2 predicts five disulfide bonds. Although PSA has some trypsin-like activity, this may be due to contamination with hK2. Both proteins have conserved active site residues HIS-41, ASP-96, and SER-189, which are common among serine proteases [12]. However, the ASP-183 residue necessary for kallikrein-specific cleavage at basic amino acid residues is conserved in hK2 but not in PSA [22]. A human kininogenase detected in seminal plasma was found to have been secreted by the prostate [32]. This kininogenase activity may be due to hK2. In fact, our study [33] and others [33] showed that hK2 is a kininogenase whereas PSA is not [34]. Note that bradykinin, the enzymatic product of hK2, can modulate many cellular activities of bone cells (both osteoclasts and osteoblasts). In addition, hK2 shows a diversified protease activity on different proteins [28,29,36], which suggests that hK2, like PSA, could play a role in tumor biology and metastasis of prostate cancer.

HK2 has multiple enzymatic actions that appear to be regulated by zinc ions and extracelluar protease inhibitors [35]. HK2 cleaves substrates C-terminal

hK2 Activation of pPSA

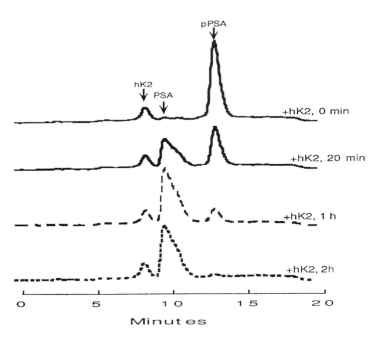

Figure 1 Enzymatic conversion of pPSA to PSA by phK2. The four chromatographs represent time series of baseline, 20 min, 1 hr, and 2 hr, showing the decrease of pPSA and increase of PSA. Data correspond to experiments described in Ref. 5. (Figure provided by Stephen Mikolajiezyk, Hybritech, Beckman Coulter.)

of single or double arginines. HK2 can activate urokinase and effectively cleave fibronectin. Protein C inhibitor (PCI) has high affinity for hK2. The high concentration of PCI in seminal fluid makes it likely that it is a regulator of hK2. The enzymatic activity of hK2 also is reversibly regulated by the concentration of Zn^2 in prostatic fluid.

Similarly to PSA, hK2 can form complexes with $\alpha 1$ antichymotrypsin (ACT) and $\alpha 2$-MG in serum [37–39]. HK2-$\alpha 2$-MG is not recognizable immunologically, whereas hK2-ACT is detectable by hK2-specific antibodies. A PSA-ACT cutoff of 2.52 ng/ml has been shown to have an increased specificity of cancer detection (1). However, hK2–ACT complexes exist in patient serum at relatively low levels. Other studies showed that hK2 can form complexes with protein C inhibitor (PCI) in seminal fluid whereas PSA does not form PSA-PCI

[40]. In addition, PSA forms complexes with alpha(1)-protease inhibitor (API), which can be detected in patient sera [41]. It has been suggested that PSA-API may have potentially clinical use, although this complex makes up only 1–8% of total immunoreactive PSA. Our studies also indicated that hK2, not PSA, forms complexes with protease inhibitor-6 (hK2-PI6) in vivo [42]. The significance of these hK2 complexes in serum remains to be determined.

Both PSA and hK2 are initially produced with a 24 amino acid leader sequence (ppPSA, pphK2), and are proteolytically cleaved into proteins with 7 amino acid leader sequences (pPSA, phK2) with subsequent activation to the mature proteins (PSA, hK2,) [37,38]. hK2 has been shown to catalyze the conversion of pPSA to PSA and autocatalyze the conversion of phK2 to hK2 [39] (see Fig. 1). This observation implicates hK2 in the regulation of these kallikrein enzymes. Our preliminary studies showed that phK2 also may be used for prostate cancer detection. These studies have suggested that serum measurements of hK2 provide information that complements PSA and free PSA in the diagnosis of prostate cancer. However, the utility of phK2 measurements in patients with prostate disease is undefined. The observation that most of the circulating form of hK2 is not bound to protease inhibitors suggests that the circulating form of hK2 is enzymatically inactive. Both phK2 and degradation products of hK2 do not bind to the protease inhibitors, ACT or α2-macroglobulin [39,43]. Saedi et al. [44] reported that phK2 was detected in higher levels in patients with benign prostatic hyperplasia (BPH) and prostate cancer than in normal males and females. It was compelling to develop a highly sensitive phK2 immunoassay to explore the possibility that phK2 could be used as a marker for prostate cancer.

III. TISSUE STUDIES

Darson et al. [6] have shown that hK2 expression correlates better than PSA with the malignant status of prostate tissue. Using immunohistochemical techniques, they evaluated 257 radical prostatectomy specimens. The intensity and extent of the epithelial cytoplasmic immunoreactivity were greater in cancer than high-grade PIN, and greater in high-grade PIN than in benign epithelium (see Fig. 2). In contrast, PSA and PAP staining were most intense in benign tissue and showed lower intensity in PIN and cancer. However, the expression of neither hK2 nor PSA was predictive of cancer recurrence. More recently it was shown that both hK2 and phK2 are expressed in primary prostate cancer tissue and lymph node metastases [45]. The expression of hK2 incrementally increased from benign epithelium to primary cancer to lymph node metastasis, whereas phK2 was expressed to the greatest extent in primary cancer. Therefore, tissue expression of these three markers appears to be regulated independently in benign epithelium, adenocarcinoma, and lymph node metastases.

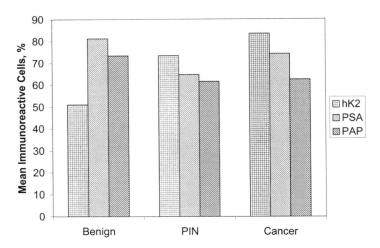

Figure 2   Increase in intensity of hK2 staining in prostate cancer compared to PIN and BPH contrasted with the decreased intensity of PSA and prostate acid phosphates (PAP) staining. (Generated from data in Ref. 6.)

IV.   ANALYTIC ASSAYS FOR hK2 IN SERUM

The concentration of hK2 in serum from normal men is in the low ng/L range; therefore, highly sensitive assays are needed. The concentration of PSA typically is 30–100 times higher than hK2, so hK2 assays also must have very low cross-reactivity with PSA. Immunometric or "sandwich" assays generally have been used to achieve this high sensitivity and high specificity. The key to specificity is the selection of at least one of the paired antibodies with low cross-reactivity with PSA. As an alternative, blocking antibodies that bind to PSA but not hK2 can be used to inhibit the reactivity of PSA in samples.

Both the precursor form (phK2) and complexed forms of hK2 have been found in prostate cancer serum using Western blots. Grauer et al., using a monoclonal antibody that reacts with both free and complexed hK2, developed a method for concentrating hK2 using immunoaffinity enrichment [51]. Western blots with monoclonal antibodies specific for phK2, hK2, and ACT showed that both phK2 and hK2-ACT were present in the serum of a patient with advanced prostate cancer. This documentation of the existence of phK2 and hK2-ACT in circulating blood led to increased interest in sensitive immunoassays to measure these forms of hK2.

Piironen et al. developed an immunofluorometric assay for hK2 using two antibodies that cross-react with both hK2 and PSA [46]. PSA immunoreactivity was blocked by preincubation with a monoclonal antibody specific for PSA, yielding a cross-reactivity of less than 1%. This assay had a detection limit of only 100 ng/L: more than one-half of the male specimens measured were undetectable. They found PSA/hK2 ratios in the range of 10–50. Subsequent improvements in the assay allowed detection down to 10 ng/L [47]. This refined assay has approximately equimolar reactivity, with the hK2-ACT complexed form having only a 6% bias compared to free hK2. Their results show that 81–96% of circulating hK2 is free or noncomplexed. This is in marked contrast to PSA, in which most of the immunoreactive PSA is complexed to ACT.

Finlay et al. developed a sandwich microtiter plate assay using two monoclonal antibodies specific for hK2 [48]. The assay detection limit is 120 ng/L with 0.5% cross-reactivity with PSA. The assay reacts 3.5-fold better with free hK2 than with hK2-ACT. The average values were quite high (370 ng/L for women and 330 ng/L for men). Higher values were found in men with benign prostate hyperplasia and prostate cancer.

We have developed an automated immunometric assay for hK2 with a detection limit of 1.5 ng/L using two monoclonal antibodies against hK2 [47]. Both monoclonal antibodies used in this assay were developed using recombinant hK2 and were selected not to cross-react with PSA. The final assay has cross-reactivities of 0.008% for PSA and 0.0009% for PSA-ACT. This assay predominantly measures free hK2: the molar cross-reactivity with hK2-ACT is only about 3%. However, on a practical basis this assay gives results similar to total hK2 assays because most of the circulating hK2 is not bound to ACT. We found a moderate correlation ($r = 0.55$) between hK2 concentrations and PSA concentrations, with PSA/hK2 ratios between 30 and 80.

Black et al. devised a two-step enzyme-linked immunosorbent assay (ELISA) assay for hK2 using a monoclonal antibody specific for hK2 in combination with an antibody against PSA [50]. This assay has a detection limit of 6 ng/L with a PSA cross-reactivity less than 0.2% at high levels. They also found a small correlation ($r = 0.44$) between hK2 and PSA concentrations. However, they found an average slope of only 2.5 in comparing concentrations of PSA and hK2. Individual subjects had PSA/hK2 ratios ranging from 0.1 to 34. Part of this difference in hK2 levels may be due to the lack of a universal standard for hK2. Prior to the development of a standard for PSA, assays for PSA differed significantly.

Saedi et al. developed a dual monoclonal immunofluorometric assay for phK2 [44]. This assay uses a monoclonal antibody specific for phK2 paired with a monoclonal antibody that reacts with both phK2 and hK2. It has < 0.1% cross-reactivity with hK2, pPSA, and PSA. The analytic sensitivity is about 20 ng/L, with a biological detection limit of 40 ng/L. They found undetectable levels in normal men and women, compared to elevated levels in some men with benign hypertrophy and some men with prostate cancer. Subsequently, we have created a semiautomated assay for phK2 with a detection limit of 2 ng/L, which shows that a substantial portion of circulated hK2 is phK2 (unpublished data).

V. CLINICAL UTILITY OF hK2 MEASUREMENTS

Each of the published studies has shown that serum concentrations of hK2, phK2, and hK2-ACT are elevated in some patients with prostate cancer. However, given the widespread use of PSA and free PSA measurements, the marginal utility from knowing that these markers are elevated is minimal because this information duplicates information provided by PSA measurements. Therefore, much of the focus for clinical research is to identify ways in which hK2 measurements can supplement the PSA and free PSA information.

A major application of PSA measurements is the early identification of prostate cancer. Serum PSA measurement and digital rectal examination (DRE) are typically performed annually in men over 50 years (or younger if there are other risk factors). However, the diagnosis of cancer requires tissue, which usually entails a prostate biopsy. Because of the morbidity and inconveniences associated with biopsy, a risk vs. benefit decision must be made regarding when to proceed with biopsy after obtaining results of the initial screening tests. This is a complex decision that should incorporate the concerns of the patient and his family, but generally it is recommended that men with abnormal DRE and men with PSA concentrations > 10 ng/mL should undergo follow-up prostate biopsy. Men with normal DRE and low PSA concentrations generally are considered to have low risk of prostate cancer and typically are screened annually. The limit for "low" PSA is not well defined, but generally is in the range of 2–8 ng/mL; sometimes age-dependent limits are used. PSA values below 2 ng/mL seldom are pursued, although significant prostate cancer does occur in some men with PSA concentrations this low. In the early detection of prostate cancer there are therefore two major opportunities for using hK2 measurements: identification of men with borderline elevated PSA who have increased risk for prostate cancer for whom prostate biopsy would be recommended; and identification of men with low PSA concentrations who are at increased risk of prostate cancer.

A large clinical study using stored sera from 937 men with histologically confirmed cancer or noncancer diagnoses evaluated the utility of hK2 measurements to complement PSA and free PSA for differentiating cancer from noncancerous disease [52]. The ratio of hK2/free PSA provided additional specificity for cancer detection. Figure 3 illustrates the advantage of this ratio for patients with borderline test values of PSA and percentage free PSA. Overall, there is a 23% chance of cancer when the PSA concentration is 4–10 ng/mL and a 13% chance when it is 2–4 ng/mL. Percentage free PSA can be used to categorize

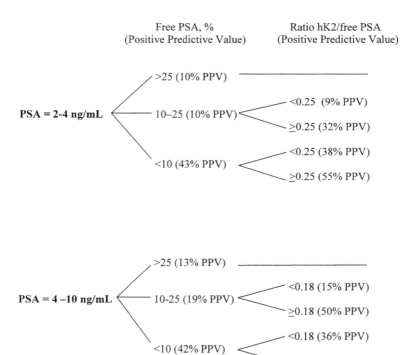

Free PSA, %
(Positive Predictive Value)

Ratio hK2/free PSA
(Positive Predictive Value)

>25 (10% PPV)

PSA = 2-4 ng/mL

10–25 (10% PPV)

<0.25 (9% PPV)

≥0.25 (32% PPV)

<10 (43% PPV)

<0.25 (38% PPV)

≥0.25 (55% PPV)

>25 (13% PPV)

PSA = 4 –10 ng/mL

10-25 (19% PPV)

<0.18 (15% PPV)

≥0.18 (50% PPV)

<10 (42% PPV)

<0.18 (36% PPV)

≥0.18 (62% PPV)

Figure 3 Improved specificity of free PSA and hK2 for detection of prostate cancer. The ratio of hK2/free PSA improves the positive predictive value (PPV) for each category of PSA and free PSA. (Adapted from data in Ref. 50.)

these patients into risk groups that have chances of cancer between 10 and 43%. hK2 measurements can be used subsequently to categorize these patients further into groups that have cancer risks between 9 and 62%. Used together, PSA, free PSA, and hK2 measurements would allow detection of many men with prostate cancer, and require fewer prostate biopsies.

Another study by Kwiatkowski et al. evaluated the utility of hK2 in improving differentiation between prostate cancer and benign hyperplasia for men with PSA values between 4 and 10 ng/mL [26]. The median hK2/free PSA ratio was 0.139 for prostate cancer and 0.075 for BPH. The specificity of this ratio was 60.3% at a 94.4% sensitivity, compared to a specificity of only 27.6% for percentage free PSA.

A third study by Magklara et al. also showed that the hK2/free PSA ratio adds specificity for cancer detection [27]. At 95% specificity, hK2/free PSA ratio identified 25% of patients with prostate cancer.

VI. CONCLUSIONS

Human glandular kallikrein is similar to PSA in many ways, but it has several unique features that may help to identify men at higher risk of prostate cancer. Further studies are needed to define more fully the metabolic roles of hK2, its proforms, and complexed forms. These new markers may help to identify subsets of men with prostate cancer for whom selective treatment regimens may be more beneficial. Many questions remain, but the initial studies are promising and truly worthy of further investigations.

ACKNOWLEDGMENTS

This work was supported in part by grants from Hybritech Inc., NIH (CA70892), and the T.J. Martell Foundation.

REFERENCES

1. CY-F Young, PE Andrews, BT Montgomery, DF Tindall. Tissue-specific and hormonal regulation of human prostatic-specific glandular kallikrein. Biochemistry 31: 818–824, 1992.
2. P Henttu, P Vihko. Prostate-specific antigen and human glandular kallikrein: Two kallikreins of the human prostate. Ann Med 25:157–164, 1994.
3. A Doherty, G Smith, L Banks, T Christmas, RJ Epstein. Correlation of the osteoblastic phenotype with prostate-specific antigen expression in metastatic prostate cancer: Implications for paracrine growth. J Pathol 188(3):278–281, 1999.
4. RT McCormack, HG Rittenhouse, JA Finlay, RL Sokoloff, TJ Wang, RL Wolfert, MD Lilja, JE Oesterling. Molecular forms of prostate-specific antigen and the human kallikrein gene family: A new era. Urology 45:729–744, 1995.
5. A Kumar, SD Mikolajczyk, AS Goel, LS Millar, MS Saedi. Expression of pro form of prostate-specific antigen by mammalian cells and its conversion to mature, active form by human kallikrein 2. Cancer Research 57:3111–3114, 1997.
6. MF Darson, A Pacelli, P Roche, HG Rittenhouse, RL Wolfert, CY Young, GG Klee, DJ Tindall, DG Bostwick. Human glandular kallikrein 2 (hK2) expression in prostatic intraepithelial neoplasia and adenocarcinoma: A novel prostate cancer marker. Urology 49(6):857–862, 1997.
7. HG Rittenhouse, JA Finlay, SD Mikolajczyk, AW Partin. Human kallikrein 2 (hK2)

and prostate-specific antigen (PSA): Two closely related, but distinct, kallikreins in the prostate. Crit Rev Clin Lab Sci 35:275–368, 1998.

8.   PJ Littrup. Prostate cancer screening: Appropriate choice? Cancer 74:2016–2022, 1994.

9.   TA Stamey, N Yang, AR Hay, JE McNeal, FS Freiha, E Redwine. Prostate specific antigen as a serum marker for adenocarcinoma of the prostate. N Engl J Med 317: 909–916, 1987.

10.   H Lilja. Significance of different molecular forms of serum PSA. The free, non-complexed form of PSA versus that complexed to −1 antichymotrypsin. Urol Clin North Am 20:681–686, 1993.

11.   AM Zhou, PC Tewari, TB Bluestein, GW Caldwell, FC Larsen. Multiple forms of prostate-specific antigen in serum: Differences in immunorecognition by monoclonal and polyclonal assays. Clin Chem 39:2483–2491, 1993.

12.   PH Riegman, P Klaassen, JA van der Korput, JC Romijn, J Trapman. Molecular cloning and characterization of novel prostate antigen cDNA's. Biochem Biophys Res Commun 155(1):181–188, 1988.

13.   P Henttu, O Lukkarinen, P Vihko. Expression of the gene coding for human prostate-specific antigen and related hGK-1 in benign and malignant tumors of the human prostate. Int J Cancer 45(4):654–660, 1990.

14.   N Heuze, S Olayat, N Gutman, ML Zani, Y Courty. Molecular cloning and expression of an alternative hKLK3 transcript coding for a variant protein of prostate-specific antigen. Cancer Res 59(12):2820–2824, 1999.

15.   TJ Wang, HJ Linton, HG Rittenhouse, RL Wolfert. Western blotting analysis of antibodies to prostate-specific antigen: Cross-reactivity with human kallikrein-2. Tumor Biol 20(Suppl 1):75–78, 1999.

16.   C Becker, I Wigheden, H Lilja. Characterization of epitope structure for 53 monoclonal antibodies against prostate-specific antigen. Tumor Biol 20(Suppl 1):13–17, 1999.

17.   GM Yousef, CV Obiezu, LY Luo, MH Black, EP Diamandis. Prostase/KLK-L1 is a new member of the human kallikrein gene family, is expressed in prostate and breast tissues, and is hormonally regulated. Cancer Res 59(17):4252–4256, 1999.

18.   SA Stephenson, K Verity, LK Ashworth, JA Clements. Localization of a new prostate-specific antigen-related serine protease gene, KLK4, is evidence for an expanded human kallikrein gene family cluster on chromosome 19q13.3–13.4. J Biol Chem 274(33):23210–23214, 1999.

19.   SD Mikolajczyk, LS Millar, A Kumar, MS Saedi. Prostatic human kallikrein 2 inactivates and complexes with plasminogen activator inhibitor-1. Int J Cancer 81(3): 438–442, 1999.

20.   M Hara, Y Koyangi, T Inou, T Fukuyama. Some physicochemical characteristics of gamma-seminoprotein, an antigenic component for human seminal plasma. Jpn J Legal Med 25:322–324, 1991.

21.   GM Yousef, EP Diamandis. The new kallikrein-like gene, KLK-L2—molecular characterization, mapping, tissue expression, and hormonal regulation. J Biol Chem 274(53):37511–37516, 1999.

22.   I Abdalla, P Ray, V Ray, F Vaida, S Vijayakumar. Comparison of serum prostate-

specific antigen levels and PSA density in African-American, white, and Hispanic men without prostate cancer. Urology 51(2):300–305, 1998.

23. CYF Young, PE Andrews, BT Montgomery, DJ Tindall. Tissue-specific and hormonal regulation of human prostate-specific glandular kallikrein. Biochemistry 31: 818–824, 1992.

24. C Lee, M Keefer, ZW Zhao, R Kroes, L Bey, K Lui, J Sensibar. Demonstration of the role of the prostate-specific antigen in semen liquefaction by two-dimensional electrophoresis. J Androl 10:432–438, 1989.

25. CS Killian, DA Corral, E Kawinski, RI Constantine. Mitogenic response of osteoblast cells to prostate-specific antigen suggests an activation of latent TGF-β and a proteolytic modulation of cell adhesion receptors. Biochem Biophys Res Commun 192:940–947, 1993.

26. MK Kwiatowski, F Recker, T Piironen, K Pettersson, T Otto, M Wernli, R Tscholl. In prostatism patients the ratio of human glandular kallikrein to free PSA improves the discrimination between prostate cancer and benign hyperplasia within the diagnostic ìgray zoneî of total PSA 4 to 10 ng/mL. Urology 52:360–365, 1998.

27. A Magklara, A Scorilas, WJ Catalona, EP Diamandis. The combination of human glandular kallikrein and free prostate-specific antigen (PSA) enhances discrimination between prostate cancer and benign prostatic hyperplasia in patients with moderately increased total PSA. Clin Chem 45:1960–1966, 1999.

28. TO Morgan, SJ Jacobsen, WF McCarthy, DJ Jacobson, DG McLeod, JW Moul. Age-specific reference ranges for serum prostate-specific antigen in black men. N Engl J Med 335:304–310, 1996.

29. JE Oesterling. Age-specific reference ranges for serum PSA. N Engl J Med 335(5): 345–346, 1996.

30. CG Roeluborn, GJ Pickens, JS Sanders. Diagnostic yield of repeated transrectal ultrasound-guided biopsies stratified by specific histopathologic diagnoses and prostate specific antigen levels. Urology 47:347–352, 1996.

31. TA Stamey, N Yang, AR Hay, JE McNeal, FS Freiha, E Redwine. Prostate specific antigen as a serum marker for adenocarcinoma of the prostate. N Engl J Med 317: 909–916, 1987.

32. R Sawyer, JJ Berman, A Borkowski, GW Moore. Elevated prostate-specific antigen levels in black men and white men. Mod Pathol 9(11):1029–1032, 1996.

33. BC Charlesworth, CYF Young, VM Miller, DJ Tindall. Kininogenase activity of prostate-derived human glandular kallikrein (hK2) purified from seminal fluid. J Androl 20:220–229, 1999.

34. EP DeAntoni, ED Crawford, JE Oesterling, CA Ross, ER Berger, DG McLeod, F Staggers, NN Stone. Age- and race-specific reference ranges for prostate-specific antigen from a large community-based study. Urology 48:234–239, 1996.

35. J Lovgren, K Airas, H Lilja. Enzymatic action of human glandular kallikrein 2 (hK2): Substrate specificity and regulation by Zn^2 and extracellular protease inhibitors. Eur J Biochem 262:781–789, 1999.

36. JE Oesterling, SJ Jacobsen, CG Chute, HA Guess, CJ Girman, LA Panser, MM Lieber. Serum prostate-specific antigen in a community-based population of healthy men: Establishment of age-specific reference ranges. JAMA 270(7):860–864, 1993.

37. A Shibata, AS Whittemore, K Imai, LN Kolonel, AH Wu, EM John, TA Stamey, RS Paffenbarger. Serum levels of prostate-specific antigen among Japanese-american and native Japanese men. J Natl Cancer Inst 89(22):1716–1720, 1997.

38. MS Saedi, MM Cass, AS Goel, L Grauer, KL Hogen, T Okaneya, BY Griffin, GG Klee, CY Young, DJ Tindall. Over-expression of a human prostate-specific glandular kallikrein, hK2, in E. coli and generation of antibodies. Mol Cell Endocrinol 109(2):237–241, 1995.

39. MF Darson, A Pacelli, P Roche, HG Rittenhouse, RL Wolfert, MS Saedi, CYF Young, GG Klee, DJ Tindall, DG Bostwick. Human glandular kallikrein 2 expression in prostate adenocarcinoma and lymph node metastasis. Urology 53:939–944, 1999.

40. MC Charlesworth, CYF Young, GG Klee, MS Saedi, SD Mikolajczyk, JA Finlay, DJ Tindall. Detection of a prostate-specific protein, human glandular kallikrein (hK2), in sera of patients with elevated prostate specific antigen levels. Urology 49: 487–493, 1997.

41. GG Klee, MK Goodmanson, SJ Jacobsen, CYF Young, JA Finlay, HG Rittenhouse. RL Wolfert, DJ Tindall. Highly sensitive automated chemiluminometric assay for measuring free human glandular kallikrein-2. Clin Chem 45:800–806, 1999.

42. WJ Catalona, JP Richie, FR Ahmann, MA Hudson, PT Scardino, et al. Comparison of digital rectal examination and serum prostate specific antigen in the early detection of prostate cancer:results of a multicenter clinical trial of 6,630 men. J Urol 151: 1283–1290, 1994.

43. MK Brawer, MP Chetner, J Beatie, DM Buchner, RL Vessella, PH Lange. Screening for prostatic carcinoma with prostate specific antigen. J Urol 147:841–845, 1992.

44. MS Saedi, TM Hill, K Kuus-Reichel, A Kumar, J Payne, SD Mikolajczyk, RL Wolfert, HG Rittenhouse. The precursor form of the human kallikrein 2, a kallikrein homologous to prostate-specific antigen, is present in human sera and is increased in prostate cancer and benign prostatic hyperplasia. Clin Chem 44(10):2115–2119, 1998.

45. MF Darson, A Pacelli, P Roche, HG Rittenhouse, RL Wolfert, MS Saedi, CYF Young, GG Klee, DH Tindall, DG Bostwick. Human glandular kallikrein 2 expression in prostate adenocarcinoma and lymph node metastases. Urology 53(5):939–944, 1999.

46. T Piironen, J Lovgren, M Karp, R Eerola, A Lundwall, B Dowell, T Lovgren, J Lilja, K Pettersson. Immunofluorometric assay for sensitive and specific measurement of human prostatic glandular kallikrein (hK2) in serum. Clin Chem 42:1034–1041, 1996.

47. C Becker, T Piironen, J Kiviniemi, J Lilja, K Pettersson. Sensitive and specific immunodetection of human glandular kallikrein 2 (hK2) in serum. Clin Chem 46(2): 198–206, 2000.

48. JA Finlay, CL Evans, JR Day, JK Payne, SD Mikolajczyk, LS Millar, K Kuus-Reichel, RL Wolfert, HG Rittenhouse. Development of monoclonal antibodies specific for human glandular kallikrein (hK2): Development of a dual antibody immunoassay for hK2 with negligible prostate-specific antigen cross-reactivity. Urology 51: 804–809, 1998.

49. GG Klee, MK Goodmanson, SJ Jacobsen, CYF Young, JA Finlay, HG Rittenhouse,

RL Wolfert, DJ Tindall. Highly sensitive automated chemiluminometric assay for measuring free human glandular kallikrein-2. Clin Chem 45(6):800–806, 1999.

50. MH Black, A Magklara, CV Obiezu, DN Melegos, EP Diamandis. Development of an ultrasensitive immunoassay for human glandular kallikrein with no cross-reactivity from prostate-specific antigen. Clin Chem 45:790–799, 1999.

51. LS Grauer, JA Finlay, SD Mikolajczyk, KD Pusateri, RL Wolfert. Detection of human glandular kallikrein, hK2, as its precursor from and in complex with protease inhibitors in prostate carcinoma serum. J Androl 19(4):407–411, 1998.

52. AW Partin, WJ Catalona, JA Finlay, C Darte, DJ Tindall, CYF Young, GG Klee, DW Chan, HG Rittenhouse, RL Wolfert, DL Woodrum. Use of human glandular kallikrein 2 for the detection of prostate cancer: Preliminary analysis. Urology 54(5): 839–845, 1999.

17
Prostate Specific Membrane Antigen

Eric H. Holmes
*Northwest Biotherapeutics, Inc. and Northwest Hospital,
Seattle, Washington*

Prostatic cancer is the most common cancer in men in the United States, and the second most common cause of death by cancer. Prostate cancer incidence and mortality have declined in recent years, mainly through the benefits of increased screening. Nevertheless, current projections indicate that there will be 180,400 new cases of prostatic cancer diagnosed in the United States in 2000, and 31,900 deaths [1]. Early diagnosis and accurate staging of prostate cancer are critical for effective treatment and management of the disease. Effective treatment options exist for organ-confined disease. However, few useful treatment options exist for metastatic disease and most treatments are directed at palliative care [2]. This is particularly true after androgen ablation therapy has become ineffective and the tumor has become hormone resistant [3,4]. Improvement in this clinical reality requires that new diagnostic and treatment strategies be developed to make optimal use of existing markers and technologies and continue the search for new ones. A potentially clinically useful prostatic marker is prostate specific membrane antigen (PSMA) [5,6]. Although PSMA has been known directly or indirectly since 1987, the most informative applied studies have been conducted in the past 5 or 6 years.

I. PHYSICAL PROPERTIES AND EXPRESSION OF PSMA

PSMA is a 750 amino acid type II transmembrane glycoprotein expressed on the surface of prostatic epithelial cells. The amino acid composition of PSMA indicates a protein molecular weight of approximately 84,000. However, PSMA migrates in a sodium dodecyl sulfate (SDS) gel with an apparent molecular weight of 110–120 kDa, indicating that it is highly glycosylated through use of 10 potential N-linked glycosylation sites in the protein. Analysis of this carbohydrate substitution indicates that *in vivo*-derived forms of PSMA contain N-linked complex type structures with few or no O-linked structures present [7].

PSMA was identified using the monoclonal antibody 7E11.C5 and has been shown to be highly prostate specific [5,8–13]. PSMA expression is increased in association with disease progression and in hormone-refractory tumors [8,14,15]. As described more fully below, weak expression of PSMA has been observed outside the prostate in brain, salivary gland, and small intestine tissues by genetic, immunohistochemical, and protein expression data [5,8–13,16]. Antibody 7E11.C5 immunoreactive protein has been shown to be increased in the serum of prostatic cancer patients with the use of enzyme-linked immunosorbent assay (ELISA) and Western blot tests [17–20].

The PSMA gene spans about 60 kb genomic DNA and consists of 19 exons that have been mapped to chromosome 11p11–p12 [21]. A nonidentical homologous gene exists on chromosome 11q14 [21]. A 1244 nucleotide portion of the 5′ region of the PSMA gene was found to drive the expression of the firefly luciferase reporter gene on prostate but not breast-derived cell lines [21]. This is generally consistent with another report in which the promoter region for PSMA was cloned and shown to promote expression in both prostatic and nonprostatic cell lines. However, increased transcription was not as great in nonprostatic cell lines [22]. No significant effect was seen with either dihydrotestosterone depletion or supplementation upon PSMA-promoted transient expression in LNCaP cells.

Because PSMA is an integral membrane protein (unlike soluble markers such as PSA or hK2), along with its strong tissue restriction to normal and malignant prostatic epithelial cells, it is particularly useful for cell-based diagnostic or therapeutic strategies.

II. TISSUE LOCALIZATION OF PSMA

A. Immunohistochemical Data

PSMA expression as defined by 7E11.C5 antibody staining was examined by Horoszewicz et al. [5] in connection with antibody characterization using immunohistochemical analyses of frozen sections from a variety of normal and malignant human tissues, as well as immunoreactivity to cultured human cell lines. These results indicated nearly complete antibody binding specificity to prostatic tissues or cells: 25/27 tissue specimens from normal and benign prostates as well as prostatic cancer stained positive with 7E11.C5. Immunostaining was restricted to epithieal cells of the prostate and no staining of stromal components was seen

[5]. This report also noted a difference in the staining intensity of normal compared with neoplastic epithelium. Strong staining of prostatic cancer tissues was most often observed; normal and hypertrophic prostatic tissues showed weak to moderate staining. No staining was observed in 26 specimens from 11 different nonprostatic human tumor types. Weak reactivity with 7E11.C5 was seen in 2/14 normal human kidney specimens. This was characterized by weak, poorly defined, diffuse, and uneven staining on the inner surfaces and in the lumen of some of the Henle's loops [5]. This reactivity was reduced by blocking fixed sections with bovine serum albumin (BSA) or gelatin and it was unclear whether this represented truly specific staining. No staining was observed in 108 specimens from 27 other normal human organs. A follow-up study confirmed prostate reactivity of the 7E11.C5 antibody, but also noted weak reactivity with cardiac muscle, proximal kidney tubules, and sweat glands. Positive staining of a subset of skeletal muscle cells was also observed [10].

A subsequent immunohistochemical evaluation of PSMA expression in normal and malignant human tissues was conducted using formalin-fixed, paraffin-embedded tissue specimens [12]. These results were similar to those of earlier studies [5,10]. Staining was observed in normal and hyperplastic prostate glands and in 33/35 primary prostate tumors [12]. Staining was also observed in 7/8 cases of prostatic cancer lymph node metastases and 8/18 bone metastases. Staining of normal human tissues was observed only in kidney tubules, duodenum, and colon. No staining of tissues derived from the nervous system was observed. An interesting finding was that staining of blood vessel endothelial cells restricted to the region of the tumor was observed in 8/17 renal cell carcinomas, 7/13 transitional cell carcinomas, and 3/19 colon tumors. In these cases, no staining of tumor cells themselves was observed [12]. Staining of tumor vascular endothelial cells by anti-PSMA specific antibodies has been confirmed in other studies. Liu et al. reported staining of vascular endothelial cells from a variety of tumors by anti-PSMA specific monoclonal antibodies [23]. Larger follow-up studies utilizing immunohistochemical staining, RT-PCR, and in situ hybridization resulted in the conclusion that PSMA expression was characteristic of tumor-associated neovasculature but was absent in normal vascular endothelia [24,25].

A detailed immunohistochemical analysis of whole-mount prostate specimens after radical prostatectomy has been conducted utilizing 7E11.C5 immunoreactivity [26]. In this study of 184 cases of previously untreated patients with pathological stage T2N0M0 adenocarcinoma at the Mayo Clinic, intense cytoplasmic immunoreactivity for PSMA was observed in all cases [26]. The number of cells staining was lower in the benign epithelium (mean, 69.5%) and prostatic intraepithelial neoplasia (PIN) (mean, 77.9%) than in adenocarcinoma (mean, 80.2%). Basal cells were stained only rarely and no staining was observed in stroma, urothelium, or vasculature. Adenocarcinomas were most intensely stained and the highest-grade cancers showed staining of almost every cell. There was greater staining heterogeneity of lower-grade cancers. In contrast, immunoreactivity with antibodies specific for PSA decreased from benign epithelium (mean, 81.2%) to PIN (mean, 64.8%) or adenocarcinoma (mean, 74.2%) [26].

A complementary study was conducted by these investigators involving 232 previously untreated patients with lymph node-positive prostatic adenocarcinoma who underwent bilateral pelvic lymphadenectomy and radical retropubic prostatectomy at the Mayo Clinic [27]. Immunohistochemical analysis using antibody 7E11.C5 was conducted on associated benign prostate tissue, the prostatic adenocarcinoma, and the lymph node metastases. Cytoplasmic immunoreactivity for PSMA was observed in all cases of benign epithelium or cancer, and in 98% of the lymph node metastases. The number of cells stained was lowest in benign epithelium (mean, 46.2%), increased in both cancer (mean, 79.3%) and in the lymph node metastases (mean 76.4%). Intensity of staining was greatest in the primary cancer and lowest in the lymph node metastases [27]. Despite other studies showing staining of tumor vascular endothelium [12,23], both of these studies at the Mayo Clinic reported no staining of prostatic tumor capillary endothelial cells [26,27].

A recent immunohistochemical study utilizing a different anti-PSMA monoclonal antibody, PM2J004.5, indicated that it reacted with a significantly greater percentage of prostatic cells in benign epithelium and prostatic cancer with greater staining intensity than did the 7E11.C5 antibody [15]. Studies have indicated that the 7E11.C5 antibody is specific for a linear protein sequence epitope composed of the first six amino acids from the N-terminal of PSMA, which is distributed on the cytoplasmic side of the membrane [28]. This epitope is a very short distance to the membrane-spanning region of the protein [6]. The PM2J004.5 antibody also binds to an epitope expressed on the intracellular portion of PSMA [29]. Other anti-PSMA antibodies specific for extracellular epitopes have been shown to provide even higher staining intensity than observed with either 7E11.C5 or PM2J004.5 [29]. Thus, it is likely that antibodies specific for less cryptic epitopes on PSMA may generally provide improved performance compared to 7E11.C5 or PM2J004.5 in both diagnostic and therapeutic applications, particularly wherein interaction with viable cells is critical.

B. Ribonuclease Protection Assay Data

PSMA expression in human tissues as defined by ribonuclease protection assays in an evaluation of prostate tissue and 11 other human-derived tissue types indicated that PSMA expression was overwhelmingly restricted to the prostate [14]. Only weak evidence for extraprostatic expression of PSMA mRNA was observed in human brain and salivary tissues. In particular, no PSMA mRNA expression was detected in kidney, supporting the observation of Horoszewicz et al. [5] that their observed immunoreactivity with kidney may be nonspecific.

C. Western Blot Data

An initial Western blot analysis of the 7E11.C5 immunoreactive protein demonstrated the presence of a 100 kDa protein band present in cultured LNCaP cells, LNCaP xenografts, normal prostatic tissue, benign prostate hyperplasia (BPH), prostatic carcinomas, and normal seminal plasma [30]. Other broader Western blot studies of PSMA expression using the 7E11.C5 antibody have been conducted with tissue extracts derived from 12 normal, benign, and malignant prostatic tissues, as well as seminal fluid. These results were compared to analyses of 11 other nonprostatic human tissue types [9]. These results yielded very similar conclusions, indicating high prostate specificity of PSMA. For example, staining of a 100–120 kDa protein band corresponding to PSMA from prostatic tissues was observed that was not detected in the majority of nonprostatic tissues that were examined. Low but significant staining in brain, salivary gland, and small intestine was observed [9].

D. ELISA Data

A dual antibody sandwich ELISA has been developed and used to test the expression of PSMA at a protein level in normal and malignant human tissues [16]. Very high levels of PSMA were found to be present in normal and malignant prostatic tissues. Low levels of PSMA were observed in membranes from ovary and breast. Negligible levels (200–500-fold lower than found in prostatic tissues) were found in membranes from skin, liver, large and small intestine, and kidney. Thus, at a protein level, quantitation by sandwich ELISA indicates PSMA to be overwhelmingly prostate specific.

E. Expression of PSM'

An mRNA coding for a truncated form of the PSMA gene, termed PSM', has been identified [31]. The coding sequence for PSM' is missing the first 57 amino acids from the N-terminal of PSMA through use of an alternate initiation site. Results indicate that the PSM' mRNA may predominate in normal prostatic tissues, whereas full-length PSMA is higher in prostatic cancers [31]. PSM' was first identified at a protein level by Western blotting with a monoclonal antibody specific for an extracellular epitope [32]. Subsequently, PSM' was purified by immunoaffinity chromatography from LNCaP cells and shown by amino acid sequence analysis to be composed of amino acids 60–750 [33]. The difference from the expected aa 58–750 structure may be due to a tryptic-like cleavage at Lys[59].

III. ENZYMATIC ACTIVITIES OF PSMA

PSMA has been reported to have carboxypeptidase activity by virtue of its N-acetylated α-linked dipeptidase (NAALADase) and folate hydrolase activity [34–36]. NAALADase cleaves the neuropeptide N-acetylaspartylglutamate to yield N-acetylaspartate and glutamate and has been cloned from a rat brain cDNA library [34]. Studies of the enzyme activity of brain NAALADase and PSMA indicate that they are remarkably similar, although the V_{max} for PSMA was lower than for the brain enzyme [35]. Folate hydrolase is localized in brush border membranes of proximal small intestine and functions in cleaving glutamate residues from folate [36]. The apparent low level of expression of PSMA in brain, salivary glands, and small intestine is most probably related to these biochemical activities. Based on expression data at both the mRNA and protein levels, PSMA is clearly expressed at much higher levels in prostatic epithelial cells. However, despite these observations, the specific biochemical function of PSMA in prostatic tissues is presently not determined.

Overall, these results indicate that PSMA is a highly prostate-restricted epithelial cell marker. Its membrane-bound character and increased expression with disease progression make it a particularly attractive marker for histological prognostic evaluation.

IV. ProstaScint SCANS

Primary extraprostatic spread or failure after prostate cancer treatment can occur locally at the prostatic fossa and/or metastasize to regional and/or distant lymphatics and/or bone [37]. Noninvasive diagnostic tools such as computed tomography (CT) or magnetic resonance imaging (MRI) are sensitive to the size of lymph nodes but cannot detect the presence of prostatic cancer cells [38]. One means to target lymph node metastases directly is the ^{111}In-labeled murine IgG_1 monoclonal antibody 7E11.C5 (ProstaScint) scan [39,40]. This immunoscintigraphic scan recognizes PSMA expression chiefly in lymph nodes and the prostate bed [41].

Multiple investigators have studied the sensitivity and specificity of the ProstaScint scan in patients with prostate cancer who underwent conventional CT or MRI scanning, surgical or needle biopsies, or show rising serum PSA after radical prostatectomy [41–52]. Table 1 illustrates the results from 637 ProstaScint scans in detecting primary or recurrent prostate cancer that spread locally or to

Table 1 Comparative Analysis of Results of ProstaScint Scan Studies

Reference	No. patients	Sensitivity (%)	Overall specificity (%)	PPV (%)	NPV (%)	AUC	Accuracy (%)
Babian [43]	19	44	86	50	83	NA	76
Hinkle [50]	51	75	86	79	NA	NA	81
Chengazi [49]	35	92	NA	NA	NA	NA	NA
Haseman [44]	14	86	43	60	75	NA	NA
Khan [42]	27	94	36	NA	NA	NA	NA
Polascik [48]	198	62	80	66	76	0.71	NA
Ulchaker [45]	38	55	NA	NA	NA	NA	NA
Elgamal [51]	100	89	67	89	NA	NA	89
Manyak [52]	152	62	72	62	72	NA	NA
Pooled results	637	73.2	67.1	67.7	76.5	0.71	82

AUC, area under receiver operator characteristic curves; NA, not available; NPV, negative predictive value; PPV, positive predictive value.

the lymph nodes. In these pooled results, ProstaScint had a sensitivity of 73% and an accuracy of 82%. In contrast, the sensitivity of conventional CT scanning ranges from about 4 to 15% in these patient groups [38,46,52], similar to the 15% sensitivity reported for MRI [52]. The ProstaScint scan may be superior to positron emission tomography (PET) scans for identifying recurrent disease in the prostate [44]. The ProstaScint scan is also useful in determining, prior to treatment, whether prostate cancer will recur or has spread to other parts of the body [47,48]. Khan et al. have reported that salvage radiotherapy was more likely to lead to a durable complete PSA response in men with prostate cancer who had failed to respond to radical prostatectomy and had a negative ProstaScint scan outside the pelvis compared with those who had a positive scan [47]. ProstaScint was more predictable than prognostic tables in predicting lymph node involvement prior to lymphadenectomy in 198 prostate cancer patients with clinical stage T2–T4 [48]. In this study, the area under the receiver operating characteristic curve was 0.71 and 0.60; the positive predictive value was 66% and 46%, respectively. Repeat ProstaScint scans in patients have shown that the initial and consecutive scans were consistent in 79% of patients, whereas in 21% there were skip metastases [53]. In this series 24/100 patients showed progression by both scan and PSA, 10/100 showed progression by scan alone, 49/100 showed no change, and 17/100 showed a remission related to adjuvant therapy.

Although ProstaScint has been shown to increase the detection of early disease spread in patients with prostatic cancer, recognition of metastatic tumor sites can be difficult, especially if the involved nodes are near blood vessels.

One means to address this has been a dual isotope method involving a single simultaneous ^{111}In-MAb and Tc-99m red blood cell (RBC) SPECT acquisition of the pelvis and abdomen 5 days after injection [54]. The Tc-99m RBC vascular component is subtracted from the ^{111}In-MAb component for easier identification of metastatic sites. This method resulted in increased information for staging primary and recurrent prostatic cancer compared with standard imaging procedures. Another report utilized a prostate to muscle ratio (P/M ratio) in evaluating results of ProstaScint scans among postprostatectomy/radiation therapy patients [55]. A P/M ratio above 3.0 correlated with the majority of positive biopsy regions, whereas a P/M ratio below 3.0 was found in negative biopsy cases.

Although no staging modality has been ideal in the diagnosis of local recurrence or regional or distant soft lymph node metastases of prostate cancer, ProstaScint has contributed to diagnosis and has complemented and often exceeded the diagnostic ability of conventional modalities [38,41–52,56–58]. Given the epitope specificity of the 7E11.C5 monoclonal antibody used in the ProstaScint scan (see below and [28]), it is likely that a superior scan with enhanced sensitivity would be possible through use of an alternative monoclonal antibody specific for an epitope within the extracellular domain of PSMA.

V. PSMA-SPECIFIC MONOCLONAL ANTIBODIES

Initial identification and characterization of PSMA relied on the use of the 7E11.C5 antibody developed by Horoscewicz et al. [5]. As discussed previously, the binding epitope for this antibody is composed of the first six amino acids from the PSMA N-terminal [28]. This places the epitope on the cytoplasmic side of the plasma membrane in an isolated environment in live prostatic epithelial cells. These physical restrictions severely limit the potential of this antibody for *in vivo* diagnostic or therapeutic applications. To obtain optimal diagnostic and therapeutic use of PSMA as a target antigen, new antibodies needed to be developed that are specific for extracellular epitopes in the PSMA molecule.

The first such antibody was prepared by immunization of mice with a peptide segment from the C-terminal portion of the protein [32]. Subsequently, a significant number of additional antibodies have been produced by multiple investigators. These are specific for extracellular protein epitopes [23,24,59–62]. Anti-PSMA antibodies that have been developed can be grouped into two general categories: those specific for linear amino acid epitopes such as 7E11.C5 and those specific for protein conformational epitopes. Such conformational epitopes arise when amino acids from differing parts of the protein come together in three-dimensional space. In contrast to linear sequence epitope antibodies, conformational antibodies have the property of binding only to PSMA in a native conformation [61,62]. These antibodies do not recognize denatured PSMA. Related to this property is their strong ability to bind to PSMA expressed on live cells. Comparative analyses of live cell binding with linear vs. conformational epitope antibodies uniformly demonstrates that antibodies specific for conformational protein epitopes are much more efficient in binding live prostatic cells [61,62]. This is an ideal property for clinical diagnostic and therapeutic applications in which viable cancer cells are targeted directly without the need to rely on a by-stander effect.

Clinical applications involving second-generation antibodies specific for extracellular epitopes on PSMA are beginning to be explored. Initial work has focused on the murine J591 antibody [23] and its humanized counterpart huJ591 [63]. This antibody is specific for a linear sequence epitope present in the extracellular domain of PSMA [23,63]. Results from a phase I biodistribution trial indicate selective localization to bone or soft tissue disease with no localization to sites other than prostatic cancer sites using the murine J591 antibody [64]. Of 21 evaluable patients, 18/21 had positive bone scans. Of these, 14/18 demonstrated antibody localization to tumor. In this group, 5/21 had soft tissue disease by CT scanning, and 4/5 showed antibody localization to soft tissue. Initial clinical studies were reported to be underway utilizing the humanized J591 antibody.

A panel of fully human monoclonal antibodies highly specific for the extracellular domain of PSMA have been developed [62]. Five of six of these antibodies, all human IgG$_1$, bind to protein conformational epitopes and demonstrate high-affinity binding to live prostatic cancer cells *in vitro*. Figure 1 shows a flow cytometric analysis of human anti-PSMA monoclonal antibodies demonstrating strong binding to live LNCaP cells. The combination of a highly tissue/tumor-specific integral membrane protein target and specific human monoclonal antibodies that optimally bind to antigen expressed on the extracellular surface of live cells are ideal for therapeutic antibody strategies. Major issues to consider with respect to both humanized and fully human therapeutic monoclonal antibodies involve evaluation of the antibody with optimal *in vivo* performance characteristics including clearance rates of a given antibody, extent to which they may elicit a humoral response in patients, and efficiency of tumor localization [65,66]. The availability of multiple potential targeting antibodies is significant and likely will yield one or more candidates whose properties are optimal for *in vivo* diagnostic and/or therapeutic applications.

VI. CLINICAL APPLICATION OF PSMA RT-PCR

RT-PCR detection of circulating prostatic cancer cells in patients with occult micrometastatic cancer in nonprostatic sites has been studied by numerous investigators using PSMA, as well as PSA and hK2, as molecular targets. A careful review of this approach has recently been published [67]. The goal of this ap-

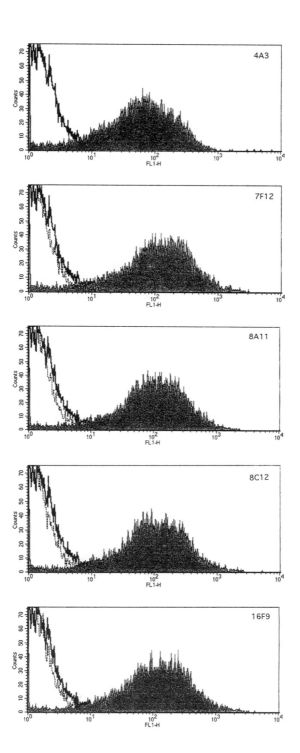

proach is to improve current staging modalities for diagnostic and prognostic purposes. RNA is isolated from cells derived from patient peripheral blood, bone marrow, or lymph nodes and amplified using gene-specific primers either directly or in a more sensitive "nested" PCR protocol. PCR results are most often visualized after gel electrophoresis and ethidium bromide staining. The high sensitivity of RT-PCR detection is both its greatest strength and weakness. RT-PCR is capable of detecting one prostatic cell in 5–10 ml peripheral blood [68–71]. Consequently, technical variations, sampling error, and sample handling are among the most significant hurdles to overcome in assessing its potential and comparing results between investigators.

A major goal of the use of RT-PCR for molecular staging of prostate cancer is to establish a test in which patients with pT2 disease is RT-PCR assay-negative, while patients with advanced disease (pT3) are positive. This result requires that the assay have a low incidence of false-positive results and also will identify a high percentage of patients with known metastatic disease. Numerous studies have been conducted (reviewed in [67]) defining the rate of false-positive results in cancer-free men. Although exceptions exist, most studies predict a false-positive rate of about 1% in PSMA RT-PCR. Among individuals with known metastatic disease, overall clinical sensitivity of PSMA RT-PCR is 70%; however, this varies from 39% to 91% between laboratories [67]. The basis for this range in variation is unknown and may relate to lab-to-lab technical differences.

Ultimately, the question is whether the assay can be used productively to help stage organ-confined cancer preoperatively. The proposition is that circulating prostatic cells would not be present in patients with clinically organ confined cancer. Positive RT-PCR evidence would point to the existence of circulating occult micrometastases from more advanced disease. A study by Okegawa et al. [72] utilizing peripheral blood from patients demonstrated that PSMA RT-PCR could preoperatively differentiate organ-confined disease from extraprostatic disease. Combined data from PSA and PSMA RT-PCR have also been shown to correlate with pathological stage with a sensitivity of 67% and a specificity of 91% in predicting extracapsular disease [73]. Despite these successes, most other reports failed to detect statistically significant correlations [67].

Variations in tissue sources or markers for RT-PCR may be important. For example, PSA RT-PCR analyses of bone marrow aspirates show promise in correlating with pathological stage [74,75], and freedom from biochemical failure

---

Figure 1 Flow cytometric analysis of PSMA-specific HuMab binding to LNCaP and PC3 cells. Closed histogram, binding to LNCaP cells; dotted line histogram, Binding to PC3 cells; solid line histogram, irrelevant human IgG$_1$ binding to LNCaP cells. The antibody designation is indicated in each panel.

[74]. RT-PCR of RNA from lymph node tissue may also be useful to detect micrometastatic spread that cannot be detected by pathological examination. In a small study using PSA RT-PCR on lymph node tissue, Deguchi et al. [76] demonstrated that all lymph nodes tested with histologically proven micrometastases were RT-PCR-positive. In a retrospective study using nodes from cancer patients that were histologically negative, 16/57 (44%) were positive, 14/16 (89%) of which failed biochemically after 5 years [77]. Similar differences in incidence of RT-PCR-positive tests among pathologically normal lymph nodes have been reported in prospective studies. However, long-term follow-up will be required to determine if positive RT-PCR results correlate with metastases [78]. RT-PCR studies of lymph nodes from stage T2 prostate cancer patients indicated that 2/18 (11%) with stage pT2a and 5/20 (25%) with stage pT2b cancer were positive. All seven patients with RT-PCR positive lymph nodes had biochemical recurrence after radical prostatectomy [79]. Further work involving a larger number of patients with a longer follow-up period is needed.

Regardless of whether RT-PCR is conducted using PSMA, PSA, or hK2 as the marker, current methodology is not adequate to detect all of those with metastases [67]. It is also apparent that for patients with early disease, the proportion with an RT-PCR-positive signal is higher than the number who will actually progress. Thus, a positive RT-PCR signal may not imply occult micrometastases in patients during the early disease stage. Likewise, among patients with known metastases, sensitivity is currently lacking and a substantial portion of these metastases are not discovered by current protocols. The answer is likely not to be increased analytical sensitivity but rather improved protocols to address these problems.

One means potentially to improve detection sensitivity and specificity involves enrichment of circulating epithelial cells in peripheral blood using magnetic immunobeads, followed by RNA isolation and PSMA RT-PCR. In a study of prostatic cancer patients with metastatic and nonmetastatic disease, 11/25 (44%) of patients with metastatic disease and 1/21 (5%) with nonmetastatic disease were positive [80]. Among patients with metastatic disease, 10/13 (77%) patients in clinical progression were positive, compared with 1/12 (8%) patients with responding or stable disease who were positive. There was a correlation with PSMA PCR positivity and high serum PSA levels. No control subjects without prostatic cancer tested positive in this study. These data suggest that improvements in assay protocols may allow more reliable clinical assessments to be made.

VII. ANALYSIS OF THE OCCURRENCE OF PROSTATIC CELLS IN BODILY FLUIDS BY FLOW CYTOMETRY

Another means to monitor enrichment of prostatic cells in bodily fluid specimens involves application of cell fractionation and/or flow cytometry. This methodology would be applicable to complex cellular mixtures such as semen or blood. The first step is to isolate or label total epithelial cell populations using, for example, immunomagnetic beads or fluorescent antibodies to a panepithelial cell marker such as cytokeratin 8/18 [81]. In a second step utilizing a different fluorescently labeled antibody to a prostatic cell membrane marker such as PSMA, the prostatic cell fraction present in the total epithelial cell population can be identified and quantitated. In a flow cytometric analysis of prostatic cells in semen from prostatic cancer patients, a clear difference in the ratio of PSMA:cytokeratin 8/18-expressing cells was found between patients with prostate cancer and samples from healthy normal individuals. Prostatic cancer specimens were marked by an increased proportion of PSMA-expressing cells among total epithelial cells with a mean PSMA/cytokeratin ratio of 0.57. In contrast, significantly fewer PSMA-expressing epithelial cells were present in semen specimens from individuals without evidence of disease. A mean PSMA/cytokeratin ratio of 0.11 was obtained for this group [81].

In addition, serial semen specimens were analyzed for a patient with stage T1a prostate cancer after treatment with an antiandrogen. After completion of the medication period, this patient's disease progressed clinically as noted by increasing serum PSA and more extensive disease upon rebiopsy [81]. This was coincident with increasing PSMA/cytokeratin ratios from 0.36 to 0.83 during this period. These results demonstrate that prostate cells present in semen could potentially be useful in the clinical diagnosis and monitoring of prostate cancer, and perhaps reduce the number of biopsies that are conducted each year based on an abnormal DRE and serum PSA values.

VIII.   USE OF PSMA AS AN IMMUNOTHERAPY TARGET

Presently available treatment modalities are inadequate for metastatic prostatic cancer [82,83]. Androgen ablation therapy is often used to control tumor growth. In time, hormone-refractory tumor cells generally emerge and continue to grow. Radiation therapy and chemotherapy have not been effective in the treatment of hormone-refractory prostatic cancer. Development of new treatment strategies is required. One such strategy involves immunotherapy: the patient's own immune system is stimulated to kill cancer cells. Active immunotherapy for prostate cancer has been studied utilizing antigen-presenting dendritic cells loaded with peptide fragments from PSMA [84].

Generation of an immune response begins with the sensitization of helper (T_H) and cytotoxic (CTL) T-cell subsets through interactions with antigen-presenting cells (APC). These interactions include specific binding of T-cell surface glycoproteins, termed T-cell receptor, to an antigenic peptide bound by the major histocompatibility (MHC) protein on the APC [85]. The most efficient antigen-presenting cells studies to date are dendritic cells (DCs) [86].

A phase I clinical trial utilizing autologous dendritic cells loaded with two 9-amino-acid peptides derived from the amino acid sequence of PSMA was conducted in 51 patients with metastatic hormone-refractory prostate cancer [87]. These patients were organized into five treatment groups receiving, according to their treatment: four or five infusions of PSMA peptides alone (PSMA-P1 and a second peptide derived from the PSMA primary sequence containing the HLA-A2 motif, PSMA-P2), autologous DCs, or DCs pulsed with either PSMA-P1 or -P2, respectively. Infusions of all substances were well tolerated by all study participants and no toxicity was observed. The results of this clinical trial showed that increased T-cell proliferation in response to antigen was most frequently observed in the groups infused with peptide-pulsed DCs. Of this group of patients, 7/51 were partial responders to the treatment based upon National Prostate Cancer Project (NPCP) criteria coupled with a 50% reduction in serum PSA values, 5 of which were in the two groups receiving autologous DCs plus peptide. The duration of response was variable between 100 days (one patient) to more than 200 days of observation (four patients) [88]. All responders also had improvements in secondary signs including weight gain, relief of pain, and good performance status.

A subsequent phase II trial involving 107 subjects in three treatment groups was conducted [89–91] that involved 66 patients with hormone-refractory metastatic prostatic cancer. The hormone-refractory patients were organized into two groups. The first group (33/66) were previous phase I study participants who requested enrollment in the phase II trial (group A-I). A second group were newly accrued patients (group A-II). Group B patients included 41 patients with earlier stage disease with evidence of local recurrence after failure of a primary treatment. A total of six infusions of autologous DCs pulsed with two PSMA-derived peptides (PSM-P1 and PSM-P2) were given at 6 week intervals. With each infusion, half of each study group received a 7 day course of GM-CSF by subcutaneous injection as a systemic adjuvant.

Among group A-I patients, 9/33 were identified as partial responders based upon NPCP criteria and a 50% reduction in PSA [89]. No significant change in disease status was observed in 11/33 patients and 13/33 patients demonstrated disease progression. This phase I/II study covered an average total period of 613 days. Survival of more than 600 days (median survival, 608 days) was observed for 12/19 patients with stage D_2 hormone-refractory metastatic prostatic cancer [88].

Among group A-II patients, 8/25 showed disease regression (two complete and six partial responders), 1/25 exhibited no change, and 16/25 progressed [90]. Ten of 37 group B patients were partial responders, 1/37 was a complete responder, 8/37 showed no significant change, and 18/37 progressed [91]. Thus, 19/62 (31%) evaluable patients in these later groups showed a partial or complete response. No significant difference in clinical response was observed with those patients also receiving subcutaneous GM-CSF injections. Continued patient follow-up in these groups suggests that the majority of the responses identified in the various groups appear to be durable [92].

Further immunotherapy clinical studies utilizing dendritic cells loaded with PSMA are underway. It is possible that this strategy may provide additional therapeutic means to treat advanced hormone refractory prostatic cancer effectively.

IX. SUMMARY

The highly prostate-restricted and membrane-bound character of PSMA makes it an ideal target for clinical diagnostic and therapeutic applications in the treatment and management of prostatic cancer. Considerable progress has been made in defining the expression patterns of PSMA and in developing improved methods and reagents for detecting or targeting PSMA-expressing cells. These improved technologies are beginning to be used and should lead to more effective and economical diagnosis, staging, and treatment of the disease.

ACKNOWLEDGMENTS

Supported in part by funds provided by Northwest Biotherapeutics, Inc.

REFERENCES

1. RT Greenlee, T Murray, S Bolden, PA Wingo. Cancer Statistics, 2000. CA Cancer Clin 50:7–33, 2000.
2. G Aus, J Hugosson, L Norlén. Need for hospital care and palliative treatment for prostate cancer treated with noncutative intent. J Urol 154:466–369, 1995.
3. ED Crawford, MA Eisenberger, DG McLeod, JT Spaulding, R Benson, FA Dorr, BA Blumenstein, MA Davis, PJ Goodman. A controlled trial of Leuprolide with and without flutamide in prostatic carcinoma. N Engl J Med 321:419–424, 1989.
4. H Lepor, A Ross, PC Walsh. The influence of hormonal therapy on survival of men with advanced prostatic cancer. J Urol 128:335–340, 1982.
5. JS Horoszewicz, E Kawinski, GP Murphy. Monoclonal antibodies to a new antigenic marker in epithelial prostatic cells and serum of prostatic cancer patients. Anticancer Res 7:927–936, 1987.
6. RS Israeli, CT Powell, WR Fair, WD Heston. Molecular cloning of a complementary DNA encoding a prostate-specific membrane antigen. Cancer Res 3:227–230, 1993.
7. EH Holmes, TG Greene, WT Tino, AL Boynton, HC Aldape, SL Misrock, GP Murphy. Analysis of glycosylation of prostate specific membrane antigen derived from

LNCaP cells, prostatic carcinoma tumors, and serum from prostate cancer patients. Prostate Suppl 7:25–29, 1996.

8. M Kawakami, J Nakayama. Enhanced expression of prostate-specific membrane antigen gene in prostate cancer as revealed by in situ hybridization. Cancer Res 57: 2321–2324, 1997.

9. JK Troyer, ML Beckett, GL Wright Jr. Detection and characterization of the prostate-specific membrane antigen (PSMA) in tissue extracts and body fluids. Int J Cancer 62:552–558, 1995.

10. AD Lopes, WL Davis, MJ Rosenstraus, AJ Uveges, SC Gilman. Immunohistochemical and pharmacokinetic characterization of the site-specific immunoconjugate CYT-356 derived from antiprostate monoclonal antibody 7E11-C5. Cancer Res 50:6423–6429, 1990.

11. MJ Rosenstrous, WJ Davis, AD Lopes, C D'Aleo, S Gilman. In vitro and in vivo reactivity of anti-prostate monoclonal antibody immunoconjugate 7E11.C5.3-GYK-DTPA. Antibody Immunoconjugates Radiopharm 3:54, 1990.

12. DA Silver, I Pellicer, WR Fair, WD Heston, C Corgon-Cardo. Prostate-specific membrane antigen expression in normal and malignant human tissues. Clin Cancer Res 3:81–85, 1997.

13. GL Wright Jr, M Grob, C Haley, et al. Upregulation of prostate-specific antigen after androgen deprivation therapy. Urology 48:326–334, 1996.

14. RS Israeli, CT Powell, JG Corr, WR Fair, WD Heston. Expression of the prostate-specific membrane antigen. Cancer Res 54:1807–1811, 1994.

15. SS Chang, VE Reuter, WDW Heston, LS Grauer, PS Gaudin. Short term neoadjuvant androgen deprivation therapy does not affect prostate specific membrane antigen expression in prostate tissues. Cancer 88:407–415, 2000.

16. RL Sokoloff, KC Norton, CL Gasior, KM Marker, LS Grauer. A dual-monoclonal sandwich assay for prostate-specific membrane antigen: Levels in tissues, seminal fluid, and urine. Prostate 43:150–157, 2000.

17. GP Murphy, EH Holmes, AL Boynton, GM Kenny, RL Ostenson, SJ Erickson, RJ Barren. Comparison of prostate specific antigen, prostate specific membrane antigen, and LNCaP-based enzyme-linked immunosorbent assays in prostatic cancer patients and patients with benign prostatic enlargement. Prostate 26:164–168, 1995.

18. YP Rochon, JS Horoszewicz, AL Boynton, EH Holmes, RJ Barren, SJ Erickson, GM Kenny, GP Murphy. Western blot assay for prostate-specific membrane antigen in serum of prostate cancer patients. Prostate 25:219–223, 1994.

19. G Murphy, H Ragde, G Kenny, R Barren, S Erickson, B Tjoa, A Boynton, E Holmes, J Gilbaugh, T Douglas. Comparison of prostate specific membrane antigen, and prostate specific antigen levels in prostatic cancer patients. Anticancer Res 15:1473–1480, 1995.

20. GP Murphy, RJ Barren, SJ Erickson, et al. Evaluation and comparison of two new prostate carcinoma markers: Free-prostate specific antigen and prostate specific membrane antigen. Cancer 78:809–818, 1996.

21. DS O'Keefe, SL Su, DJ Bacic, Y Honguchi, Y Luo, CT Powell, D Zandvliet, PJ Russell, PL Molloy, NJ Nowak, TB Shows, C Mullins, H Vonder, WR Fair, WDW Heston. Mapping, genomic organization and promotor analysis of the human prostate-specific membrane antigen gene. Biochim Biophys Acta 1443:113–127, 1998.

22. D Good, P Schwarzenberger, JA Eastham, RE Rhodes, JD Hunt, M Collins, M Batzer, C Theodossiou, JK Kolls, SR Grimes. Cloning and characterization of the prostate specific membrane antigen promotor. J Cell Biochem 74:395–405, 1999.

23. H Liu, P Moy, S Kim, Y Xia, A Rajasekaran, V Navarro, B Knudsen, NH Bander. Monoclonal antibodies to the extracellular domain of prostate-specific membrane antigen also react with tumor vascular endothelium. Cancer Res 57:3629–3634, 1997.

24. SS Chang, VE Reuter, WDW Heston, NH Bander, LS Grauer, PB Gaudin. Five different antiprostate-specific membrane antigen (PSMA) antibodies confirm PSMA expression in tumor-associated neovasculature. Cancer Res 59:3192–3198, 1999.

25. SS Chang, DS O'Keefe, DJ Bacic, VE Reuter, WDW Heston, PB Gaudin. Prostate-specific membrane antigen is produced in tumor-associated neovasculature. Clin Cancer Res 5:2674–2681, 1999.

26. DG Bostwick, A Pacelli, M Blute, P Roche, GP Murphy. Prostate specific membrane antigen expression in prostatic intraepithelial neoplasia and adenocarcinoma: Study of 184 cases. Cancer 82:2256–2261, 1998.

27. SD Sweat, A Pacelli, GP Murphy, DG Bostwick. Prostate specific membrane antigen expression is greatest in prostate adenocarcinoma and lymph node metastases. Urology 52:637–640, 1998.

28. JK Troyer, Q Feng, ML Beckett, GL Wright. Biochemical characterization and mapping of the 7E11-C5.3 epitope of the prostate-specific membrane antigen. Urol Oncol 1:29–37, 1995.

29. SS Chang, VE Reuter, NH Bander, LS Grauer, WDW Heston, PB Gaudin. Characterization of multiple antibodies to prostate specific membrane antigen (PSMA) in benign and malignant tissues and tumor-associated neovasculature. Proc Am Assoc Cancer Res 40:489 (abst), 1999.

30. GL Wright Jr, Q Feng, ML Beckett, D Lopes, SC Gilman. Characterization of a new prostate carcinoma-associated marker: 7E11-C5. Antibody Immunoconjugates Radiopharmaceut 3:89 (abst), 1990.

31. SL Su, IP Huang, WR Fair, CT Powell, WD Heston. Alternatively spliced variants of prostate-specific membrane antigen RNA: Ratio of expression as a potential measurement of progression. Cancer Res 55:1441–1443, 1995.

32. GP Murphy, WT Tino, EH Holmes, AL Boynton, SJ Erickson, VA Bowes, RJ Barren, BA Tjoa, SL Misrock, H Ragde, GM Kenny. Measurement of prostate-specific membrane antigen in the serum with a new antibody. Prostate 28:266–271, 1996.

33. LS Grauer, KD Lawler, JL Marignac, A Kumar, AS Goel, RL Wolfert. Identification, purification, and subcellular localization of prostate-specific membrane antigen PSM' protein in the LNCaP prostatic carcinoma cell line. Cancer Res 58:4787–4789, 1998.

34. RE Carter, AR Feldman, JT Coyle. Prostate-specific membrane antigen is a hydrolase with substrate and pharmacologic characteristics of a neuropeptidase. Proc Natl Acad Sci USA 93:749–753, 1996.

35. CW Tiffany, RG Lapidus, A Merion, DC Calvin, BS Slusher. Characterization of the enzymatic activity of PSM: Comparison with brain NAALADase. Prostate 39:28–35, 1999.

36. JT Pinto, BP Suffoletto, TM Berzin, CH Qiao, S Lin, WP Tong, F May, B Mukherjee, WD Heston. Prostate-specific membrane antigen: A novel folate hydrolase in human prostatic carcinoma cells. Clin Cancer Res 2:1445–1451, 1996.

37. MJ Varkarakis, GP Murphy, CMK Nelson, M Chehval, RH Moore, RH Flocks. Lymph node involvement in prostatic carcinoma. Urol Clin North Am 2:197–212, 1975.

38. S Kramer, J Gorich, HW Gottfried, P Riska, AJ Aschoff, N Rilinger, HJ Brambs, R Sokiranski. Sensitivity of computed tomography in detecting local recurrence of prostatic carcinoma following radical prostatectomy. Br J Radiol 70:995–999, 1997.

39. E Sanford, R Grzonka, A Heal, M Helal, L Persky, I Tyson. Prostate cancer imaging with a new monoclonal antibody: A preliminary report. Ann Surg Oncol 1:400–404, 1994.

40. GP Murphy. Radioscintiscanning of prostate cancer. Cancer 75:1819–1822, 1995.

41. D Kahn, RD Williams, MJ Manyak, MK Haseman, DW Seldin, JA Libertino, RT Maguire. Indium-111 capromab pendetide in the evaluation of patients with residual or recurrent prostate cancer after radical prostatectomy. J Urol 159:2041–2047, 1998.

42. D Kahn, RD Williams, DW Seldin, et al. Radioimmunoscintigraphy with [111]Indium-labeled CYT-356 for the detection of occult prostate cancer recurrence. J Urol 152:1490–1495, 1994.

43. RJ Babaian, J Sayer, DA Podoloff, LC Steelhammer, VA Bhodkamkar, JV Gulfo. Radioimmunoscintigraphy of pelvic lymph nodes with [111]Indium-labeled monoclonal antibody CYT-356. J Urol 152:1952–1955, 1994.

44. MK Haseman, NL Reed, SA Rosenthal. Monoclonal antibody imaging of occult prostate cancer in patients with elevated prostate-specific antigen: Positron emission tomography and biopsy correlation. Clin Nucl Med 21:703–713, 1996.

45. J Ulchaker, E Klein, C Zippe, H Levin, D Newmann, M Ward. Indium-111 capromab monoclonal antibody: Utility in differentiating local versus distant relapse after radical prostatectomy. J Urol 157:205 (abst), 1997.

46. JK Burgers, GH Hinkle, MK Haseman. Monoclonal antibody imaging of recurrent and metastatic prostate cancer. Semin Urol 13:103–112, 1995.

47. D Kahn, RD Williams, MK Haseman, NL Reed, SJ Miller, J Gerstbrein. Radioimmunoscintigraphy with in-111-labeled capromab pendetide predicts prostate cancer response to salvage radiotherapy after failed radical prostatectomy. J Clin Oncol 16:284–289, 1998.

48. TJ Polascik, RT Gurganus, AW Partin, B Rogers, R Maguire, MJ Manyak, et al. Comparison of staging algorithms and a monoclonal antibody scan (ProstaScint) to predict lymph node involvement in high-risk prostate cancer. J Urol 159:289, 1998.

49. VU Chengazi, MR Feneley, D Ellison, M Stalteri, A Granowski, M Granoska, CC Nimmon, SJ Mather, RS Kirby, KE Britton. Imaging prostate cancer with technetium-99m-7E11.C5.3 (CYT-351). J Nucl Med 38:675–682, 1997.

50. GH Hinkle, JK Burgers, CE Neal, et al. Multicenter radioimmunoscintigraphic evaluation of patients with prostate carcinoma using indium-111 capromab pendetide. Cancer 83:739–747, 1998.

51. AA Elgamal, MJ Troychak, GP Murphy. ProstaScint may enhance identification of prostate cancer recurrence after prostatectomy, radiation, or hormone therapy: Analysis of 136 scans of 100 patients. Prostate 37:261–269, 1998.

52. MJ Manyak, GH Hinkle, JO Olsen, RP Chiaccherini, AW Partin, S Piantadosi, JK Burgers, JH Texter, CE Neal, JA Libertino, GL Wright Jr, RT Maguire. Immunoscintigraphy with indium-111-capromab pendetide: Evaluation before definitive therapy in patients with prostate cancer. Urology 54:1058–1063, 1999.
53. GP Murphy, AA Elgamal, MJ Troychak, GM Kenny. Follow-up ProstaScint(R) scans verify detection of occult soft-tissue recurrence after failure of primary prostate cancer therapy. Prostate 42:315–317, 2000.
54. JC Quintana, MJ Blend. The dual isotope ProstaScint imaging procedure: Clinical experience and staging results in 145 patients. Clin Nucl Med 25:33–40, 2000.
55. DB Sodee, RJ Ellis, MA Samuels, JP Spirnak, WF Poole, C Riester, DM Martanovic, R Stonecipher, EM Bellon. Prostate cancer and prostate bed SPECT imaging with ProstaScint: Semiquantitative correlation with prostatic biopsy results. Prostate 37:140–148, 1998.
56. GP Murphy, RT Maguire, B Rogers, AW Partin, WB Nelp, MJ Troychak, et al. Comparison of serum PSMA, PSA levels with results of cytogen-356 ProstaScint scanning in prostatic cancer patients. Prostate 33:281–285, 1997.
57. WD Figg, BA Ammerman, N Patronas, SM Steinberg, RG Walls, N Dawson, E Reed, O Sartor. Lack of correlation between prostate-specific antigen and the presence of measurable soft tissue metastases in hormone-refractory prostate cancer. Cancer Invest 14:513–517, 1996.
58. GP Murphy, MJ Troychak, OE Cobb, VA Bowes, RJ Kenny, RJ Barren, GM Kenny, H Ragde, EH Holmes, RL Wolfert. Evaluation of PSA, free PSA, PSMA, and total and bone alkaline phosphatase levels compared to bone scans in the management of patients with metastatic prostate cancer. Prostate 33:141–146, 1997.
59. GP Murphy, TG Greene, WT Tino, AL Boynton, EH Holmes. Isolation and characterization of monoclonal antibodies specific for the extracellular domain of prostate-specific membrane antigen. J Urol 160:2396–2401, 1998.
60. EH Holmes, WT Tino, TG Greene, RJ Barren, AL Boynton, GP Murphy. Development and characterization of monoclonal antibodies specific for the extracellular domain of prostate-specific membrane antigen. Cancer Biother Radiopharmaceut 13:55 (abst), 1998.
61. WT Tino, MJ Huber, TP Lake, TG Greene, GP Murphy, EH Holmes. Isolation and characterization of monoclonal antibodies specific for protein conformational epitopes present in prostate-specific membrane antigen (PSMA). Hybridoma, 19:249–257, 2000.
62. EH Holmes, D Hudson, WT Tino, MJ Huber, TP Lake. Development of human monoclonal antibodies specific for extracellular epitopes in prostate-specific membrane antigen (PSMA). 12th International Conference on Monoclonal Antibodies for Cancer, San Diego, CA, 1999, p41.
63. A Hamilton, S King, H Liu, P Moy, N Bander, F Carr. A novel humanised antibody against prostate-specific membrane antigen (PSMA) for *in vivo* targeting and therapy. Proc Am Assoc Cancer Res 39:440, 1998.
64. NH Bander. Monoclonal antibody therapy for prostate cancer. 6th Annual CaP CURE Scientific Retreat, Lake Tahoe, NV, 1999.
65. R O'Donnell, S DeNardo, XB Shi, G Mirick, G DeNardo, L Kroger, F Meyers. L6 monoclonal antibody binds prostate cancer. Prostate 37:91–97, 1998.

66. DJ Buchsbaum. Experimental tumor targeting with radiolabeled ligands. Cancer 80(suppl):2371–2377, 1997.

67. SL Su, AL Boynton, EH Holmes, AAA Elgamal, GP Murphy. Detection of extra-prostatic prostate cells utilizing reverse transcription-polymerase chain reaction. Semin Surg Oncol 18:17–28, 2000.

68. RS Israeli, WH Miller, SL Su, CT Powell, WR Fair, DS Samadi, RF Huryk, A DeBlasio, ET Edwards, GJ Wise, WDW Heston. Sensitive nested reverse transcription polymerase chain reaction detection of circulating prostatic tumor cells: Comparison of prostate-specific membrane antigen and prostate-specific antigen-based assays. Cancer Res 54:6306–6310, 1994.

69. C Cama, CA Olsson, AJ Raffo, H Perlman, R Buttyan, K O'Toole, D McMahon, MC Benson, AE Katz. Molecular staging of prostate cancer. II. A comparison of the application of an enhanced reverse transcriptase polymerase chain reaction assay for prostate specific antigen versus prostate specific membrane antigen. J Urol 153: 1373–1378, 1995.

70. S Loric, F Dumas, P Eschwege, P Blanchet, G Benoit, A Jardin, B Lacour. Enhanced detection of hematogenous circulating prostatic cells in patients with prostate adeno-carcinoma by using nested reverse transcription polymerase chain reaction assay based on prostate-specific membrane antigen. Clin Chem 41:1698–1704, 1995.

71. E Corey, EW Arfman, MM Oswin, SW Melchior, DJ Tindall, CY Young, WJ Ellis, RL Vessella. Detection of circulating prostate cells by reverse transcriptase-polymerase chain reaction of human glandular kallikrein (hK2) and prostate-specific antigen (PSA) messages. Urology 50:184–188, 1997.

72. T Okegawa, K Nutahara, E Higashihara. Preoperative nested reverse transcription-polymerase chain reaction for prostate specific membrane antigen predicts biochemical recurrence after radical prostatectomy. Br J Urol 84:112–117, 1999.

73. Y Zhang, CD Zippe, F Van Lente, EA Klein, MK Gupta. Combined nested reverse transcription-PCR assay for prostate-specific antigen and prostate-specific membrane antigen in detecting circulating prostatic cells. Clin Cancer Res 3:1215–1220, 1997.

74. DP Wood Jr, ER Banks, S Humphreys, JW McRoberts, VM Rangnekar. Identification of bone marrow micrometastases in patients with prostate cancer. Cancer 74: 2533–2540, 1994.

75. DP Wood Jr, M Banerjee. Presence of circulating prostate cells in the bone marrow of patients undergoing radical prostatectomy is predictive of disease free survival. J Clin Oncol 15:3451–3457, 1997.

76. T Deguchi, M Yang, H Ehara, S Ito, Y Takahashi, Y Nishino, S Fujihiro, T Kawa-mura, H Komeda, M Horie, et al. Detection of micrometastatic prostate cancer cells in lymph nodes by reverse transcriptase-polymerase chain reaction. Cancer Res 53: 5350–5354, 1993.

77. RA Edelstein, AL Zietman, A de las Morenas, RJ Krane, RK Babayan, KC Dallow, A Traish, RB Moreland. Implications of prostate micrometastases in pelvic lymph nodes: An archival tissue study. Urology 47:370–375, 1996.

78. AC Ferrari, NN Stone, JN Eyler, M Gao, J Mandeli, P Unger, RE Gallagher, R Stock. Prospective analysis of prostate-specific markers in pelvic lymph nodes of patients with high-risk prostate cancer. J Natl Cancer Inst 89:1498–1504, 1997.

79. T Okegawa, K Nutahara, E Higashihara. Detection of micrometastatic prostate cancer cells in the lymph nodes by reverse transcriptase polymerase chain reaction is predictive of biochemical recurrence in pathological stage T2 prostate cancer. J Urol 163:1183–1188, 2000.

80. RA Ghossein, I Osman, S Bhattacharya, J Ferrara, M Fazzari, C Cordon-Cardo, HI Scher. Detection of prostate specific membrane antigen messenger RNA using immunobead reverse transcriptase chain reaction. Diagn Mol Pathol 8:59–65, 1999.

81. RJ Barren, EH Holmes, AL Boynton, A Gregorakis, OE Cobb, CL Wilson, H Ragde, GP Murphy. A method for identifying prostate cells in semen using flow cytometry. Prostate 36:181–188, 1998.

82. C Mettlin. Changes in patterns of prostate cancer care in the United States: Results of American College of Surgeons Commission on Cancer Studies, 1974–1994. Prostate 32:221–226, 1997.

83. WK Oh, PW Kantoff. Management of hormone refractory prostate cancer: Current standards and future prospects. J Urol 160:1220–1229, 1998.

84. BA Tjoa, GP Murphy. Progress in active specific immunotherapy of prostate cancer. Semin Surg Oncol 18:80–87, 2000.

85. RM Zinkernagel, PC Doherty. Restriction of in vitro T cell-mediated cytotoxicity in lymphocytic choriomeningitis within a syngeneic or semiallogenic system. Nature 248:701–702, 1974.

86. SC Knight, AJ Stagg. Antigen-presenting cell types. Curr Opin Immunol 5:374–382, 1993.

87. G Murphy, B Tjoa, H Ragde, et al. Phase I clinical trial: T-cell therapy for prostate cancer using autologous dendritic cells pulsed with HLA-A0201-specific peptides from prostate-specific membrane antigen. Prostate 29:371–380, 1996.

88. BA Tjoa, SJ Erickson, VA Bowes, H Ragde, GM Kenny, RC Cobb, OE Ireton, MJ Troychak, AL Boynton, GP Murphy. Follow-up evaluation of prostate cancer patients infused with autologous dendritic cells pulsed with PSMA peptides. Prostate 32:272–278, 1997.

89. BA Tjoa, SJ Simmons, VA Bowes, H Ragde, M Rogers, A Elgamal, GM Kenny, OE Cobb, RC Ireton, MJ Troychak, ML Salgaller, AL Boynton, GP Murphy. Evaluation of phase I/II clinical trials in prostate cancer with dendritic cells and PSMA peptides. Prostate 36:39–44, 1998.

90. GP Murphy, BA Tjoa, SJ Simmons, J Jarisch, VA Bowes, H Ragde, M Rogers, A Elgamal, GM Kenny, OE Cobb, RC Ireton, MJ Trotchak, ML Salgaller, AL Boynton. Infusion of dendritic cells pulsed with HLA-A2-specific prostate-specific membrane antigen peptides: A phase II prostate cancer vaccine trial involving patients with hormone- refractory metastatic disease. Prostate 38:73–78, 1999.

91. GP Murphy, BA Tjoa, SJ Simmons, H Ragde, M Rogers, A Elgamal, GM Kenny, MJ Troychak, ML Salgaller, AL Boynton. Phase II prostate cancer vaccine trial: Report of a study involving 37 patients with disease recurrence following primary treatment. Prostate 39:54–59, 1999.

92. BA Tjoa, SJ Simmons, A Elgamal, M Rogers, H Ragde, GM Kenny, MJ Troychak, AL Boynton, GP Murphy. Follow-up evaluation of a phase II prostate cancer vaccine trial. Prostate 40:125–129, 1999.

Index